Apricots and Oncogenes

Apricots and Oncogenes

On Vegetables and Cancer Prevention

Eileen Jennings

McGuire & Beckley Books
Cleveland

TO THE READER: It is advisable to consult a physician about all matters concerning your health including making substantial changes in your diet. The suggestions in this book concern only possible ways to reduce the risk of cancer and are not concerned with the treatment of cancer.

Printed in the United States of America

ISBN 0-9635890-3-2

Library of Congress Catalog Card Number: 93-77061

McGuire & Beckley Books
P.O. Box 770445
Cleveland, Ohio 44107

Contents

Preface

Not many of us care to spend much time thinking about the cancer statistics—most of the time we are far too busy with our daily work, our plans and ambitions, our social obligations to worry about something that may not happen. So if it does, it does; what could you do to prevent it, anyway? Yet all too often we are forced to pause and grieve for a while when a friend or relative develops this illness. One out of four in the United States encounters cancer during his or her lifetime. One out of nine or ten women develops breast cancer.

Research is finally showing us a way to improve this situation. During the last few years scientists have found a broad body of evidence that shows there are factors in vegetables that can and do prevent the development of cancer of many types, including breast cancer. Some of the research has appeared in bits and pieces in the newspapers, always with the same kind of warning: this is preliminary, more research is needed.

Scientists who are familiar with the whole story are not so cautious. They are excited about the overall evidence that better diet can prevent a substantial fraction of the cases of cancer, and they are excited about testing the idea in long-range human trials by giving specific substances to volunteers.

Human trials require many years and are very expensive to set up and monitor. Some trials are already in progress; a few small ones have been finished. I believe we should not wait any longer to take full advantage of this simple method for improving our own future health. The benefits of better diet begin early, and keeping more vegetables in the diet is an intelligent measure we can take to turn the research results to our own favor.

Chapter 1

Vitamin A in the News

The astonishing scientific finding that our vegetable intake has a bearing on the development of the dread disease, cancer, first hit the headlines in November of 1981. Persuasive results from a study on diet and health at a factory in Chicago had been set down in a medical journal for all to see. The word spread lightly through the newspapers and magazines that doctors had found that men who ate more vegetables were less likely to develop lung cancer, even if they were longtime smokers. (" . . . A carrot a day keeps the doctor away.") Then the story faded out from the news, and those doctors and scientists who were interested continued to scrutinize the evidence while they planned more studies to find out how important these results might be. And the public did not fully realize that the answer to one of our most perplexing health problems had been found.

The research on lung cancer in Chicago was part of a nineteen yearlong study of a large group of men working at the Western Electric Company. The study was not the first to show lower incidence of lung cancer linked to higher levels of beta-carotene from vegetables, but it was one of the largest and longest running studies ever done and it included an important factor that was absent in other studies. The detailed dietary survey that the men and their wives participated in allowed the scientists to differentiate between the effects of vitamin A itself and the effects of the vitamin A precursor, beta-carotene, in the diet.

The results were most striking for the five hundred or so men in the group who smoked for more than thirty years, and in whom the incidence of lung cancer was several times higher than in the five hundred nonsmokers. The thirty-year smokers with low amounts of beta-carotene in their diet had eight times more lung cancer cases than thirty-year smokers with high levels of beta-carotene in their diet.

Then, in the following year, an unusual report on vitamin A came from London, from a field of research that would seem to be far removed from concerns about human health. Vitamin A prevented the growth of new tissue in an experiment involving salamanders, lending support to other work showing anticancer effects of vitamin A. A biologist at the National Institute for Medical Research described experiments on limb regeneration in the axolotl stage of a small salamander. This amphibian can grow a new leg if one is cut off during the early stages of its development. The axolotl does this by allowing some blastemal cells at the site of the cut to reassume the undifferentiated state of the developing organism (similar to a growing cancer) and begin again to grow. The new tissue normally responds to some little-known factors of positional information or cell surface conditions on nearby cells that tell it that a leg is needed here, and a proper new limb is produced from a type of blueprint in the blastemal cells, a phenomenon known as pattern formation. But if the experimental animals were kept in a dilute solution of vitamin A instead of in tap water, development of the new leg was delayed until the vitamin A was removed! This is a most fascinating result because some characteristics of cancer cells resemble the undifferentiated cells of developing new tissue. If vitamin A can inhibit growth of a new amphibian limb, might it also have some effects in preventing the initiation of cancer?

These two scientific studies evoked recollections of earlier stories on the vitamin. Some years ago research reports began to appear that showed that vitamin A or its relatives could inhibit experimental cancer in animals. For instance, a report in 1977 told how a chemical related to vitamin A could prevent bladder cancer in animals that had been given a potent chemical carcinogen.

I also recalled that during the 1950s popular magazines carried photographic stories about an almost mythical people who lived in a valley high in the Himalayas in isolation from the rest of the world, who enjoyed freedom from heart disease and cancer, and who commonly lived to very old age as a result. The Hunzas consumed large amounts of apricots, an excellent source of beta-carotene. They also worked very hard to raise their crops and had little fat in their diet. Is it true that they were able to avoid cancer and did the beta-carotene have anything to do with it?

Now, since 1988 there are full page ads in popular magazines listing fourteen ongoing studies that will try to answer these questions about beta-carotene as a possible aid in avoiding cancer. The ads are placed by Hoffmann-LaRoche Inc., the pharmaceutical manufacturer that makes synthetic beta-carotene and has studied vitamin A and related compounds for many years. There are no conclusions in the ads—it's too early to know the results of the fourteen studies. But the ads serve to remind us that the National Research Council has recommended in 1982 and again in 1989 that we ought to consume plenty of green and yellow vegetables and little fat if we want to reduce the risk of cancer.

My lifelong interest in human nutrition, biochemistry, and the cancer problem came to focus on vitamin A and its precursor, beta-carotene, as many reports were published in recent years describing new research linking low incidence of cancer with high dietary intake of beta-carotene. These reports are especially intriguing because they have the potential to open a new perspective on the problem of why cancer develops—a new perspective that can be immediately useful to people who like to take care of their health.

The new reports prompted me to search for more information. Since I have worked in chemistry—in medical research and in industrial chemistry—for many years, it was easy for me to find the information in the medical literature. My goal was to find out: how much do they really know about vitamin A and cancer? I found that there is a wealth of research results on the subject scattered throughout the scientific literature. Epidemiologists (medical specialists who study the correlations between environmental factors and the incidence of disease) have found convincing evidence that people who consume more vegetables develop cancer less often than their neighbors who eat few vegetables. Some of their studies will be described. There has also been a great deal of research on the effects of vitamin A in animals and in cells in culture, but this work will not be described here, in the interest of brevity.

Many people in the medical research community are aware of the potential for protective effects from beta-carotene in reducing the incidence of cancer, or at least carcinomas, but for them to make a strong recommendation to consume more carotene is still a dubious step. The reasons come from the many uncertainties—the great difficulties in proving dietary effects in human populations, the well-known toxicity of vitamin A if excessive amounts are consumed, and the research results that indicate there are probably several protective factors that are supplied by fruits and vegetables. For instance, vitamin C and a B vitamin, folic acid, also have anticancer effects. The safest and wisest thing for us to do, then, is to eat more of the most nutritious foods, and indeed, we see specific advice in this regard in advertising and in magazine articles.

About eighty per cent of cancers that occur in adults are carcinomas and this is the type of cancer that has been linked to diet. Some of these cases of cancer are closely associated with tobacco, heredity, or a few other specific initiating factors, but the majority of the carcinomas cannot be blamed on anything in particular. Cancer research during the past twenty years points to various types of damage to the chromosomes such as mutations as the cause of these cases of cancer. These mutations are not the kind that are inherited; they occur during adult life as rare, small errors during DNA replication, as new cells are continuously produced in many tissues to replace old cells. If a sufficient number of critical genes in one cell are damaged as a result of such errors in DNA replication, the cell can become malignant. The vegetable part of our diet contains vitamins that help prevent this from happening.

The recent research into relationships between cancer incidence and diet in people around the world is generating evidence for a new hypothesis about how cancer develops, and this is the idea that cancer is to a considerable extent a deficiency disease, caused by the mutations that can happen at any time but which are more likely when there is a deficiency of folic acid in the diet, and by deficiencies of the other critically important factors found in vegetables, the most important of which is beta-carotene.

This book will summarize some of the recent studies on human diet and cancer with some of the history of vitamin research. Included is a section on the toxic effects of vitamin A should excessive amounts be ingested. The emphasis here will be on vitamin A itself, historically a mysterious unknown factor that was needed for life and for vision and, as its distribution in various chemical forms in nature was discovered and its effects on all aspects of normal development were found out, a fascinating subject that continues to draw curious minds to its study, rather than on the scientists who have followed this path. The scientists have been finding out more and more details about the vitamin A story in a continuous effort since 1913, when vitamin A was discovered. Some have used great imagination in their research; others have labored patiently using technical expertise to make their discoveries, but all must be gratified to see how the most recent research into the role of vitamin A as a gene regulator promises important and exciting discoveries still to be made.

The subject of vitamins and human health is complex and this book is not meant to be a complete review. I will try only to give the reader an overview of a few fascinating areas of science in hopes of conveying a sense of how difficult it is to set exact rules for maintaining one's own precious health, in hopes of providing a glimpse of the complexities of the chemical world within us, and in hopes of entertaining the reader's natural curiosity with a few details of the scientific endeavor.

A note on terminology: in this book "carotene" and "beta-carotene" are used interchangeably, and "vitamin A" is a general term that includes several forms of the vitamin. There is a glossary of vitamin A terminology and structural formulas of vitamin-related substances for the interest of those readers who may be chemically inclined.

Chapter 2

The Hunza River Valley

The relation between diet and health has concerned those who serve in medical fields since ancient times. Hippocrates wrote that everything we eat has an effect on the body. Physicians ever since have tried to develop dietary advice for their patients by drawing on their observations in their practices and the teachings of the master practitioners. Prescribing the best way to eat is no easy task. One of the interesting things about human nutrition is our ability to survive in regions as different as the Tropics and the Arctic. Our basic food requirements can be obtained in Indonesia or in Alaska. The human digestive system and metabolic functions are so adaptable to different environments that some populations thrive on diets that are nearly all meat and animal products, while other people do equally well on diets that are all vegetable. How can we determine whether one dietary style has greater benefits than another?

One way to find out if our health can be improved by changes in diet is to study in detail the dietary customs and the health successes and failures of people with differing diets. We may not find scientific proof for health effects related to diet, but we can expect to find suggestions that could be tested further. The study of people in other lands—their diet, life styles, and customs—has long occupied explorers, scientists, and armchair travelers. One subject a researcher might like to pursue in puzzling out how other people fare, is the question of their health problems, and how they compare with our own. But researchers face a difficult task when they attempt to analyze the health problems in some other countries. People who live in remote areas cannot always be studied by modern methods. They may not have access to medical diagnosis or record-keeping practices that could be used for reliable research and discussions of their health history. So, our understanding of their health successes and failures is limited. Nevertheless, some reasonable suggestions based on observations of people in distant locations have been put forward by physicians and scientists who would like to help us improve our own health. One of the most valuable suggestions is that plenty of vegetables and other high-fiber natural foods may confer improved health and well-being and greater freedom from chronic diseases, including cancer.

The people of Hunza in central Asia are a population who consume a high-fiber diet of vegetables, fruit and whole grains, and who have been greatly admired for their apparent good health and long life. They live in one of the most remote areas of Asia, in a valley in the Karakoram mountains that was extremely difficult to visit until a road went through in 1960. Many travelers visited Hunza in earlier decades and brought back glowing tales of a country free of diseases, where the people enjoyed marvelous good health, good dispositions, and had unusual endurance. Westerners have wondered whether these stories were true and whether the people of Hunza had some secrets for better health.

The Karakoram range in central Asia contains twenty-three peaks over twenty thousand feet high including K2 (Mt. Godwin Austen), second highest in the world after Mt. Everest. Part of the rooftop of the world, the Karakorams stretch along the northernmost reaches of Pakistan between the Hindu Kush mountains to the west in Afghanistan and the Himalayas to the east. The Karakorams stand on the modern-day border between Pakistan and China. Alexander the Great traveled near the southern border of the mountains after his campaign through Afghanistan, and on the northern side of the Karakorams, caravans on the old Chinese Silk Road wound through the deserts of Sinkiang.

The province of Hunza lies on the southern slopes of the Karakoram range, in what is now northern Pakistan. Beginning in the late eighteenth century when the British arrived in the area and continuing to recent years, the people of Hunza have been the object of interest and admiration by western explorers because of their good health and also because of their wonderfully picturesque, terraced farms and apricot orchards.

The farms and orchards thrive because of the people's hard work and because of the river that supplies the valley with water. The glacier-fed Hunza River begins in the snow-packed heights of the Karakorams and carries mountain silt and melted snow to the Gilgit River and thence to the Indus River that arises to the east in Tibet and flows southward through the length of Pakistan to the Arabian Sea near Karachi. The people of Hunza call the river water "glacier milk" because of the heavy loading of silt and the murky grey color. They consider it to be a beneficent source of good health and good crops.[1]

The river is certainly the source of their livelihood, as without it there would be no farms and no Hunza. All crops in Hunza are watered by irrigation. A miles-long system of aqueducts and water channels built of stone directs water from the higher levels to the man-made terraced fields. The Hunza River valley is one to four miles wide and approximately one hundred miles long, home to twenty-five thousand (as of the mid-twentieth century) Hunzukuts, as they prefer to be called, who make their living by farming. The valley is steep sided, rocky, temperate in climate, and dominated by spectacular mountains.

Superb photographic essays in *National Geographic Magazine* have shown us views of green terraces planted with grains and bounded with whitish stone walls above and below which rise like steps from the narrow valley bottom toward the steep sides of stark, grey-brown mountains. Cloudlike clusters of white-blossoming apricot trees arranged in irregular fashion along the terraces give an illusion of softness to the landscape in spring.

Natural vegetation is sparce. Rain is almost nonexistent. Some willows, birch, and poplars grow in Hunza, and shrubs. The grass available for sheep and goats is sufficient for only small flocks.

Baltit, the capital of the Hunza district, is reached by jeep from Gilgit, a city in northern Pakistan, on a road built only in 1960. Prior to that, Baltit was reached by a treacherous mountain trail, only the first part of which was negotiable by jeep. Early travelers went by foot or on horseback and contended with avalanches, deep snows in winter, and a suspension bridge over the raging Hunza River on a trip of sixty-seven miles that could take Westerners several days.

Even though Hunza is one of the most inaccessible of regions, the area was not completely isolated from outside influence. Caravans going from Chinese Turkestan to India or Afghanistan passed over the Karakorams in former times and legend has it that the Hunzukuts did their share of toll-taking on the caravans. A tyrannical ruler of the area, Safdar Ali Khan, made so much trouble for travelers during his five-year rule in the late nineteenth century that the English sent an expedition to Hunza from India in 1891. The ruler fought and fled, and the Hunzukuts have stuck to farming ever since.

The Hunzukuts have lived in this remote area for about two thousand years according to their legends. They are handsome people, of Mediterranean mien, or Persian. The men wear traditional white wool rolled-brim hats, and long wool coats over cotton shirts and trousers. The women complement their outfits with fancy silk-embroidered caps and embroidered silk scarves imported from China.

Houses are two- to four-room affairs made of stone, with flat roofs constructed from poplar timbers and earth. The roofs have a square hole near the middle over the hearth or cooking pit that allows some of the smoke from the fire to escape. Fireplaces are not known. Eye irritation from the smoky houses is a common problem, especially during the cold winters when people remain indoors. The ground floor has a partially roofed anteroom for the animals (a few sheep and goats), a large living room with the fire pit, raised benches for sitting and sleeping, large cupboards for storage, and a large storeroom for food. An upstairs may have another room and a storeroom.

The custom is that everyone in Hunza moves to the upper level of the house on the same day in the spring and they cook for the rest of the summer on the roof. In any event, the flat roof is the place for summer sitting outdoors and for drying apricots.

Emily Lorimer's marvelously detailed book about her and her husband's fourteen-month stay in Hunza in the village of Aliabad in 1935 has complete descriptions of the Hunzukuts' houses, as well as details on many aspects of their daily lives. She describes how they manage to conserve irrigation water in the hot summer weather and how they avoid polluting the water supply. She says, "I made great friends with the family who worked just below us (I have named them in my notebook Household No. 1), and I felt quite sad when their wheat harvest was over—it was so convenient just to run down and join them in sight of our own windows. They asked me, however: "Won't you come home and sit in our shade?" Of course I accepted with delight. It was just a few steps along the Dala [water channel] and down one of the little lanes, half path, half watercourse. . . . I didn't, however, go up on to the roof, but on into a larger courtyard where there was a pool in the corner at which their washing is done. They would not dream of polluting the running water by washing themselves or their clothes in it as it flows by; they draw off what they want for these purposes into a separate pond of their own. . . . I got into a walled-in shady garden full of fruit trees—apples, mulberries, peaches, apricots, and vines. It is incredible how luxurious mere shade is at such a temperature. It wasn't remotely like a garden in our sense. The earth was bare without one blade of grass or green, and was all cut up into little beds round each precious tree, with banks between them, so that the water could be directed to each tree as desired, when it was No. 1's turn to have water at all." [2]

Lt. Colonel David L. R. Lorimer and his wife, from England, spent fourteen months in Hunza in 1934-1935 in order to further refine their knowledge of the unwritten language of Hunza, Burushaski, the origins of which were a mystery to scholars. Lorimer at this time was on a military pension, having been formerly in the Indian Army and the Foreign and Political Department of the Government of India during the years when India was governed by England. Lorimer had learned the Hunza language during his 1920-25 assignment as Political Agent in Gilgit and, later on, was to publish a dictionary and a grammar of the language.

For the Lorimers, a trip back to Hunza was a bonus adventure, the frosting on the cake after a long career in government service. They had enjoyed learning the language and culture of the Hunzukuts whom they had met in Gilgit but duties had not allowed them to learn as much as they would have desired. In retirement, they scraped up enough funds by securing a fellowship for language study, and packed up their typewriters and other gear for the long trip from England to the Hunza River valley. The trip from Srinagar in Kashmir to Hunza required long days an steep mountain trails, crossing rushing mountain streams, and crossing a snow-filled mountain pass. Illnesses, trail accidents and other hardships never damaged their plucky spirits or their determination to accomplish their work.

They were welcomed in Hunza by the Mir, or ruler, and given a vacant house to use while they studied the local language and traveled about getting acquainted with their new neighbors. Visitors to Hunza are always welcomed cheerfully. The Hunzukuts are renowned as alert, intelligent, hard workers and everyone works in the fields. They claim to be descendants of soldiers of Alexander the Great of Macedonia who reached this part of Asia in the fourth century B.C.

(In 326 B.C. Alexander the Great of Macedonia arrived with a huge retinue in the area now known as northern Pakistan in the eighth year of his twelve-year expedition to conquer the Persian Empire. His goals included consolidating the Greek and Persian peoples, governing responsibly, and combining local religions and customs with the Greek idea of the city-state. Eighty of his soldiers married Persian women of noble birth in a mass marriage ceremony coincident with one of his marriages and, after his death at the age of thirty-two in Babylon, the story of his life became the stuff of legend and lesser rulers across Asia claimed to be his descendants. Alexander had reached the Indus River and gone a little way further. He had intended to add India to his new empire, and indeed defeated the Indian king, Porus, in a battle near the Jhelum River, but his troops were taken aback at the prospect of further battles with war elephants and decided for him that it was time to return home.)

From wherever and whenever they arrived, the people of Hunza have remained in their valley, building terraced fields and aqueducts and growing grains, vegetables and fruits, and they have especially cherished their wonderful apricots and their silty glacial river. Land for farming is scarce and the population grows slowly but steadily. The Hunza men joke that they cannot move to another region because their women won't live where the apricot does not thrive. The Hunzukuts work hard but they cannot produce as much food as they really need. Food is rationed carefully during the winter, but the people suffer famine every spring after the winter stores have been depleted and prior to the barley harvest at the end of June.

The grains grown in Hunza are barley, winter wheat, millet and buckwheat. The fields yield two crops; millet is planted after barley is havested in early July and buckwheat is planted after the winter wheat is harvested.

The Hunza women make a flat bread called chapatties from their milled grains. Lorimer describes the procedure: flour and a little water are kneaded in a shallow wooden tray and small lumps of dough are rolled thin with a small rolling pin. These are cooked briefly on a hot iron griddle. In older times hot stones were used for cooking.

Vegetables are boiled or eaten raw. Since firewood is scarce, only small amounts of water are used for cooking, and food is not cooked very long. Tea and salt are commonly used.

John H. Tobe, who visited Hunza in 1959, described a typical day's menu in Hunza. Breakfast was fresh or boiled apricots and chapatties, followed by a midmorning lunch of boiled vegetables, dried apricots and chapatties, a midday meal of apricot soup (made from dried apricots), and dinner of boiled or raw vegetables, fruit and chapatties.[3]

The apricots and the grains were obviously their staples, and the Hunzukuts took good care of their apricot trees. Mrs. Lorimer reported seeing the method for removing grubs from the trees early in March. The family that owned a tree used long sticks with curved iron knives on the ends to remove twigs that held a cocoon containing a grub that was known to devour the leaves. The cocoons were all removed this way, and burned.

John Clark was another visitor who described the Hunzukuts' methods of caring for the apricot trees.[4] The Hunzukuts knew how to graft different varieties of apricots to the strongest roots. Trees were topped when they were about fifty years old and allowed to grow for another fifty years. Fully mature trees were large and produced a great quantity of fruit. The fruit was harvested by children climbing the trees and shaking branches. Which meant that soil contaminated the harvest. Clark thought this was probably the cause of cases of bacillary dysentery common in Hunza. The apricot seeds were also used. Seeds were cracked and the kernels were eaten if they were sweet (from grafted trees). Bitter kernels from wild trees were ground and kneaded by hand, warmed, and an oil was separated for use in lamps. Some writers have said the oil was also used in cooking but this is uncertain. John Clark and Emily Lorimer said only that the extracted oil was used for lamps and occasionally as a hair dressing.

Lorimer explained more about the daily life of the Hunzukuts than other visitors have done, and published a wealth of her own photos. Her easy rapport with the women and children as they worked at threshing barley, spinning wool, herding the few cows to and from grassy strips each day, and watching craftsmen work helped her and her husband with their mission to learn the intricacies of the language and study the life style. Her account of the friendly and unselfconscious generosity of the Hunzukuts is so convincing that the reader of her story is as charmed by the happy Hunzukuts as she was.

Franc Shor, later on an editor at *National Geographic,* and his wife, Jean, traveled to Hunza in the spring of 1952. They had met the Mir of Hunza, Mohammed Jamal Khan, on an earlier trip to Asia[5] and they were made welcome on a return visit. This Mir, who ruled from 1945 into the 1970s, knew English well, liked to explain the history and way of life in Hunza, and welcomed visitors who braved the mountain trails. He thus helped provide us with a written and pictorial record of Hunza before the influences of modern Pakistan reached the valley.

The Shors' account of their visit[6] includes wonderful photographs of the treacherous mountain trails, the suspension bridge over the raging river, and the houses and fields of the Hunzukuts. The Shors tell of a seventy-eight year-old Hunzukut who walked sixty-five miles in a day over the mountain trails to bring a message to them in Gilgit from the Mir in Baltit.

The sixty-five mile trip from Gilgit in northern Pakistan to Baltit, the village capital of the Mir of Hunza, began with a thirty mile mountain road, negotiable by jeep, to the village of Chalt. From there it was two days on a narrow mountain trail either on foot or on horseback to the village of Najir. One crossed the river on a suspension bridge to continue on to Baltit.

In their one-week stay in Baltit, the Shors learned much about the Hunzukuts' crops, cultivation techniques, and the importance of apricots in the diet. They show a photo of a pile of dried apricots in the Mir's storeroom, left over from the previous year's harvest. Apricot trees are so important that they can be given away separately from the land on which they grow. A daughter might be given a particular apricot tree to care for and harvest for her lifetime even after she marries and moves to another village.

The Shors visited in spring and so could see that the Hunzukuts did not grow quite enough food to feed themselves well all year. In addition to grains and apricots, the Hunzukuts grew potatoes, carrots, turnips, beans, peppers, pears, cherries, apples, mulberries and walnuts. Most families kept a few sheep and goats and slaughtered only one or two animals a year, at the late October harvest festival.

In December 1954, Lowell Thomas Jr. and his wife, Tay, piloted their single-engine Cessna from Karachi to Gilgit en route to Hunza. They were on an extended flying tour of Africa and Asia and also published photos and accounts of their travels in *National Geographic Magazine*.[7] From Gilgit they traveled the treacherous mountain trails by jeep and on horseback to Baltit. Visiting in the chill of December they became aware of the scarcity of firewood in the valley. Although they stayed only three days with the Mir in his palace, their report is valuable for the spectacular photos of the mountains and the valley.

Why did so many explorers go to Hunza and write about it in the early part of this century? There were a variety of reasons. Some went to climb mountains, some went in service to the British Empire, some went to photograph the scenery, and some went for scholarly and other personal missions.

Visitors to Hunza were always impressed by the endurance and apparent good health, as well as the amiability, of the Hunzukuts. European explorers in the 1920s and 1930s wrote favorably about the hard-working, always cheerful and willing Hunzukuts, whom they employed as porters and whom they found to be charming companions on strenuous treks over the mountains.[8]

In the early part of the century a British medical officer, Sir Robert McCarrison, spent several years stationed in the Gilgit Agency, an area that included Hunza, and he was much impressed by the Hunzukuts. He considered the Hunzukuts to be unusually healthy and, later in his career, he lectured widely and wrote enthusiastically about the healthy Hunzas. He said, "Their nerves are as solid as cables and sensitive as the strings of a violin."[9]

McCarrison assumed that diet was the main reason for their good health. He knew that goiter and cretinism were common problems in northern India but the Hunzukuts did not suffer from these problems. McCarrison described the Hunzukuts as being resistant to "all kinds of degenerative and pestilential diseases" that afflicted other peoples in the area. He considered them to be unusually fertile, long-lived, with excellent nervous systems, and free of digestive diseases. He said, "Indeed, their buoyant abdominal health has, since my return to the West, provided a remarkable contrast with the dyspeptic and colonic lamentations of our highly civilized communities." - 1921. McCarrison never saw a case of cancer in Hunza.

In 1959 John H. Tobe spent a month in Hunza for yet another purpose. He hoped that a study of the Hunzukuts' diet and cultivation methods would yield some secrets to greater health and vitality. Tobe was a nurseryman from Niagara, Ontario who was keenly interested in organic gardening, in health matters in general, and in folk medicine.

While in Hunza, staying with the Mir, he questioned a young resident physician, Dr. Mohammed Yusuf Khan, who claimed that "gallstones, renal calculi, coronary heart disease, hypertension, valvular lesions, [thyroid disorders], mental deficiencies, cancer, poliomyelitis, arthritis and diabetes are absolutely unknown in Hunza."[3]

Tobe gave consideration to all the possibilities he could think of as to the secrets of the Hunzukuts' good health—returning everything to the soil, apricot oil, glacier milk, lots of sunshine—but admitted that he did not learn the answers to his questions while in Hunza. He thought the general quality of the fruits, vegetables, and grains in Hunza was not as good as in North America.

In the story of the Hunzukuts it seems we have the makings of a myth. No cancer, no heart disease, long life and happiness. Is this all possible, is it all true? Well, the part about no cancer and no coronary heart disease does seem to be true from all accounts that are available to us. As for long life, we know there were no records kept on mortality rates. John Clark's book[4] includes an informal survey he took on the number of deaths among close relatives of his craft school students in Hunza in 1950. Nine teenage boys were able to list twenty-five deaths among their immediate families, which seems to be a lot. As we shall see, Clark had the opportunity to observe much illness during his stay in Hunza, also.

The early books on Hunza were sometimes written in a style of romantic exaggeration. An example is J.I. Rodale's book, *The Happy Hunzas.*[8] Rodale's book was written to promote organic gardening. Rodale had first learned about organic farming and composting from the writings of Sir Albert Howard, who had developed the methods in India beginning in 1905. While working as a government scientist for several decades, Howard showed how a wide variety of crops could be grown more productively when compost farming is used. Howard's recommendations were adopted with good results on farms and plantations all over the world. Rodale made a thorough study of the many advantages of maintaining a high-humus soil, and tried out the compost methods on a farm in Pennsylvania. Rodale had also accepted, on the basis of a couple of brief stories and without thinking to ask for scientific evidence, the notion that organically grown food could ward off infectious diseases. When his own health improved (fewer headaches and colds) after he shrugged off his job as a magazine editor and bought the farm, he was convinced that organically grown food provided benefits for human health. He set out to advocate organic farming through his publications.

Rodale read everything he could about Hunza because the stories from Hunza told of an especially healthy community where all available plant and animal wastes were returned to the soil. Rodale assumed that crops were more nutritious in Hunza. The stories he relates told by travelers who had visited Hunza give an exaggerated picture of their good health. As we will see, the Hunzukuts were strong and hard working and free of cancer and heart disease, but they did in fact suffer from infectious diseases.

Sir Robert McCarrison's career is discussed at length in Rodale's book. McCarrison spent 1904-1911 as the Gilgit Agency surgeon. He realized that there were several characteristics of the Hunza way of life that were much different from Western ways of the times and were possible explanations for their good health. He listed breast-feeding of infants, the diet of "unsophisticated foods," avoidance of alcohol, and a life of vigorous exercise.

Sir Robert's early medical career was full of adventures. As a young fellow (twenty-five years old) he discovered that a three-day fever prevalent in India was caused by the bite of the sandfly. In the Gilgit Agency one of the great mysteries for McCarrison was why the Hunzukuts should be spared from goiter and the more serious associated condition, cretinism, while these conditions were common in neighboring valleys and parts of India, as they were in many inland regions of the world. Iodine had been used to cure goiter in Switzerland soon after its discovery in 1811, but toxic overdoses gave iodine therapy a bad reputation for a full century; so the study of goiter epidemiology continued. McCarrison made a careful study of the correlation between goiter incidence rates and water pollution in villages along the Gilgit River, and proved by experiments on himself and on volunteers that drinking polluted water could induce goiter. He made an accurate conclusion when he ascribed the Hunzukuts' freedom from goiter to one of their most obvious differences from their neighbors, which was their scrupulous avoidance of polluted water.

After his seven years at Gilgit, McCarrison became director of nutrition research for India, a position that enabled him to experiment with dietary variations in laboratory animals and with various methods of fertilizing crops. His dietary studies showed how much different the animals' well-being could be when their diets varied as much as human diets vary. Financial cutbacks by the government at the outbreak of World War I ended his research in India sooner than he would have liked. Later on, back in England, he lectured and wrote several books on thyroid disorders and on the role of vitamin deficiency and poor diet in the common human condition of ill health. In England, his patients included many sickly children and older people with gastrointestinal complaints who all lacked the vegetables and whole grains they sorely needed in their diet, in spite of the greater abundance of food available in England compared to Hunza. In England, he saw patients who avoided vegetables because they were "difficult to digest" and avoided fruit because "it carried infection," and who suffered from ill health while they continued to consume diets containing much starch, sugar, and fats. McCarrison was convinced by his observations in England and his experience in India of the crucial importance of vitamin-rich foods and unrefined foods as one indispensable factor for maintaining health and vitality. Through his books and lectures McCarrison sought to educate the public in better ways to plan their diets.

J.I. Rodale had some further ideas on reasons for the Hunzukuts' success. His chief speculations derived from their custom of returning everything to the soil and on the possibility of beneficial limestone minerals in their irrigation water. Not much information is available about the composition of the water and the silt in the Hunza River. The mountains are considered to be granite (silicates), although John Clark did find a large area of marble (limestone) in his geologic survey. Whether the Hunza River water contains especially beneficial minerals is unknown, but the Hunzukuts certainly did return everything to the soil. Lorimer and Clark both described the necessary custom of collecting every bit of dung from the animals, since manure was the only fertilizer available.

John Clark had a reason for going to Hunza that was different from the other visitors' reasons. Clark was an American geologist who had served in the U.S. Army as reconnaissance engineer with General Joseph W. Stilwell in Sinkiang, China in 1944, working on the nine thousand mile survey of trails and roads in western China. He saw firsthand the brutal ambitions of the Russian communists in Asia as they took over Chinese villages and knew firsthand the difficulties of accomplishing change by working with local officials. He believed help from the West would be needed to improve education and living standards so that people would be better prepared to decide their own future governments. After the war, he undertook a personal mission to central Asia to try to improve the self-reliance and standard of living of one small group of worthy people. His aim was to set up a craft school and possibly other money-making endeavors, help start new crops, and try to encourage new ways of independent thinking as a deterrent to the spread of communism. A preliminary scouting trip in 1948 through Pakistan and into Chinese Turkestan (Sinkiang) taught him that the Chinese government was still undergoing disruptive spasms of restructuring and would probably not allow a stranger to stay and work. His second choice was the state of Hunza where he thought the young people especially were sufficiently ambitious to learn new ways and poor enough to benefit from the little help he might be able to give them.

Lacking funding, he returned to the U.S. to teach for a while at the University of Michigan while he raised money through a research foundation for a one-man expedition to Hunza. He hoped his undertaking (called "a one-man Marshall Plan" by William O. Douglas) would serve as a demonstration project for more extensive Western efforts to halt communism in Asia.

Clark spent twenty months in Hunza in 1950-51, and the detailed account of his experiences was published in 1956.[4] Apparently, by the time he wrote his book, he had become aware of others' efforts to advertise the unusual good health and happiness of the Hunzukuts, and he was vexed by what seemed to be promotion of a myth of a perfect way of life in Hunza. His own sojourn in Hunza had shown him that life in Hunza included problems of hardship, scarcity, infectious diseases and yearly bouts with famine.

His book and Lorimer's are the most objective and accurate accounts of life in Hunza. They both spoke the language of Hunza and lived in the villages for considerable periods, although both lived in better circumstances than the Hunzukuts since they brought money and could purchase food, hire horses, and hire workers. Their books are complementary since each concentrated on different aspects of daily life.

Clark and the Hunzukuts communicated in a combination of Burushaski, Urdu, and Uzbek. Blessed with keen perception and total recall, Clark produced a fascinating story of the interplay of personalities from different cultures trying new endeavors while sometimes hampered by tradition and difficult circumstances.

The Mir of Hunza appreciated Clark's intention of setting up a dispensary in Baltit—the nearest medical help at the time was in Gilgit, a three day journey away—and lent him an unused former residence to use as a home and office in return for his medical services. The Mir also arranged for Clark to purchase food while in Baltit, further enabling Clark to concentrate on his dispensary, setting up a craft school for boys, and doing some geological surveys as a favor to the Pakistani government.

The dispensary turned out to be a major part of Clark's work in Hunza. Patients arrived every morning and, with the help of two boys whom he hired and trained, he diagnosed and treated impetigo, ascariasis, sores and boils, trachoma, ringworm, malaria, and an epidemic of bacillary dysentery in one village. His own malaria recurred at times. One woman with tuberculosis was too far advanced to be helped. A small boy covered with sores and near death from being unable to eat recovered by the gradual application of sulphathiazole to the sores.

Clark took with him to Hunza iodine, potassium permanganate to sterilize water, merthiolate, magnesia, sulphathiazole, penicillin, drugs for malaria, undecylenic acid for fungus infections, and other medicines. His medical training was "a minor in anatomy, a year's college course in first aid and public health, and some very practical information from doctors of Billings Hospital in Chicago, Johns Hopkins in Baltimore and the United Mission Medical Council."

Clark treated more than five thousand people during his stay in Hunza. He commented in an article in *Natural History* magazine on the different types of illnesses seen there compared to the common illnesses in the West.[10] He saw many cases of staph infections and, in addition to the diseases mentioned above, he saw mild cases of rickets and scurvy. Heart disease was rare and he never observed cancer. Clark's medical training was meager, but his careful observations on the health problems of the patients he saw tell us there were several types of infectious diseases and parasites and some incidence of deficiency disease in Hunza.

Clark also made a few interesting observations on farming techniques. He had taken vegetable seeds to Hunza and had the school boys plant a vegetable garden using a new method—raised rows for planting between shallow ditches for irrigating. The Hunzukuts were accustomed to using broadcast planting and irrigated by flooding a field. The Hunzukuts were already familiar with potatoes (introduced by the British), melons, carrots, cucumbers and peppers. Clark described the construction of the terraced fields. Some of the man-made terraces in the valley had retaining walls twice as high as the terrace was wide. Terraces were constructed by building a retaining wall from rocks, flooding the pool and allowing the silt from the river to settle in the pool. Water was drained and the pool was reflooded. In two years enough silt was collected to create a terrace. Clark says, "This is certainly the most desperate expedient of land-starved people anywhere on earth, yet visitors have written about Hunza as the land where everyone has "just enough" and there are no poor!"

Manure was the only fertilizer used in Hunza, applied to the fields four times in a season. In summer the sheep and goats were moved to higher summer pasture and were corralled every night for milking by a few men and boys from each village. Butter and dried manure were hauled back to the village. The pasture land was so meager that only a few animals could be kept by each family.

The Hunzas seem to have encouraged the story of their good health and longevity—perhaps as a mild form of rivalry with neighboring provinces. John Clark thought the myth of their longevity was probably an exaggeration. He found out for himself that the Hunzukuts were very casual about giving precise answers to his questions on their age, at least the young people he worked with and had a chance to become friends with. He thought the elderly people he treated were probably not more than about seventy-five years old from looking at the amount of wear on their teeth.[10]

In the early 1970s Dr. Alexander Leaf visited Hunza because of his interest in medical problems of the elderly. Leaf was a professor at Harvard University Medical School and Chief of Medical Services at Massachusetts General Hospital. He traveled to three locations around the world where people were thought to commonly live to very old age. These were the Andean village of Vilcabamba in Ecuador, Abkhazia in the Caucasus in the USSR, and Hunza. Leaf wanted to talk to some of the very old, try to verify their ages, and see for himself how they lived. In Abkhazia he interviewed some old people and was able to verify their ages from their recollections of historical events. In Hunza he photographed one man alleged to be 110 years old, but he was not able to actually verify any unusual ages in Hunza. He was impressed by the physical fitness of many of the elderly people there.

Dr. Leaf[11] cites the study by a Pakistani nutritionist and chemist, Dr. S. Maqsood Ali, who interviewed fifty-five men in Hunza and found an average caloric intake of only 1923 Calories per day. This included 50 grams of protein, 36 grams of fat, and 354 grams of carbohydrate. Most oil in the diet was from apricot seeds. Meat and dairy products comprised only 1 1/2 % of the total calories. There was no obesity and no signs of undernutrition.

By 1974 modern civilization was getting a little closer to Hunza. Sabina and Roland Michaud, French writer-photographers, went by jeep the entire sixty-seven miles from Gilgit to Baltit and found a small hotel being built in Baltit. They met the same Mir Mohammed Jamal Khan who had ruled Hunza since 1945, but who was now pensioned in retirement by the government of Pakistan and the bitter observer of progress arriving inexorably in the Hunza River valley.[9] The new road from Gilgit to Baltit, built in 1960, allowed importation of flour, kerosene, margarine, and a few hand-powered sewing machines. Younger Hunza men had begun enlisting in the Pakistani army, bringing some cash back home to Hunza along with a taste for tobacco, sweets and such treats of civilization. The Michauds stayed several weeks in Baltit and in Shimshal and found that the Hunzukuts still lived a spare existence, keeping modest herds and using the same methods of cooking and farming as ever.

What can we conclude from the story of Hunza? Their low-calorie, restricted diet and their strenuous life style seem to have protected them from some of the health problems of richer societies. The prevalence of infectious diseases seen by John Clark and ignored or not observed by other writers leads us to listen skeptically to the claims or myths of perfect health—the earlier stories were probably incomplete. Their fat intake of only 17% of total calories is now thought to be an ideal level we should aim for to reduce the risk of atherosclerosis.

Whether their high intake of beta-carotene from apricots and vegetables provided protection from cancer is a question that cannot be answered until more populations around the world are studied.

Chapter 3

The Hawthorne Works

Beginning in the 1970s medical scientists have stepped up their efforts to study more and more populations around the world for details on the relationship between diet and disease, and they have found that people who are in the habit of frequently eating vegetables are less likely to develop cancer than their neighbors who eat vegetables less often. The reason for this result is not yet completely understood, but a new emphasis on the value of vegetables is growing as a result of this research. There are several components of vegetables that are good candidates for being the active principles that help prevent this disease. Vitamin A, vitamin C, folic acid, and fiber all have functions in metabolism that theoretically could help prevent cancer. There are a few other components of vegetables that also may help; and in addition, there are traditional dietary and food preparation customs that are important in determining whether or not cancer is common in certain populations.

The study of people's diets in relation to the incidence of cancer received a tremendous boost in the 1980s from a provocative article on the possible involvement of beta-carotene in cancer prevention that appeared in 1981 in the British scientific journal, *Nature*. The article suggested that the consumption of beta-carotene-containing vegetables and fruits is related to low risk for several types of cancer. This suggestion came from a handful of reports on human diets and cancer that were scattered through the scientific literature and from experimental work on animals and cells that demonstrated cancer-inhibiting activity of vitamin A. The article spelled out the types of studies that would need to be done in order to find out whether the suggestion was a valid one.

Long-term studies on diet would be especially useful inasmuch as cancer is thought to be a condition that develops slowly over many years. A few long-term studies on diet were already underway. A long-term study in Japan had been started in 1965, a study of several thousand Norwegians who lived in either Norway or Minnesota was set up in 1964, and a nineteen year-long study in Chicago at the Western Electric Company had been started in 1957. The study in Chicago was a large, carefully designed project that was meant to test the idea that dietary habits are related to heart disease. As it turned out, the study produced striking results on the relation between diet and lung cancer in addition to results on diet and heart disease.

The Hawthorne Works of the Western Electric Company was a very large manufacturing plant located in a densely populated, close-in suburb of Chicago. Built in 1904 on a 115-acre, prairie site on the outskirts of Chicago, the plant became over the years a giant industrial complex that was also a social and recreation center for its thousands of employees. During some periods of its history, the plant employed more than forty thousand people doing light assembly work or heavy shop work or clerical work. The plant produced telephones and other communication equipment, and some home appliances.[1]

The Hawthorne Works was also the site of some famous industrial research studies in the 1920s and 1930s that dealt with the effects of working conditions such as improved illumination on workers' productivity. In those studies the expected results were found and some unexpected results showed up, as well. The unexpected results were that workers' output increased when illumination went up *and* when illumination went down. The productivity of the constant-illumination control group also went up in both experiments due to the increased attention from outsiders. When a group of workers was studied during several years of periodic changes in working conditions—such as changing the scheduled hours and breaks, catering lunches and allowing more freedom—their productivity went up due to the altered nature of the supervision rather than due to changes in the working conditions. The workers' preferences and opinions were solicited by the people doing the experiments as they searched together for better ways to do the work. The workers found that their ideas contributed to production improvements and found that they were involved as a group with the new supervision rather than being at odds with supervision. Their involvement paid off in higher productivity.[2]

In the twenty year-long study on dietary habits and workers' health that was started in 1957 at the Hawthorne Works, some unexpected results were found again. This time a study that was set up with coronary heart disease in mind yielded some interesting information on lung cancer incidence in cigarette smokers when the results were all in.

The Western Electric Study, as it was called, was designed and carried out by a group of physicians, dieticians, and epidemiologists from the University of Illinois College of Medicine and Presbyterian-St. Luke's Hospital in Chicago, with the encouragement of the medical department of the Western Electric Company.[3] Coronary heart disease was a major unsolved national health problem in the 1950s. Doctors had strong suspicions that the problem was largely due to such factors as overweight, lack of exercise, cigarette smoking, hereditary lipid problems, serum cholesterol level and blood pressure, but there were other factors such as the contribution of dietary fat to serum cholesterol level that were controversial and difficult to pin down.

Studies in several countries had failed to show correlation between diet and serum cholesterol, but studies of this type are very difficult to do. There are always some second thoughts on how the dietary survey could have been done more accurately, some second thoughts on other factors in people's lives that could have influenced the results and were not included in the survey.

The Western Electric Study was designed to use very careful dietary survey methods to try to find out whether saturated fatty acids, polyunsaturated fatty acids or cholesterol intake was related to serum cholesterol level or to future coronary heart disease. Two thousand men from the Hawthorne Works were enrolled in the Western Electric Study through a selection process where men between forty and fifty-five years of age who had been employed there for at least two years and who had no known heart disease were invited at random to participitate in a health survey. The doctors' main interest in coronary heart disease was not disclosed and no medical advice was offered by the professionals doing the health survey.

The voluntary participants were given thorough medical exams at the beginning of the study with interviews on family history and physical activity on and off the job. Two dietary interviews, one year apart, were done by trained dieticians at the beginning of the study. Medical exams were done annually until 1969.

Since the study population was mostly of similar cultural background and eating habits, very careful analysis was needed in order to discriminate between what might be minor variations in diet among the participants. The dietary interviews included detailed questions on the usual eating habits during the week and the frequency of eating 195 specific foods during the past month. Questionnaires on food preparation were filled out by the men's wives.

Dietary surveys are acknowledged to give only an approximation of actual diet; so the dieticians did a repeat interview one year after the first to get additional data, and they believed their data were reasonably accurate. The next step was to calculate the amounts of fat in the diet. Foods have been analyzed for fats, protein, carbohydrate, vitamins and minerals by food chemists, and the results of these analyses are collected and published, often by government agencies. From the known chemical composition of foods, each man's diet was calculated for milligrams of cholesterol consumed and for saturated and unsaturated fatty acid calories as a percentage of total calories consumed.

The men in the Western Electric Study consumed rich diets. Their average daily intake was about 3170 Calories, which included 118 grams of protein, 152 grams of fat, and 304 grams of carbohydrate. Forty-three percent of their total calories came from fat, including both animal fat and vegetable fat. In the 1950s, diets high in fat and cholesterol were common in the United States heartland. Awareness of the links between high-fat diet, cholesterol in the diet, and coronary heart disease was beginning to spread through the population, though, and the men at the Hawthorne Works did change their eating habits somewhat after finding out their initial serum cholesterol levels, because of this new awareness.

Four years and five months into the study at the Hawthorne Works, eighty-eight new cases of coronary heart disease (angina pectoris or heart attack) had been diagnosed in the group and statistical evidence began to show the relation of coronary heart disease to some observable characteristics in the men such as cigarette smoking, chest discomfort, high serum cholesterol level, and high blood pressure. Other studies had also shown some of the same relationships. No relation of coronary heart disease to diet was noted at this point.[3]

It is interesting to reflect on the difficulties of proving cause and effect relationships when studying human populations. One way to address a problem is to do a prospective study, meaning to determine the characteristics of a population before illness strikes and monitor changes in health status over a period of time. The individuals in the population will have different values for their cholesterol level, blood pressure, servings of vegetables per day, or whatever factor is being evaluated, and these differences may or may not correlate with development of an illness. Statisticians who help design and analyze such studies look for associations (correlations) between measurable characteristics in a population and outcomes of a diagnostic test. At the end of the study the statisticians use the laws of probability to calculate the chance of random association between the measured characteristic and various outcomes. For instance, what is the probability that blood pressure higher than a certain value would be associated with double the usual heart attack rate simply from mere chance? If an association occurs in the group being studied in spite of a probability of less than one out of twenty from mere chance ($p < .05$), the association is said to be "statistically significant." This would be a preliminary type of proof that the characteristic is related to the outcome; it may not be a direct cause of the outcome, as it could also be indirectly related.

If a study is very long lasting, statisticians know that all manner of factors can interfere with interpretation of the mathematical conclusions. During the last few decades for instance, the growing awareness of the importance of diet, exercise, and other life style factors has led many of us to make an effort to change some of our old habits in order to improve our present and future well-being. Some of this occurred in the Western Electric Study and occurs in other long-range studies. Prospective studies where the participants are followed for several years are considered to be the most reliable way of analyzing the relation between life style and health, but even this type of reliable study is not foolproof—people do change their eating habits from time to time, or their environments can change, and these possibilities are always considered by the interviewers running the studies.

Twenty years after the initial interviews at the Hawthorne Works, a final accounting of the vital status of the Hawthorne study group was done to find out who had died from coronary heart disease. The statistics showed very small, but statistically significant, associations between fat intake and serum cholesterol and between dietary cholesterol and death from coronary heart disease.

A report of these results was published in the *New England Journal of Medicine*[4] and was the subject of a front page article in the *New York Times* the same day. (Several of the general-interest, scientific and medical journals distribute advance copies of their journals to newspapers as an aid to journalists who want to keep the public informed of the latest news. These technical journals can often be found in the public libraries as well as in university libraries.)

So, the idea that fat in the diet can contribute to coronary heart disease gained a little more scientific backing from the Western Electric Study. This was an unexpectedly involved biochemical subject because of the complicated nature of cholesterol metabolism. Cholesterol circulates in the blood included in several types of lipoproteins which vary according to eating habits, a recent meal, exercise habits, hereditary conditions, and even vary with stress levels and the seasons of the year. Besides using cholesterol absorbed from food, the cells of the body make new cholesterol using breakdown products of fatty acids, carbohydrates, and protein. All of these factors are variable to some extent among individuals and vary from time to time in a particular individual.

For these reasons and others, the question of whether dietary fats are related to serum cholesterol in large groups of freely eating individuals was very difficult to answer definitively and many large studies were done in the 1960s and 1970s. The studies usually left some questions unanswered and some doubts in the minds of the medical scientists. On the other hand, it had been easy to demonstrate for years, in controlled clinical trials, that serum cholesterol levels could be lowered through dietary changes that included lower fat intake. In clinical trials, individuals would be tested at regular intervals while adhering strictly to prescribed diets and would show decreases in their serum cholesterol levels.

This problem had difficulties similar to the related question of whether lowering serum cholesterol would actually reduce the incidence of heart attacks. This aspect of the cholesterol story was also difficult and expensive to demonstrate with certainty.[5] So, it wasn't until the 1980s that the strategy of eating less fat and cholesterol in order to reduce the risk of heart disease became finally uncontested and could be recommended by physicians without any reservations. In the meantime, the mortality rate from heart attack declined 30% from the mortality rate in the 1950s, thanks to great progress in medical care such as Emergency Medical Service, Medicare, coronary care wards, anticlotting drugs and cholesterol-lowering drugs, blood pressure drugs, and surgery, and thanks to changes in life style such as quitting smoking, exercising, and controlling weight.

The cholesterol study at the Hawthorne Works was reported in a January, 1981 issue of the *New England Journal of Medicine* and became part of the vast medical literature on the consequences of cholesterol in the diet.

Just two months later a most provocative article appeared in the British scientific journal, *Nature*, which would motivate new labors by the scientists working on the Western Electric Study and would inspire extensive new research efforts into diet and disease. The new research would focus on the relation between vitamin A in its different natural forms and cancer in man, a possible connection that had been tested in only a few studies at that time and which had not been analyzed for its biologic complexity and possible significance.

In an article entitled "Can dietary beta-carotene materially reduce human cancer rates?" Peto, Doll, Buckley and Sporn brought together ideas and research results from several fields to point out the intriguing new evidence that linked green and yellow vegetables to reduced risk for cancer.[6]

Sir Richard Doll and Richard Peto, who are epidemiologists at Oxford University in England, had just finished preparing a major study of cancer risk factors in the United States—a study that was commissioned by the Congressional Office of Technology Assessment.[7] In this study, Doll and Peto had given much consideration to the possible role of diet as one of the twelve types of environmental factors that could be examined as possible causes or contributing causes of cancer. Epidemiologists had been aware for many years that populations in different parts of the world had different rates and different types of cancer, and differing diets were thought to be part of the explanation; but identifying which dietary changes might be important was problematical. Doll and Peto had found several studies from the 1970s that showed lower levels of circulating vitamin A in cancer patients than in controls. And several studies on diet had shown lower amounts of green vegetables in the diets of cancer patients compared to controls. These studies lead them to give serious consideration to the possibility that some form of vitamin A could be important for cancer prevention.

For their article on the possible role of beta-carotene, the epidemiologists recruited Michael B. Sporn of the National Cancer Institute, whose areas of expertise include the biochemistry and anticancer effects of vitamin A-related compounds in animals. In their article in *Nature,* Peto, Doll, Buckley & Sporn reviewed some of the basic metabolism of vitamin A and pointed out the gaps in our knowledge about beta-carotene and cancer. Anticancer effects had been observed in animals when compounds related to retinol were tested, but it was uncertain whether beta-carotene would have similar effects.

(Vitamin A is found in foods in two forms, retinol and beta-carotene. Retinol is found in animal foods such as egg yolk, milk fat, liver, and cod liver oil. Beta-carotene is found in fruits and vegetables. Beta-carotene is partly converted to retinol in the wall of the small intestine during digestion.)

The article in *Nature* by PDB&S (as I shall call them for the rest of this chapter) became a landmark in the development of the idea that vitamin A-related compounds might help prevent cancer in man. The authors are among the most highly regarded scientists in their fields. In an eight-page article they reviewed previous studies on vitamin A intake and cancer incidence in man and pointed out that the studies seemed to show that beta-carotene from vegetables, rather than retinol from milk and eggs, was related to lower incidence of cancer. They described the types of studies that would be needed to check on this possibility, and explained how fairly brief (perhaps five year-long) prospective intervention trials using beta-carotene as a dietary supplement might very well demonstrate beneficial effects on cancer rates if such effects are to be found.

PDB&S found eight published studies, going back to 1941, where the level of vitamin A in the blood was tested in recently diagnosed cancer patients and was compared with the level in other patients. All eight studies showed slightly lower levels of circulating vitamin A in the cancer patients. This result was a puzzle that would require further research, as the level of circulating vitamin A (retinol) does not change much from dietary changes but, rather, is maintained at a steady level by the liver.

PDB&S found twenty studies where dietary intake of beta-carotene was estimated through the use of questionnaires, either in prospective studies like the Western Electric Study or in retrospective studies where people with cancer and people without cancer were questioned about their diets during the previous years. In general, it was found that people who fell into the class of highest beta-carotene consumption were only 59% as likely to develop cancer as people who consumed lower levels of beta-carotene; but, as explained by PDB&S, the nature of the errors from using questionnaires makes it likely that the true difference between the high and low groups is greater than this.

With twenty studies to think about, all pointing in the same direction, we begin to see an interesting story. Even with the acknowledged uncertainty inherent in asking people to recall how often they eat various foods, the results become convincing when study after study shows that people who eat more green and yellow vegetables have lower rates of many types of cancer.

As pointed out by PDB&S, we cannot tell from these studies whether beta-carotene is providing some anticancer effect, or whether some other component of the vegetables is responsible for the trend of lower cancer incidence in big vegetable eaters. It is also possible that big vegetable eaters eat less of something else in the diet that contributes to the development of cancer. Because of this uncertainty, PDB&S made vigorous suggestions that prospective intervention trials using beta-carotene as a dietary supplement should be done in order to answer this question.

PDB&S knew that many large studies have been done where researchers collected blood samples for testing and froze part of each sample for later tests, and collected health data or dietary information at the same time in order to do long-range studies for various purposes. One of the suggestions made by PDB&S in their 1981 article was that researchers in possession of dietary information or frozen serum samples and long-term health statistics might be able to search their databases for information on beta-carotene or vitamin A intake and cancer incidence over the years.

The Western Electric Study with its detailed dietary surveys and nineteen year follow-up on two thousand men was exactly the type of study needed, and in fact PDB&S were aware of the potential use of the Western Electric Study for further analysis.

The suggestion from the British epidemiologists was taken up quickly by the Chicago epidemiologists. This group in 1981 had just completed their twenty year check on causes of death in the Western Electric Study, and now they sent questionnaires to all the survivors to inquire about any diagnoses of cancer during the past years. At the same time, the dieticians went back to work on the 1958 dietary information to calculate how much of the men's vitamin A intake consisted of retinol from animal foods such as milk, butter, eggs, and liver, and how much consisted of beta-carotene from fruits and vegetables. The carotene intake could only be estimated for each man, however, because the original detailed surveys had been replaced with dietary information in terms of consumption of food groups—for instance, vegetables as a group, soups, and fruits.

Nevertheless, the dieticians made estimates for the carotene intakes by averaging the carotene contents of the thirteen vegetables they had included in the original survey.[9]

The statisticians then placed the men in order from highest to lowest according to either their carotene intake or their retinol intake. The two thousand men were then divided into four groups, or quartiles, each quartile containing the same number of individuals, and the statisticians counted the number of cases of lung cancer or other carcinomas in each quartile. The men in the highest quartile had a carotene intake more than three times higher than the men in the lowest quartile.

When the data were analyzed, the results showed a highly significant association between high intake of carotene and low incidence of lung cancer, and in those men who had smoked for more than thirty years, the risk of lung cancer was eight times higher if they were in the lowest quartile for carotene intake than if they were in the highest quartile.

The results were published in November, 1981 in the British journal, *The Lancet*.[8] This paper by the Chicago epidemiologists was also the subject of stories in the *New York Times* and in popular magazines.

The statistical calculations on the data from the Western Electric Study showed no significant association between carotene intake and other types of cancer, only between carotene and lung cancer. Also, there was no association between higher retinol intake (that is, vitamin A from animal foods such as milk, butter, and eggs) and lower incidence of cancer. So, the Western Electric Study with its careful dietary analysis and long-term follow-up turned out to be an important milestone in the developing hypothesis that vegetables contain some cancer-preventing propety, at least as far as lung cancer was concerned. (A few years later these men's diets were studied in connection with another hypothesis, namely, that vitamin D or calcium can protect against colon cancer. The study showed that more calcium and vitamin D in the diet were definitely associated with low risk for colon cancer.)

Earlier dietary surveys had also shown protective effects of vegetables against the risk of lung cancer. In Norway, a mail survey was done in 1964 to question a sample of the general population about their diet and about their smoking habits. The aim was to compare respiratory and cardiovascular illnesses in Norwegians with the same illnesses in Britons and in brothers and sisters of Norwegians who had migrated to the United States. Norway has a cancer registry which covers the entire country and all diagnosed cases are eventually reported to the registry.

In 1973 Erik Bjelke of Norway, who had worked and studied in the United States, realized that the surveys could be used to look into the question of whether vitamin A was related to lung cancer incidence. Bjelke got this idea from experiments in laboratory animals at the Chicago Medical School which were published in 1967 and had shown that vitamin A could slow or prevent the development of experimental cancer of the respiratory tract.

Dr. Bjelke analyzed the incidence of lung cancer in more than eight thousand of the men who had responded to the Norwegian survey and found thirty-six cases of lung cancer.[10] This was a rather small number of cases, but when the relationship of cases to vitamin A intake was analyzed, Bjelke thought the results were so dramatic that he published the results early on in hopes that others might search their data to see if the same results would be found by other researchers.

The amount of vitamin A in the diet of the eight thousand men was estimated from the answers to the dietary questionnaire. The dietary questionnaire did not give a complete picture of all possible dietary sources of vitamin A. The estimated vitamin A intake came mostly from the milk and carrots items on the questionnaire, which means this study calculated vitamin A intake as a blend of retinol and beta-carotene from milk and beta-carotene from carrots.

When the Norwegian men were divided into high and low vitamin A consumers, the risk of lung cancer in the high vitamin A consumers was only 31% as great as in the low vitamin A consumers. The incidence of lung cancer was associated with the amount of cigarette smoking, of course, but at all levels of smoking, those in the high vitamin A group had much lower incidence of lung cancer than the men in the low vitamin A group.

The results were later confirmed in a longer-lasting study in a larger group of men and women in Norway several years later. When the individual foods on the questionnaire were analyzed, only milk, carrots, cabbage and tomatoes showed protective effects. A vitamin C index did not show protective effects.

A study of life style factors of lung cancer victims in Singapore was also carried out in the 1970s. The study included a few questions on dark green leafy vegetables, and this study also turned up a surprising result.

A high rate of lung cancer in Chinese women had been noticed in several parts of the world including the republic of Singapore, where the population is 77% Chinese. The reasons for the high rate of lung cancer were a mystery. One of the pecularities of the situation was that many of the cases among Cantonese women were a type of lung cancer called adenocarcinoma, which is not very common in most countries.

In an effort to find some explanations, the researchers went into the hospitals in Singapore to talk to lung cancer patients.[11] They conducted interviews with 233 lung cancer patients and, as controls, they interviewed 300 patients who were hospitalized for other reasons, but not for any smoking-related illnesses. The questions they asked had to do with a variety of environmental and dietary factors. The researchers had a few tentative ideas about factors that might be important in the etiology of lung cancer in addition to smoking. For instance, occupational history was included because there was some thought that talc used for dusting bales of rubber might lead to lung cancer. (The packing and shipping of natural rubber is one of the major industries on the Malay peninsula.) The practice of burning incense in the home was questioned as this custom would be expected in some of the more traditional Chinese families, and incense was known to contain carcinogens. Whether or not the patient cooked using hot oil for stir-frying, and with what type of fuel, was questioned because it was thought that use of kerosene might produce hotter oil and more aerosols containing carcinogens than old-fashioned, wood-fired cooking does. The patients' history of cigarette smoking and opium smoking was carefully documented.

The frequency of eating dark green leafy vegetables such as Chinese mustard greens and kale was questioned because these are sources of nitrate and there is a hypothesis that nitrate in foods might lead to the production of mutagenic nitrosamines and nitrosamides which might cause cancer. However, the findings on the consumption of green vegetables were the opposite of what would be expected if the nitrate in greens were a danger. (This should not be taken to mean that nitrosamines are not a cause of cancer. Experimental work with animals and epidemiological studies in humans clearly show that preformed nitrosamines do cause cancer of the upper gastrointestinal tract and the nasopharynx. People who eat a lot of pickled or salted fish or pickled vegetables consume too much nitrosamine and are at higher risk for these cancers.)

When the results of the interviews in Singapore were analyzed, it was found that cigarette smoking and the total quantity of tobacco smoked during the lifetime correlated with increased risk of lung cancer, as was expected. Opium smoking also increased the chances of having lung cancer. Burning incense in the home, especially while sleeping, increased the risk of lung cancer, perhaps due to carcinogens in the smoke. Too few rubber packers were found among the hospital patients interviewed to calculate whether this occupation led to a significantly increased risk. No evidence was found to connect cooking chores with increased risk. A significant association was found between higher economic status and increased risk of lung cancer; the researchers puzzled over this result but could not think of an explanation.

The researchers were surprised to find that when the green vegetable consumption was divided into two classes, those who ate green vegetables more often had less than half the risk for lung cancer as did those who ate these vegetables less often. The lower risk for lung cancer was found among those who ate more than three servings per week of at least three of these vegetables: mustard greens, kale, eggplant and long beans. Other vegetables had also been questioned during the interviews but this selection of only four vegetables served the statisticians' purpose of being representative of the overall vegetable content of the diet.

The researchers realized that this result agreed with results of the Norwegian study published two years earlier in 1975 and might contribute to a new hypothesis on involvement of vitamin A in preventing cancer.

This type of study comparing data on patients with data on nonpatients who are matched as closely as possible as to age, sex, and other background characteristics is called a retrospective, case-control study. It has advantages and disadvantages as a method for epidemiological study. One advantage is that data can be acquired and analyzed in only a few months, in contrast to the five or ten years or more that have been the rule in long-term prospective studies. A disadvantage is that people who are sick enough to be in a hospital or who have been diagnosed to have a serious illness may not feel well enough to endure lengthy questioning and may be too distracted to take much interest in accurate answers for the interviewers.

Nevertheless, case-control studies are widely used and much thought and effort goes into minimizing the biases, or discrepancies, that might be in the data.

After all these epidemiological studies showing less frequent lung cancer in people who ate more vegetables, it is interesting to try to trace back the sequence of events to search for the origins of the idea that vitamin A or beta-carotene might be important for preventing cancer.

Modern substantiation for the idea seems to have arisen from the results of observational epidemiology on the one hand and from laboratory tests of vitamin A supplements in experimental cancer in hamsters on the other hand.

When PDB&S proposed further testing of beta-carotene in 1981, there were already several dietary studies where people were asked about their diets, usually without any thought for testing any particular hypothesis. When the results of the surveys were inspected for various types of relationships, consumption of leafy green vegetables and yellow-orange vegetables stood out as a factor associated with lower incidence of some types of cancer.

During the early part of this century, when vitamin A was discovered, the effects of vitamin A on animals were studied, and one of the chief observations (after the findings that vitamin A was needed for reproduction and for vision) was the requirement for vitamin A in maintenance of normal epithelial tissues. In experiments that were published in 1925 and are still cited in modern reviews on vitamin A metabolism, Wolbach and Howe, of Boston, studied groups of rats maintained on diets that included either butter as a source of vitamin A or else lard (no vitamin A) in place of butter. The rats that were deficient in vitamin A suffered numerous pathological changes including wasting of many glands, loss of stored fat, and conversion of normal epithelial tissues into abnormal proliferating, keratinizing epithelium in many internal organs of the animals.[12] (Epithelial tissue is a major type of tissue throughout the body, and is a major part of the linings of the respiratory and digestive tracts and the various glands, as well as skin. Most cases of cancer in adults begin in epithelial tissue.)

A lack of vitamin A caused so many defects in epithelial tissues of animals that scientists during the 1930s tried to find specific explanations for the effects and tried to determine whether vitamin A was an important factor in the growth of neoplastic tissues in animals, but the results were mostly rather ambiguous. Referring to these efforts, Burk and Winzler of the National Cancer Institute were prompted to suggest in 1944: "Taken as a whole, the relationship between vitamin A and malignant growth appears to be a rather nebulous one. . . . However, sufficient evidence has accumulated which makes it desirable to seek further a peculiar and perhaps specific relationship between vitamin A and malignant growth." [13]

During the 1960s Dr. Umberto Saffiotti, who was at the Chicago Medical School at the time, was studying experimental lung cancer in hamsters. He was able to produce tumors in the respiratory tract by giving the carcinogen, benzpyrene. He knew vitamin A played a role in maintenance of normal tissue in the respiratory tract; so in experiments carried out to study the mechanism of action of carcinogens, he fed one group of hamsters large doses of vitamin A in the form of retinyl palmitate in addition to the benzpyrene treatment. These animals developed markedly fewer tumors in the respiratory tract than the animals treated with benzpyrene alone. [14]

Other scientists had also demonstrated anticancer effects of vitamin A in animal experiments in the early 1960s, and in earlier years a few studies in several countries using vitamin A-deficient animals showed that more tumors developed in the deficient animals than in those on the normal diet. Sporn, of the PDB&S team, knew from his own studies and those of other researchers that vitamin A-related compounds were necessary to prevent precancerous changes in animal tissues and that vitamin A could even cause reversal of some of these changes.

These early studies on animals that hinted that vitamin A might protect against cancer were known to the epidemiologists who studied human cancer in the 1970s. Erik Bjelke knew about the hamster experiments on vitamin A when he decided to inspect the Norwegian dietary surveys to see if they could be used to estimate vitamin A intake. Laboratory researchers studying the effects of carcinogens in animals also knew about the hamster experiments, but they had encountered an obstacle in their attempts to inhibit the cancer process by giving animals large doses of vitamin A. This was the toxicity caused by large doses of vitamin A in its retinol form. It wasn't until PDB&S pointed out the apparent benefits of carotene-containing foods (vegetables)—which are never toxic—that scientists realized that vitamin A could be both safe and effective and began testing the hypothesis that carotene-containing vegetables could help prevent cancer in man.

Sir Richard Doll and Richard Peto of the PDB&S team got involved in the vitamin A question when they accepted the task of reviewing available data on cancer risks and summarizing the status of trends in cancer incidence and mortality in the United States. An earlier survey by the National Cancer Institute had concluded that cancer rates were increasing rapidly, and doubts about this conclusion had prompted the Congressional Office of Technology Assessment to seek another opinion. Doll and Peto's studies of the possible environmental factors that might influence cancer rates led them to the exciting possibility that eating *more* of some foods might be beneficial. The article by PDB&S in *Nature* in 1981 generated tremendous interest among cancer researchers and helped start an avalanche of new studies on the possibility that beta-carotene might play a role in cancer prevention, and also on its puzzling mode of action. The focus of attention has remained on the likelihood that vegetables help prevent cancer because of their carotene content, although there are other factors in the vegetables that might be just as important as carotene for cancer prevention.

Chapter 4

Study After Study

We have seen impressive statistics in the last chapter which showed the apparent effects of vegetables in helping to protect cigarette smokers from the most common forms of lung cancer. Be that as it may, one wonders whether beta-carotene or other components of vegetables can help prevent other types of cancer. After all, we well know by now that cigarette smoking is hazardous and should be avoided. If only the most common forms of lung cancer show reduced incidence from beta-carotene, and not other types of cancer, the role of vegetables would not be a very important story to tell, because we know that most forms of lung cancer could have been avoided by simply not smoking.

But we know very little indeed about measures we might take to avoid the other major types of cancer. One would like to know whether epidemiological studies of the types described in the last chapter have found reduced risk for any other common types of cancer. Is there any evidence that people who eat a lot of green and yellow vegetables are less likely to develop cancer of the colon, of the prostate, of the breast, or of the ovary, for instance? Does beta-carotene help protect only certain tissues against the carcinogenic effects of tobacco, or are there more general stabilizing effects of beta-carotene that work to prevent malignancies in other parts of the body? Does it matter whether the cancer cells were initiated by environmental carcinogens or by some kind of error in the maintenance of normal properties of the cells?

In this chapter I will describe briefly more of the studies that have been done in recent years to try to find the answers to the question of whether vegetables in the diet help to reduce the incidence of carcinomas. When PDB&S published their article in *Nature* in 1981, the evidence for vitamin A or beta-carotene being important in this respect was extremely intriguing—today it is far more compelling. The data have already convinced many people who are familiar with the field that vitamin A or beta-carotene has a definite preventive effect against cancer at many sites in the body.

Conferences have been held to discuss the research results on cancer and nutrition, and cancer and vitamin A, and to discuss the types of research still needed. Clinical trials have been started in the 1980s to find out whether taking extra beta-carotene or other vitamin A-related compounds will have an effect on the cancer statistics. Until a few of these controlled clinical trials are finished and analyzed, there will be some doubt as to the extent of beneficial effects that can be obtained by including more beta-carotene in the diet. In the meantime, the reader can browse here through some of the many epidemiological studies from around the world and judge for himself whether eating more beta-carotene-containing vegetables should be part of his own dietary strategy.

The reader may wonder about the meaning of the word "carcinoma" used above. Doctors use carcinoma to mean cancer that arises in any of the epithelial tissues of the body, which include mucous membranes, linings of various ducts and tracts, and glands, as well as the skin. About 80% of the cases of cancer are carcinomas. Cancer that arises in other types of tissue is *not* called carcinoma. The other types of tissue are connective tissue (for instance, bone and bone marrow), nerve tissue, and muscle.

First we will look at a few more retrospective case-control studies on lung cancer. Lung cancer has been the subject of more studies in relation to vegetables than any other type of cancer. Also, the question of whether vitamin A can inhibit cancers arising in glandular tissues— an important question in relation to the extent of the benefits that might be expected from consuming more vitamin A—was first brought up by some puzzling results in the studies on the different types of lung cancer. Additional studies on diet and lung cancer were needed to ferret out the whole story.

Many epidemiological studies have been done at Roswell Park Memorial Institute. Roswell Park Memorial Institute in Buffalo, New York is one of the major centers for cancer research and cancer treatment in the United States. It was started in 1898 and was the first such center where the staff devoted full time to study of the cancer problem.

Beginning in 1957 and continuing to 1965, all patients admitted to RPMI were interviewed before admission on matters of dietary history, smoking history, and other personal information. The interviews followed a questionnaire format and the interviews were completed before the patients were diagnosed; so the interviewer did not know what the patients' outcome would be. (Many patients turned out to have a variety of disorders other than cancer.) Scientists at RPMI and the State University of New York at Buffalo have used the data from the interviews to study the risk factors associated with cancer.

A study on lung cancer showing beneficial effects of vitamin A was published by epidemiologists at RPMI in 1979. Among men who had been heavy smokers, the risk of lung cancer was seen to be 2.4 times higher in those who had little vitamin A in the diet compared to those who consumed a lot of vitamin A. In the older heavy smokers (presumably long-time smokers), the increased risk was even greater (four times higher). Light smokers also had different risks depending on their dietary vitamin A, with the differences in risk being smaller. When the 292 lung cancer patients and 801 controls were combined and then separated into three groups depending on how much vitamin A was in their diets, there was a graded effect, or dose-dependent effect, through the three groups showing increasing risk with decreasing vitamin A level.

When the scientists analyzed the dietary histories for fat, protein, vitamin C and carbohydrate intake levels, they found no relation between these nutrients and the risk of lung cancer. Whether the patients were from rural areas or urban areas made no difference, either.

The dietary surveys at RPMI did not include all possible sources of vitamin A in the diet, but did include many vegetables and milk. The reduced risk of lung cancer was seen when milk alone or carrots alone was considered, similar to the Norwegian study, as well as when the total vitamin A from the dietary questionnaire was used in the calculations, lending credence to the conclusion that it was the vitamin A content of the diet which was responsible for the reduced risks rather than some other nutrient in the food items on the questionnaire.

Curtis Mettlin et al., "Vitamin A and Lung Cancer," *J. Natl. Cancer Inst. 62*, 1435 (1979).

A somewhat larger study using much more detailed and sophisticated analysis was done a few years later at Roswell Park Memorial

Institute. This time the effects of smoking and the effects of diet were analyzed for three of the main histological types of lung cancer, separately.

The most common type of lung cancer in smokers is squamous cell carcinoma arising in the lining of the lungs. Some cancers are small cell carcinoma of the lung arising from endocrine (hormone-secreting) cells in the lung. A less common type is adenocarcinoma arising in the glands in the lung that secrete mucus. Adenocarcinoma is a type of lung cancer that occurs in nonsmokers as well as in cigarette smokers. In this RPMI study, all three types were strongly associated with the amount of cigarette smoking, but only the squamous cell and small cell types appeared to be inhibited by high intake of vitamin A.

As in the earlier study, there was a decreasing incidence of the squamous cell and small cell types as the intake of vitamin A went from low to medium to high. Out of the 1521 men in the study (cases and controls), the group with the high vitamin A intake had only 69% as much chance of having squamous cell carcinoma and 56% as much chance of having small cell carcinoma as the group with a low intake of vitamin A. This was after adjusting for variations in age and pack-years of cigarettes smoked. But the less common adenocarcinoma occurred with the same frequency in low, medium, and high vitamin A consumers, which made it appear that vitamin A would not prove to be associated with the risk of this glandular type of cancer.

Out of 465 lung cancer cases in the study, 33 were non-smokers. No association was found between lung cancer and vitamin C in the diet.

The scientists felt that caution should be used in the interpretation of their results. They did not think they had found strong enough evidence to make any great claims for beneficial effects from diet at this point, and they thought there could be a variety of explanations for the observed inverse association between vitamin A and risk of lung cancer.

> Tim Byers et al., "Dietary Vitamin A and Lung Cancer Risk: An Analysis by Histologic Subtypes," *Amer. J. Epidem. 120*, 769 (1984).

Epidemiologists from the National Cancer Institute studied the vitamin A intake of lung cancer cases among men in New Jersey and found a very significant risk reduction associated with dark yellow-orange and dark green vegetables. More than sixteen hundred cases and controls were interviewed about the frequency of eating forty-four foods that provide most of the vitamin A in the American diet. The subjects were asked to try to remember the frequency of eating each food about four years earlier, before becoming ill. The interviews included questions that enabled the scientists to determine how much of the vitamin A was retinol from dairy products, eggs, liver, fortified cereals, or vitamin supplements, and how much of the vitamin A was carotene from vegetables and fruits. The interviewers also asked questions about vitamin C-containing foods and cruciferous vegetables, and questions about smoking history, occupation, and exposure to hazardous materials.

(Cruciferous vegetables are especially interesting as potential cancer-preventing foods. These vegetables contain indoles, which induce increased production in the body of one of the many enzymes that can detoxify the natural toxins found in foods. Cruciferous vegetables in the diet have been consistently correlated with lower risk for colon cancer and several other types of cancer. The cruciferous vegetables include cabbage, Brussels sprouts, broccoli, turnip and several others—see chapter 11. Many of these are excellent sources of beta-carotene and folic acid, as well. Folic acid is a B vitamin that may help prevent cancer by preventing the chromosome damage that is thought to be involved with cancer initiation.)

About 60% of the cases and controls in the New Jersey study were interviewed directly. The remainder of the cases and controls had died or become incapacitated; so the wife or a child was interviewed instead. The controls were selected with an eye for matching the cases as closely as possible for smoking history, age, education, high-risk occupations, and area of residence.

The results of the study showed no association between total vitamin A in the diet and the risk of having lung cancer, and no association with retinol or vitamin A supplements. (Supplements are usually retinyl palmitate or retinyl acetate; only recently has beta-carotene been included in multivitamins.) However, the consumption of carotenoid-containing vegetables (dark green and dark orange vegetables) was associated inversely with risk of lung cancer after controlling for level of cigarette smoking. When the group was divided into short-term and long-term smokers, little benefit was seen in the short-term smokers or in those who had quit some years earlier, but among current smokers, those who were in the highest quartile for dark green and orange vegetables in the diet had half the risk of lung cancer as those in the lowest quartile.

Counting overall vegetables in the diet, those in the lowest quartile ate one or less servings per day and those in the highest quartile averaged over 2.4 servings per day.

Details on the association of lung cancer with vitamin C-containing foods and cruciferous vegetables were not given in the report, except to say that they were no stronger than the association with other vegetables.

Regina G. Ziegler et al., "Carotenoid Intake, Vegetables, and the Risk of Lung Cancer Among White Men in New Jersey," *Amer. J. Epidem. 123*, 1080 (1986).

The authors of the above report discussed a major problem in calculating the carotene content of the diet. The analytical method that was used for many years to determine the amount of beta-carotene in vegetables and fruits was not specific for beta-carotene. The method did not distinguish between beta-carotene and many similar carotenoids that cannot be converted to vitamin A. Nevertheless, the results of this method were used for calculation of the vitamin A value of fruits and vegetables for the U.S. Department of Agriculture tables on Composition of Foods.

These tables have been used by epidemiologists to calculate the beta-carotene content of diets, but for many vegetables the tables give a poor estimate of the beta-carotene content. This makes it difficult to calculate the milligrams of carotene in anyone's diet, but statistical studies can still be done if servings of vegetables and fruits are counted, instead, and used for comparisons. Attempts to correlate cancer risk with intake of beta-carotene have occasionally shown poorer correlation than the correlation with servings of vegetables, and our inaccurate knowledge of beta-carotene content might be part of the explanation. Another explanation for low correlation between risk and beta-carotene is the existence in vegetables of other anticancer factors such as folic acid.

The U.S. Department of Agriculture has undertaken to re-analyze many of the fruits and vegetables using a new method of analysis (high performance liquid chromatography) which yields accurate data for beta-carotene in a food sample even when there are many other carotenoids present. The results of this undertaking will be a great improvement in the ability to calculate the carotene content in diets.

In Hawaii, some researchers at the Cancer Center of Hawaii pursued the question of whether total vitamin A, beta-carotene, or vitamin C in the diet might be protective against lung cancer. They identified all the lung cancer cases on Oahu who were diagnosed between late 1979 and the middle of 1982 by searching the records at several hospitals and by using the state-wide Hawaii Tumor Registry. Out of 627 cases found, 364 patients participated in the study. (As is true for most of these case-control studies, not all cases could be interviewed due to such reasons as refusals from the patient or the attending physician, language barriers, the patient moved away, or the patient died without leaving a close relative.) Controls for the study were recruited by means of random phone dialing and were chosen to match the cases as closely as possible in sex and age.

The interviewers used a dietary history method with a structured format that had been devised and tested for validity by nutritionists. The subjects were asked about the frequency of eating eighty-four specific foods during a typical week prior to the onset of symptoms. The interviewers also asked about vitamin supplements, about smoking history, and about occupational history.

The scientists used statistical methods to examine the relationships between lung cancer and total vitamin A (including vitamin supplements), vitamin A from foods only, beta-carotene from foods, and vitamin C from foods. The data showed an inverse relation between total vitamin A and lung cancer incidence in men but not in women. The same was true for beta-carotene. In other words, in men, the lower the vitamin A intake level, the higher the risk of lung cancer. Vitamin C intake was also tested, but since many foods that contain vitamin C also contain carotene, the vitamin C analysis was adjusted for vitamin A intake. Vitamin C did not show any protective effect.

For the entire study group—men and women, smokers and non-smokers—there was about 60% higher incidence of lung cancer in those with lowest vitamin A or carotene in the diet.

M. Ward Hinds et al., "Dietary Vitamin A, Carotene, Vitamin C and Risk of Lung Cancer in Hawaii," *Amer. J. Epidem. 119*, 227 (1984).

Some of the studies on lung cancer and diet have failed to find a protective effect of beta-carotene in women, although the effect was found in men. Why this should be true has been a puzzle. A possible explanation might involve the different pattern of histologic types of lung cancer that develop in women who get lung cancer. Lung cancer in women is more likely to be adenocarcinoma than it is in men. In many studies, adenocarcinoma of the lung occurs in nonsmokers as often as it does in cigarette smokers. In most countries only 15% of all lung cancers are adenocarcinomas, although adenocarcinoma was the type of lung cancer with unusually high incidence in the Singapore

Chinese women of Cantonese dialect, and it was found in the Singapore women who did not smoke at the same rate as in cigarette smokers. The studies in Norway and in Buffalo found no protective effect of beta-carotene against adenocarcinoma, but these studies contained only a few cases of adenocarcinoma. (The effect of vegetables on risk of lung cancer in Singapore was not calculated for the smokers and nonsmokers separately, but only for the group as a whole; so some interesting information was overlooked.)

The prefix "adeno" means glandular; so "adenocarcinoma" is a carcinoma that began in glandular tissue. In the case of the lung this means the glands that secrete mucin. The glandular tissues are derived from epithelial cells in the fetus and so are influenced by vitamin A during growth and development and may also be powerfully influenced by circulating hormones in later life. Specific hormones have long been known to aggravate certain cancers and antihormone therapy is used to treat some of these cancer cases.

For the glandular carcinomas, which include adenocarcinoma of the lung, prostate, breast, and colon, the association between high consumption of beta-carotene and lower risk is still a little uncertain. Not as many studies have been done on these types of cancer in relation to vegetable eating as have been done on lung cancer.

We have a few dietary studies on these types of cancer to describe later in this chapter, and we will have to pay close attention to the results of the beta-carotene intervention trials now underway to see whether the high doses of beta-carotene being tested will reduce the incidence of adenocarcinomas.

Scientists at the University of Southern California conducted a large case-control study during the mid-1980s to investestigate a variety of possible risk factors for adenocarcinoma of the lung in women, and one of their findings was a definite association between high intake of beta-carotene and low risk for this disease.

In addition to cigarette smoking, other factors that have been associated with increased risk of lung cancer have been passive smoking, other indoor pollutants from cooking and heating, previous lung diseases, and family history of lung cancer. Hormonal influences have also been suspected.

To study these potential risk factors as well as the beta-carotene effect, the scientists from USC conducted detailed interviews in person with 336 women who had been diagnosed to have adenocarcinoma of the lung and they interviewed an equal number of controls, matched for age and race, who lived in the same neighborhood. The cases were located through the Los Angeles County Cancer Surveillance Program.

The scientists asked detailed questions about smoking habits, about history of lung ailments such as asthma, bronchitis, pneumonia, tuberculosis or TB or lung cancer in relatives, and about reproductive history and hormone use. Information was collected on the frequencies and quantities of eating thirty-two foods that provide most of the vitamin A in the diet.

The results of the study showed the expected increase in risk for this type of cancer from cigarette smoking and also showed increased risk for those who had suffered from TB many years earlier or whose family history included cases of TB or lung cancer. (TB has been associated with this type of lung cancer in other studies, also.) Asthma, bronchitis, and emphysema were not associated with increased risk after adjusting for smoking habits. The smokier types of fuels used for cooking (coal, wood, or kerosene) were not risk factors.

The results of the study included a strong protective effect from higher levels of beta-carotene in the diet. Those in the highest quartile for beta-carotene consumption had one-half the risk for adenocarcinoma as those in the lowest quartile, after adjusting for smoking habits; and the effect of carrots was particularly striking, with those eating carrots almost every other day having one-third as high a risk as those eating carrots less than thirty times a year. Preformed vitamin A (retinol) in the diet did not show any protective effect.

Anna H. Wu et al., "Personal and Family History of Lung Disease as Risk Factors for Adenocarcinoma of the Lung," *Cancer Res. 48*, 7279 (1988).

Linda C. Koo at the University of Hong Kong studied the dietary habits of Chinese women who developed lung cancer in spite of never having smoked and found that a better diet helped prevent lung cancer, and especially reduced the risk of adenocarcinoma.

Hong Kong has an unusually high incidence of lung cancer. In men, 95% of the cases occur in smokers, but in women, at least half of the cases cannot be explained by smoking or even by "passive" smoking. This situation provided an opportunity to study the direct role of diet in lung cancer, to see whether the protective effects of vegetables or beta-carotene which have been seen in many studies on cigarette smokers also are effective in nonsmokers.

To do this Koo conducted a retrospective case-control study of 88 lung cancer cases of all histologic types and 137 controls living in the same district, none of whom had ever smoked. She collected dietary information and information on living conditions. The Chinese style of meal preparation—often several mixed dishes containing many ingredients from which the household members serve themselves at the table—led her to tabulate the dietary information in terms of frequencies of consuming certain food groups rather than specific food items.

Food groups that were included in the survey were cruciferous vegetables, leafy green vegetables, legumes, soy products, fresh fruit, fresh fish, salted fish, cured meats, fermented fish sauces or bean sauces, chili sauces and pickled vegetables. Beverages were also questioned but were found to be unrelated to risk of lung cancer.

Koo found statistically significant associations between higher levels of fresh fruit and fresh fish in the diet and lower incidence of lung cancer. Those women who ate fresh fruit at least once a day had half the risk of lung cancer as those who ate fresh fruit less than once a week; and those who ate fresh fish at least twice a day had less than half the risk as did those who ate fewer than five servings per week. (Presumably fresh fish substitutes for dried and salted fish and for smoked meat in the diet, which did not correlate significantly with the risk of lung cancer.)

The risk of adenocarcinoma or of large cell cancer was lower for those who ate more leafy green vegetables, carrots, soy products, fresh fruit and fish. Those in the bottom third for frequency of eating green leafy vegetables had three times higher risk for these types of lung cancer, and those in the bottom third for carrot consumption had six times higher risk, compared to those in the top third for frequencies of eating these vegetables.

These apparent effects of vegetables, fruits, and fish in reducing the risk of adenocarcinoma of the lung were different from the results of studies in other countries where adenocarcinoma (usually in smokers) did not seem to be associated with dietary habits. The exclusive use of nonsmokers as the study group in this small study in Hong Kong, by avoiding the powerful influence of tobacco carcinogens, was no doubt the key to clarifying a role for diet in helping to prevent this type of lung cancer.

Linda C. Koo, "Dietary Habits and Lung Cancer Risk Among Chinese Females in Hong Kong Who Never Smoked," *Nutr. Cancer 11*, 155 (1988).

One of the largest prospective studies ever done on life style, diet, and cancer mortality in the world was started in Japan in 1965. More than a quarter of a million adults, aged forty or over, were interviewed regarding their smoking, drinking and dietary habits, and their socio-economic status. The people interviewed made up most of the population of twenty-nine districts. Death certificates obtained during the next ten years in these districts provided the data for statistical comparisons between types of cancer deaths and life style factors. After ten years there had been 7377 cancer deaths in the study group.

Tremendous changes in Japanese life style have occurred since the 1950s. Cigarette smoking is widespread—75% of adult men smoke daily and lung cancer rates are increasing. Cancer of the stomach is becoming less common in spite of a statistical association between smoking and stomach cancer. Modern refrigeration has reached every household, and consumption of milk, meat, and eggs has increased considerably. One of the factors that appears to protect against the risk of stomach cancer in Japan is drinking two glasses of milk a day. Another factor that appears to protect is daily consumption of green or yellow vegetables.

Lung cancer mortality rates in the Japanese study increased according to the number of cigarettes smoked daily. For all levels of lifetime smoking habit, the mortality rates were lower for smokers who ate green or yellow vegetables daily compared to those who ate these vegetables less often. For smokers who only occasionally ate green and yellow vegetables, the mortality rate for lung cancer remained high even five years after quitting. However, in those ex-smokers who ate green or yellow vegetables daily, the mortality rate five years after quitting was almost as low as in nonsmokers.

Daily consumption of carotene-containing vegetables also was associated with lower mortality rate from prostate cancer in men under sixty-nine years of age.

Takeshi Hirayama, "Diet and Cancer," *Nutr. Cancer 1,* 67 (1979).

I have described in this chapter and the last, several studies that showed lower risks for lung cancer in people who ate larger amounts of carotene-containing vegetables. Just about all of the scientists who wrote these reports included in their discussions of the results their personal fears that people might get the idea that vegetables could prevent lung cancer, even if they continued smoking. So let's answer this question right now.

If you choose to smoke cigarettes but eat many vegetables, can you be sure you won't get lung cancer? The answer is no, no, no, no! It works like this—if you are a long-term smoker and you eat green and yellow vegetables only infrequently, your chances of getting lung cancer are approximately twenty times greater than those of a person who doesn't smoke at all.

If you are a long-term smoker and you eat lots of vegetables, your chances of getting lung cancer are approximately ten times greater than a person who doesn't smoke. Cigarette smoke is a powerful carcinogen and commonly damages the lungs and other organs in other ways besides lung cancer. Vegetables won't save you. While any prudent person, smoker or nonsmoker, will eat at least five servings daily of fruits and vegetables, doing so does not excuse you from your efforts to quit.

Cigarette smoking is associated with other types of cancer besides lung cancer. Cancer of the larynx was studied in six counties in the Houston area during 1976-1980 as part of a larger study to investigate the high mortality rate from respiratory cancers in this part of Texas.

People with laryngeal cancer were interviewed in their homes after being located through hospital records. Cases and controls—151 cases and 178 controls—were matched as to age and ethnic background. The interviewers asked about the frequency of eating forty-two food items, including most of the common carotene- and retinol-containing foods that are popular in the United States, for a period of about four years prior to the interview. Tobacco use and alcohol consumption were also questioned.

The results showed an inverse association between carotene intake and laryngeal cancer, especially in those people who had stopped smoking some years earlier. Heavy cigarette smoking proved to be a powerful risk factor for the illness, and alcohol and passive smoking were weaker risk factors. People who were in the top third of carotene intake levels had 2.3-fold lower risk of cancer of the larynx after adjusting for age, smoking, and drinking differences than people in the bottom third. High carotene intake seemed to be especially beneficial for those who had quit smoking several years earlier, as among these ex-smokers, those who were in the top third of carotene intake had six-fold reduced risk compared to ex-smokers who were low carotene eaters.

Dorothy Mackerras et al., "Carotene Intake and the Risk of Laryngeal Cancer in Coastal Texas," *Amer. J. Epidem. 128,* 980 (1988).

An epidemiological study in Louisiana showed that vegetable consumption was associated with lower risk for a different type of cancer, mesothelioma of the lung. Mesothelioma is the type of cancer that has afflicted people who were exposed to asbestos on the job. It is not a carcinoma because the cells that became cancerous were not epithelial cells. But even in this type of cancer, there was a statistically significant lower risk in those people who habitually ate more vegetables, especially cruciferous vegetables.

Epidemiologists from the National Cancer Institute and Louisiana State University questioned cases and controls about their past diet, occupations, residences, and smoking history. People who had worked in shipbuilding, pipefitting and boilermaking, or asbestos manufacturing were considered to have been definitely exposed to asbestos. For this group there was a much higher risk for this type of cancer. Cigarette smoking was not related to risk.

Among the dietary differences between cases and controls, only carotene and cruciferous vegetables were found to be statistically significant. The cruciferous vegetables that were questioned in the study were broccoli, turnips, cabbage, Brussels sprouts, and collard, turnip or mustard greens. Those people who had one of these vegetables more than thirteen times per month had only one-fifth the risk for mesothelioma as did those who ate one of these cruciferous vegetables seven times per month or less. The epidemiologists suggested that the results of the study might provide some reason to test the effect of micronutrients (vitamins, etc.) on populations that have been exposed to asbestos.

> Mark H. Schiffman et al., "Case-Control Study of Diet and Mesothelioma in Louisiana," *Cancer Res. 48*, 2911 (1988).

A prospective study on nutrition and cancer deaths in people aged sixty-five and over in Massachusetts showed very significant benefits for these older people from eating more fruits and vegetables. Cancer is far more common in older people than in young adults, probably because it takes many years for any one cell in the body to acquire the four to six mutations in critical genes that must usually be present before a cell can become malignant. The possibility that this process might be halted, or at least slowed, by a diet rich in fruit and vegetables was dramatically suggested by the results of this study.

A representative sample of older people in Massachusetts had been interviewed in 1976 as part of a study on nutrition programs for older Americans. In 1976, the aim was to acquire general information on nutrition rather than information on intake of vitamin A or carotene in particular. Scientists from Boston later decided to use the dietary questionnaires to test the hypothesis that carotene or vegetables may be protective for cancer risk. They scored each participant's answers based on servings per week of a selection of items from the question- naire—carrots or squash, tomatoes, salads or greens, dried fruits, fresh berries or melon, and broccoli or Brussels sprouts.

The fruit and vegetable scores for the twelve hundred or so people in the group were ranked from highest to lowest and were divided into five groups (quintiles) with an equal number of individuals in each group. The number of cancer deaths in each quintile was found by ex- amination of death certificates for the five year period following the original interviews with this group. (There were 252 confirmed deaths from all causes, not counting those who died during the first year after being interviewed.) The scientists used statistical methods to calculate the relative risks through the quintiles, adjusting for other known risk factors such as age and smoking habit and adjusting for total food in- take. The results were a statistically significant trend toward lower risk of death from cancer as the fruit and vegetable score went up, with a relative risk for the highest score of only 0.3 times the risk for the lowest score. In other words, those who did not eat very many fruits and vegetables had three times higher risk of dying from cancer during the five year period as did those who ate plenty of these foods.

The scientists who conducted the study pointed out that the results of their small survey in Massachusetts are compatible with the hypoth- esis that a generous amount of green and yellow vegetables in the diet may protect against cancer, although their dietary survey was not spe- cific enough to ascribe the vegetable effect to beta-carotene rather than to some other characteristic of the diet. Nor does this type of study prove that it was diet that was responsible for the fewer cancer deaths in those who ate the better diet. Only randomized intervention trials would be able to make this determination.

> Graham A. Colditz et al., "Increased green and yellow vegetable in- take and lowered cancer deaths in an elderly population," *Amer. J. Clin. Nutr. 41*, 32 (1985)

Another recent study on older people did not find evidence for a cancer-preventing function for beta-carotene. More than ten thousand residents of a retirement community near Los Angeles (Leisure World, median age = 74 years) were surveyed as to diet and vitamin A supplement usage as well as details of their health history and smoking history. The scientists, from the University of Southern California Department of Preventive Medicine, collected information on the types of cancer cases that occurred during the next five years.

They found no evidence that any type of vitamin A protected smokers from cancer. In nonsmoking men there were some nonsignificant data that might indicate protective effects, and women with higher carotene intake had significantly fewer cases of bladder cancer. Some results on prostate cancer indicated a higher risk associated with use of vitamin supplements.

Annlia Paganini-Hill et al., "Vitamin A, b-Carotene, and the Risk of
Cancer: A Prospctive Study," *J. Natl. Cancer Inst. 79*, 443 (1987).

A small case-control study on women getting Pap tests at the Bronx Municipal Hospital Center in New York City showed a very significant correlation between abnormal tcst rcsults and low intake of beta-carotene.

Studies on laboratory animals had long ago demonstrated that vitamin A affected the condition of the cervix. Epidemiologists at Albert Einstein College of Medicine set up a study to find out whether dietary vitamin A was associated with cervical dysplasia or with carcinoma in situ. Several other risk factors for these conditions are already known, and the participants in the study were interviewed by a nurse for details of their personal history and by a nutritionist for details of dietary habits and vitamin usage. The participants were unaware of the scientists' main interest in vitamin A. The participants included eighty-two controls who had normal Pap smcars and eighty-seven cases who had cervical dysplasia, severe dysplasia, or carcinoma in situ. The participants werc taught how to keep a detailed three-day food record to itemize their actual diet, and their retinol and carotene intakes were calculated from the food records.

The eighty-seven cases ate 14% less total vitamin A and 29% less beta-carotenc than did the eighty-two controls, but this difference in aveiage intakes was not statistically significant, due to wide variation among the individuals. However, when the individuals were divided into two classes based on whether their carotene intake was above or below the median level, there was a highly significant difference between the controls and the cases with dysplasia. Being in the lower group for carotene intake meant having a greater than two-fold higher risk of having cervical dysplasia and a three-fold higher risk of having a more severe dysplasia or carcinoma in situ.

When the same calculations were done using total vitamin A (both retinol and carotene), the effects were similar but less profound, indicating that beta-carotene in the diet was more influential than total vitamin A for prevention of these conditions.

In addition, vitamin C intake was significantly different between cases and controls, and other differences in their characteristics also contributed to the risk of dysplasia.

> Judith A. Wylie-Rosett et al., "Influence of Vitamin A on Cervical
> Dysplasia and Carcinoma In Situ," *Nutr. Cancer 6*, 49 (1984).

The epidemiologists at Roswell Park Memorial Institute and State University of New York at Buffalo also studied diet in relation to the cervix. They found 513 women with cervical cancer among the patients who had completed detailed interviews and dietary questionnaires before admission. Four hundred ninety controls were selected for comparison. Many factors besides diet were analyzed in this study such as smoking, drinking, and marital history.

The scientists found that smokers had a somewhat higher risk for cervical cancer than did nonsmokers. Drinking did not have much effect on the risk. Diet did have some effects on the risk. Estimates of beta-carotene intake were made from the group's answers to the food frequency questionnaire, and there was a statistically significant trend toward higher risk of cervical cancer with lower intake of beta-carotene. No trend was seen for variation in retinol intake from meats and milk.

> James R. Marshall et al., "Diet and Smoking in the Epidemiology of
> Cancer of the Cervix," *J. Natl. Cancer Inst. 70*, 847 (1983).

The dietary database acquired at Roswell Park Memorial Institute from 1957 to 1965 has yielded a wealth of scientific findings. We have a few more of their studies to review in this chapter before we move on to some of the very exciting studies that have been done in Europe in recent years.

In the summer of 1960, when I was an undergraduate chemistry student, I had the privilege of spending two wonderful months working in an endocrinology laboratory at Roswell Park, practicing my future profession of analytical chemistry and enjoying the extensive lecture series presented by the researchers there for the staff and for the students and high school teachers who were invited in each summer to work and learn the latest new ideas in biology and biochemistry. At that time, the dietary questionnaire project was in full swing and was the subject of a little flurry of talk among the research staff in the hall-ways and in the labs.

Like most people, I thought hormones and viruses were much more interesting than diet and would surely be more important in the cau-sation of cancer than what people ate. How much more complicated the problem appears today! Today, a theory of cancer development must include oncogenes, growth factors and their receptors, G pro-teins, cell surface glycoproteins and adhesion molecules, transcription factors, angiogenesis factors, abnormal methylation of DNA, and many more cellular phenomena that were undiscovered in 1960, as well as a role for dietary factors in prevention of the cancer process at some stage.

How fortunate for us that someone had the determination to inves-tigate the complex problem of cancer etiology from every imaginable angle, including diet, so early in the game, in spite of the difficulties this entailed. Great determination was needed to carry out the dietary project. Dietary interviews can be frustrating for the researcher be-cause many people pay little attention to what they eat, especially if they don't cook. Although the researchers at Roswell Park were a lit-tle discouraged by the difficulties of getting people to recall their usual diet and were skeptical about the value of the project at the beginning, they persisted, knowing that interviews are an accepted method of in-vestigation in other fields and knowing that environment, including diet, was suspected in the etiology of cancer. Their foresight produced results that were unexpected, as the dietary project was initiated long before the vitamin A-cancer hypothesis came to light.

The Roswell Park studies showed apparent beneficial effects from vegetables for the risk of several more types of cancer in addition to those already mentioned.

The risk of having bladder cancer was found to be associated with low vitamin A intake. Among the patients seen at Roswell Park be-tween 1957 and 1965, there were 569 men and women who were found to be suffering from bladder cancer. Other risk factors that had already been implicated in this disease were smoking and certain occupations such as leather work, painting, and smelting. Coffee drinking had also been suspected by previous investigators.

The estimated vitamin A intake for the subjects in this study on bladder cancer (569 cases and 1025 controls) averaged only about 63%

of the Recommended Dietary Allowance (RDA). The questionnaire used at Roswell Park did not include all possible sources of vitamin A, however. For instance, the use of vitamin supplements was not questioned and eating liver or cod liver oil was not questioned. People who did eat any of these items would have attained a much higher level of total vitamin A in their diet, but the vitamin A would have been retinol, not beta-carotene. The Roswell Park questionnaire did cover vegetables in the American diet very well and for this reason, the effect of beta-carotene or some other vegetable component in preventing carcinomas becomes apparent from analysis using the questionnaires. The questionnaire did not give a very complete picture of the types of fruit in the diet—the frequency of eating "fresh fruit" and "citrus fruits" was asked but there were no further questions on specific fruits. This has little effect on the results for beta-carotene in American diets where green and orange vegetables provide most of our carotene; the "fresh fruit" item on the questionnaire probably contained mostly apples and bananas, which have very little carotene, and only smaller quantities of carotene-rich apricots, cantaloupe, and papaya.

When the cases and controls in the bladder cancer study were ranked from high to low for intake of vitamin A, a statistically significant, dose-dependent trend was found showing that the relative risk for cancer was twice as great among those with the lowest vitamin A intake compared to those with the highest intake. People working in high-risk occupations were distributed through the various vitamin A categories just like low-risk occupations. In other words, the vitamin A effect was not related to the high-risk occupations.

Coffee drinking was found to be associated with a slight increase in risk in men, but this might have been due to lower milk intake among coffee drinkers rather than due to the coffee itself. When either milk or carrots in the diet was analyzed separately, it was found (like total vitamin A) to be inversely related to bladder cancer.

Curtis Mettlin and Saxon Graham, "Dietary Risk Factors in Human Bladder Cancer," *Amer. J. Epidem. 110*, 255 (1979).

One study in the series from Roswell Park Memorial Institute found detrimental effects associated with higher levels of vitamin A in the diet. About three hundred men with prostate cancer were compared with controls. When all the dietary questionnaires were calculated and the estimates for several nutrients were ranked and divided into quartiles or quintiles, it was found that men who ate more meat and fish, more animal fats, more vitamin A or vitamin C had statistically significant higher risks for prostate cancer, but the dose-dependent trends through the quintiles were a little erratic, giving an appearance of uncertainty to the results.

When the cancer patients were divided into those under seventy years of age and those over seventy years, the group under seventy no longer showed any higher risk with higher intakes of any of these nutrients, but the group over seventy years of age did have significantly higher risks for higher intakes.

Similar results have been found by others. The study of Leisure World residents in California contained results that showed higher vitamin A intake in men who developed prostate cancer, and a study in Hawaii found higher risk for prostate cancer with higher intake of vitamin A in men seventy years or older. On the other hand, Hirayama's analysis of the prospective study in Japan did show protective effects from green and yellow vegetables against prostate cancer, but this was in men under the age of sixty-nine. Several other recent studies have also shown lower risk associated with more beta-carotene in the diet. The inconsistent results on studies of the possible correlation between retinol or beta-carotene and risk for prostate cancer most likely mean that vitamin A is not important in the development of this disease. Prostate cancer is one of the most common cancers in men, and the epidemiology of this disease has been studied in various parts of the world; but so far, no good explanations for its frequent occurrence have been found.

> Saxon Graham et al., "Diet in the Epidemiology of Carcinoma of the Prostate Gland," *J. Natl. Cancer Inst. 70*, 687 (1983).

Higher consumption of vegetables and fruits was associated with a much lower risk for cancer of the esophagus in the Roswell Park Memorial Institute series of studies. Cancer of the esophagus is not very common in the United States, but there are several parts of the world where it occurs much more frequently. Parts of China have very high incidence of esophageal cancer, for instance, and studies have been done there to find out if this might be caused by carcinogens in moldy vegetables or bread or by pickled vegetables, which are popular in the diet.

Regions in various parts of the world with high rates of esophageal cancer are characterized by lower socioeconomic status and poor diets, leading to the suspicion that deficiencies in the diet might somehow increase one's susceptibility to the effects of carcinogens, such as nitrosamines or carcinogens produced by molds.

The study at Roswell Park compared 147 white males with cancer and 264 controls. A significant correlation was found between the number of cigarettes smoked and risk for esophageal cancer, and an even stronger correlation was found between alcohol intake and esophageal cancer.

When the scientists calculated the frequency of eating a serving of any fruit or vegetable on the questionnaire and compared this with the risk of cancer, after controlling for smoking and drinking habits, they found that those who ate 2.7 or more servings per day had lower risk than those who ate 1.3 or less servings per day, with a difference in relative risks of almost five. A dose-dependent variation in risk could be seen as the reported vegetable frequency varied from high to low.

> Curtis Mettlin et al., "Diet and Cancer of the Esophagus," *Nutr. Cancer 2*, 143 (1981).

The association between poor nutrition and cancer of the esophagus was also shown clearly and dramatically in a study of black men in Washington, D.C. In the United States this type of cancer is more common in black people than in whites, and the mortality rates are higher in counties with lower economic status.

Epidemiologists from the National Cancer Institute studied 115 cases and 234 controls for dietary habits, including alcohol, and the usual frequency of eating thirty-one food items. An unusual aspect of the study was the researchers' use of cancer victims who had already died between 1975 and 1977. In 1979 the epidemiologists interviewed next of kin (about half were wives and half were other relatives) for the subjects and the next of kin for 234 black men who had died from other causes. The food information requested was the next of kin's recollection of dietary habits before illness struck. Only those subjects were included in the study for whom fairly complete answers to the food frequencies could be provided by the next of kin.

Food items questioned included many types of meats and fish (fresh or frozen or canned), nitrite-containing meats such as lunch meats and bacon, dairy products, various types of fruits and vegetables, and grains and potatoes.

Cancer was more common in those men with poor diets. Risk of esophageal cancer was about doubled for those men who ate small amounts of fresh or frozen meats and fish compared to men who ate larger amounts of foods in this group. The same was true for fruits and vegetables as a group and for dairy products and eggs as a food group.

For those who consumed low amounts of all three of these food groups, risk of esophageal cancer was fourteen times higher than it was for those who ate high amounts of all three food groups. These risks were calculated after adjusting for alcohol intake; alcohol was known to be a risk factor from an earlier study.

Foods that were not associated with either increased or decreased risks were nitrite-containing foods as a group, corn and cornbread, whole grain breads and cereals, and potatoes. Vitamin C intake was statistically significant in reducing risk. The high intake of fruits and vegetables that provided significant risk reduction consisted of three to six servings per day compared to less than two servings per day for the high risk group.

> Regina G. Ziegler et al., "Esophageal Cancer Among Black Men in Washington, D.C. II. Role of Nutrition," *J. Natl. Cancer Inst. 67*, 1199 (1981).

In the city of Milan in northern Italy, 105 cases of esophageal cancer were found during 1984-1985 in the large teaching hospitals there, and they were interviewed for a study of their dietary, smoking, and drinking customs. Both men and women were studied in comparison with 348 controls. The interviewers questioned the participants about their usual frequency of eating the most common foods containing vitamin A in the Italian diet.

Some expected results were found. The cases were generally from lower socioeconomic levels and were heavier smokers and drinkers. The weekly frequencies of eating carrots, green vegetables, fruits, and fish were all significantly lower in the cases than in the controls. Heavy drinking greatly increased the risk of this cancer. Those who were the heaviest drinkers and lowest carotene eaters had twenty-three times higher risk of cancer than those who were light drinkers and ate more carotene. Differences in the risk for this type of cancer could be seen at all levels of alcohol intake, depending on whether the carotene intake was high or low.

> Adriano Decarli et al., "Vitamin A and Other Dietary Factors in the Etiology of Esophageal Cancer," *Nutr. Cancer 10*, 29 (1987).

Tobacco and alcohol are also known risk factors for oral cancer (carcinoma of the lip, tongue, etc.) and, at Roswell Park Memorial Institute, these cancers were found to be less frequent in the group of patients who were in the habit of eating a little more vegetables.

425 cases and 588 controls were compared. The scientists calculated vitamin A (mostly beta-carotene) and vitamin C in the diets, and divided the study group according to their vitamin intake. Even after adjusting for cigarette smoking and alcohol consumption, there was twice as high a risk for those people consuming only 50% of the RDA for vitamin A as there was for those people consuming 84% or more of the RDA.

The statisticians emphasized that there were only rather small differences between cases and controls in nutrient intake. Because the dietary interviews were rather brief and did not include all foods containing these vitamins and are based on the patients' ability to remember how they ate before noticing symptoms of illness, one would expect that the interview method might easily have missed small correlations. The fact that preventive effects associated with vitamin A and with vegetables in general were found and were calculated to be statistically significant, means that these results must not be ignored. When these epidemiological results corroborate experiments in animals and experiments in tissue culture, we have found a very important factor indeed for prevention of carcinomas.

James Marshall et al., "Diet in the Epidemiology of Oral Cancer," *Nutr. Cancer 3*, 145 (1982).

The Roswell Park patients interviewed from 1957 to 1965 included 293 women who were newly diagnosed to have cancer of the ovary. Not all of them were studied as to vitamin A in the diet; nineteen who had nonepithelial cancer of the ovary were eliminated from the dietary study. The ovary can develop cancers in connective tissue as well as in epithelial tissue, and the epidemiologists wanted to limit their dietary study to the more common epithelial tumors.

The remaining 274 cases and 1034 controls were compared as to many characteristics of their reproductive history and other health history as well as their dietary questionnaires. Factors that were found to be not associated with the risk for ovarian cancer included marital status, religion, smoking, and educational level. The scientists found a significant risk reduction in women who had had a greater number of pregnancies.

For the dietary analysis, cases and controls were ranked for intakes of each nutrient and divided into thirds. The under-fifty age group was studied separately from the fifty to seventy-nine year-old group. Neither group had significant associations between risk and vitamin C, cruciferous vegetables, fat, protein, coffee, tea, or alcohol. The vitamin A level from fruits and vegetables (beta-carotene) *was* significantly associated with reduced risk for ovarian cancer in the under-fifty group, with a difference in relative risk of more than double for the low carotene group compared to the high carotene group; but the carotene effect did not show up in the over-fifty group of women.

The risk reduction associated with carotene-containing fruits and vegetables in the younger women was just as strong an effect as the risk reduction associated with more pregnancies. Those women in the entire study group, younger and older, who had had five or more pregnancies were only half as likely to develop ovarian cancer as women who had had two or less pregnancies. For the under-fifty group, the same risk reduction could have been achieved by eating an extra two carrots a week! This would have put them in the top third for vitamin A intake, where the incidence of ovarian cancer was low.

We will see very similar benefits from either many pregnancies or many vegetables when we review some studies on breast cancer later in this chapter.

Tim Byers et al., "A Case-Control Study of Dietary and Nondietary Factors in Ovarian Cancer," *J. Natl. Cancer Inst. 71*, 681 (1983).

A smaller case-control study on ovarian cancer was conducted in Utah in the mid-1980s. Cases and controls came from four counties in the Salt Lake City area. Ninety per cent of the cases were epithelial cancer. Participants were interviewed in their homes regarding their socioeconomic status, religion, smoking habits, pregnancy history, and consumption of 183 food items, with methods of food preparation. The scientists were interested in several dietary factors that might be related to ovarian cancer. These were total calories, protein, fats, vitamin A, beta-carotene, vitamin C, and fiber. The amounts of specific nutrients in the diet were calculated from the dietary information.

The scientists found a lower risk of ovarian cancer associated with higher income and with a greater number of full-term pregnancies. Smoking was not related to risk, and neither were protein, fat, and vitamin C.

Beta-carotene was the only nutrient that was significantly associated with lower risk for ovarian cancer. The subjects were divided into thirds according to nutrient intake levels. The group that was in the top third for beta-carotene (from green vegetables and carrots) had one-half as great a risk as the group with the lowest intake level, after adjusting for differences in age, body mass index, and number of pregnancies. There was a dose-dependent reduction in risk as the beta-carotene intake increased from low to medium to high.

Martha L. Slattery et al., "Nutrient Intake and Ovarian Cancer," *Amer. J. Epidem. 130*, 497 (1989).

Perhaps we should pause in this litany of examples to assess what these case-control studies are leading us to understand. What these case-control studies are revealing—as plainly as is possible using statistics and small populations—is a most welcome weapon against one of the most mysterious scourges of mankind, a weapon against premature death from cancer, and the grief and anxiety that strike so many families so rudely.

What the scientists would like to tell us is that they are beginning to find proof that moderately higher intake of beta-carotene, or some other component of vegetables closely associated with beta-carotene, results in demonstrably fewer cases of some of the most frustrating illnesses we have to deal with.

The scientists would like to tell us this, but they seldom do, partly because their training in skepticism and caution requires them to withhold judgment until all the facts are in. The scientists who worked on each of these studies were keenly aware of limitations in their procedures. They knew that dietary recall is only about 85% accurate. They knew their questions did not cover all factors or foods that might be important. They knew that interactions between foods or other factors that they had overlooked would give misleading results. And they worried that their questions on the diet of one year ago or four years ago might be irrelevant if the initiation of the carcinoma really happened ten or twenty years ago.

For reasons such as these, news reports of links between diet and cancer usually contain more caveats than counsel. As well they should, if it is only one small population that has been studied. But when study after study gives the same results, we do not have to ask the individual scientists to tell us the answers, or to tell us what needs to be done. We can simply look at the data and decide for ourselves.

This is what in fact the National Research Council has done during the past few years. A committee of nineteen leading scientists has examined five thousand individual studies—on both humans and animals and on other chronic diseases in addition to cancer—and one of their recommendations in a 1989 report is that we all should be eating at least five servings a day of vegetables and fruit, with emphasis on the green and yellow vegetables and citrus fruits.

The reasons for this recommendation are completely obvious after seeing the differences in risk that have been found for so many types of cancer in the studies described so far. How could we not make more effort to follow the experts' advice after seeing for ourselves the difference diet can make in the cancer statistics?

Breast cancer was another type of cancer that was studied in the Roswell Park series. Two thousand women who were found to have breast cancer were compared with 1463 age-matched controls without any known cancer. The scientists found no correlation between risk of breast cancer and the amount of vitamin C or cruciferous vegetables in the diet, or with the amount of fat in the diet.

They did find a statistically significant correlation between higher amounts of vitamin A in the diet (mostly from vegetables and fruit in the Roswell Park surveys) and lower incidence of breast cancer in women fifty-five years or older. The older women who had only about one-third of the RDA level of vitamin A in their diet had 50% higher risk for breast cancer than the small proportion of patients who consumed more than the RDA level. The association between higher vitamin A intake and reduced risk was not seen in women under fifty-five years of age.

This study was the earliest one to investigate possible association of dietary qualities other than fats with the incidence of breast cancer. A large number of studies have tried to determine whether breast cancer is more common in individuals who eat more animal or vegetable fats of various kinds ever since international studies in the 1960s showed much higher mortality from breast cancer in North America and northern Europe than in Asia. One of the best-documented differences in life style between North America and Asia has been the greater amounts of meat and fat in the American diet compared to Japan and other countries where breast cancer is less common. However, studies on breast cancer and fat in the diet of individuals have been unable to confirm unequivocally that high fat in the diet increases the risk for breast cancer. More about these dietary fat studies in later chapters.

Saxon Graham et al., "Diet in the Epidemiology of Breast Cancer," *Amer. J. Epidem. 116*, 68 (1982).

One of the most exciting studies on vegetables in the diet in relation to risk for cancer was published in the *International Journal of Cancer* in 1986. A group of epidemiologists from Athens, Greece, in cooperation with epidemiologists from Harvard School of Public Health, undertook a case-control study on diet and breast cancer by interviewing patients at three Athens hospitals.

The Greeks are a homogeneous ethnic population but they enjoy a greater variety of dietary customs than people in some other countries, so they say. According to the Food and Agriculture Organization, an agency of the United Nations, the Greeks consume twice as many vegetables and only one-third as much animal fat as do Americans. The incidence of breast cancer in Greece is lower than in the United States, being only about 60% of the rate seen in the United States, where approximately one woman in nine or ten can expect to face this illness sometime during her life. (These comparisons of rates of breast cancer incidence are consistent with most of the studies we have seen so far where the risk is about one-half when the vegetable or beta-carotene intake doubles.)

The greater range of dietary habits in Greece enabled the scientists to find statistically significant correlations between higher vegetable intake and lower breast cancer incidence by studying only 120 cases and 120 controls. When the results of the interviews were analyzed, the difference in relative risk between those in the highest and lowest vegetable groups was a difference of *ten times higher risk* in the lowest vegetable group after adjusting for age, number of children, menopausal status and several other variables.

The hospital interviews included questions on socioeconomic status, child-bearing and breast-feeding history, weight and menopausal status. This study, like other studies, did show higher incidence of breast cancer in those with fewer children or shorter duration of breast-feeding or higher socioeconomic status—hormonal effects of child-bearing and breast-feeding are possibly of some importance in reducing the risk of breast cancer, but the risk reduction from hormonal effects was much less than the risk reduction from vegetable effects in this study.

The scientists questioned the study group about the frequencies of consuming 120 food items and beverages. The study group was divided into quintiles for each of the food groups analyzed. The vegetables food group showed the strongest association with lower cancer risk ($p < 0.001$ for the trend) of any of the food groups or hormone-related items on the questionnaire. Fruits and dairy products showed a weak statistical association with lower cancer risk. Food groups that were not related to risk for breast cancer were cereals, sugars, legumes and nuts, meats and fish, fats and oils, alcohol, coffee, tea and cola.

Foods that made up the vegetable group in the questionnaire were tomatoes, cucumber, squash, onions, eggplant, cabbage, lettuce, spinach, okra, leeks, dandelion, artichoke, beets, carrots, broccoli, cauliflower, and peppers.

These results of the study in Greece are far more dramatic than the results from Roswell Park Memorial Institute. The Greek women in the highest quintile for total vegetable score had ten times lower risk than the women in the group with lowest vegetable score. The actual values, in terms of servings per week, for the highest quintile were not given in the report, unfortunately.

The scientists considered many possible sources of error in their study, but were unable to identify any reason why the results should be false. They did not attempt to ascribe the wonderful protective effect of higher vegetable intake to any particular component of vegetables, such as carotene, because they thought the effect could also be due to a variety of other nutrients or to indirect effects of vegetables on various aspects of human metabolism.

> K. Katsouyanni et al., "Diet and Breast Cancer: A Case-Control Study in Greece," *Int. J. Cancer 38*, 815 (1986).

In Italy the rate of breast cancer mortality has been increasing since 1955 for reasons that are not completely understood. In an effort to find some clues to the causes of the increase, scientists in Milan interviewed 1108 breast cancer patients, ages twenty-six to seventy-four, and for comparison they interviewed 1281 hospitalized controls who had complaints that were unrelated to cancer or hormones.

Striking reduced risk for breast cancer was found in those who ate green vegetables more often. The estimated relative risk for those who ate at least eight servings per week of green vegetables was only 40% of the risk for those who ate less than seven servings per week.

Many other statistically significant results were found in this study. Women who reported consuming higher amounts of butter, margarine, and oil had one-third higher risk than those who consumed low amounts. Women who ate seven or more servings of meat per week had one-third higher risk than those who ate only four to six servings per week. Women who drank alcoholic beverages had higher risk— three or four drinks per day doubled the risk for breast cancer compared to no alcohol. (Several other studies have also shown association between alcohol and breast cancer.)

As in many other studies, the risk of breast cancer was higher for women with more education, who had been older when first giving birth, who had had benign breast disease, or who had a mother or sister with breast cancer.

Two of the food items questioned in the interviews were liver and carrots—good sources of vitamin A. Both cases and controls reported similar frequencies of eating these items—liver was eaten about once every two weeks and carrots about once every four or five days. The scientists calculated the approximate quantities of retinol and beta-carotene in the diets using the food frequencies from the interviews and food composition tables. They found that retinol was not associated with breast cancer risk, and beta-carotene showed a significant association or not, depending on how the statistical adjustments were done.

Carlo LaVecchia et al., "Dietary Factors and the Risk of Breast Cancer," *Nutr. Cancer 10*, 205 (1987).

Because many studies on dietary fat and cancer have given inconsistent results, scientists in Australia decided to compare dietary fat and other nutrients in the diets of breast cancer patients and in women living in the same city who were not known to have cancer. Dietary intake of fats, protein, total calories, and vitamin A were studied in 451 breast cancer patients living in Adelaide, South Australia.

A 24% reduced risk of breast cancer was found in those who ate more beta-carotene and a suggestion of a one-third reduced risk was found in those who ate higher amounts of fiber.

Cases were interviewed in their homes a few months after their diagnoses. Controls of the same age were selected at random from the electoral roll and were invited to particitate in a study of life style and health. The scientists obtained information on family history, reproductive history, and menopausal status. The subjects completed a self-administered dietary questionnaire that covered 179 items and included cooking practices such as the use of sugar, salt, fat, and portion sizes. The questionnaires were used to calculate nutrient intakes. The use of vitamin supplements was not questioned.

The results of the medical history part of the investigation were similar to results of other studies. For instance, women who had never given birth had 50% higher risk of breast cancer than those who had a child before the age of twenty, a finding often seen in studies on breast cancer. The Australians found no association between the risk of breast cancer and total calories, protein, total fat, sugar, or starch in the diet. They found some evidence for higher risk in those who ate more than 400 milligrams per day of cholesterol, and they found some evidence for reduced risk in those with higher fiber intake.

The 24% reduced risk of breast cancer for those in the top two quintiles of beta-carotene intake was statistically significant, even though it was a rather small change in the risk. There was no association between retinol and risks in the total group studied.

T.E. Rohan et. al., "A Population-Based Case-Control Study of Diet and Breast Cancer in Australia," *Amer. J. Epidem. 128,* 478 (1988).

In the city of La Plata in Argentina, the incidence of breast cancer is just as high as in North America, Australia, and northern Europe. The population of La Plata is mainly people of European descent, and the diet in the region is high in meats, milk, cheese, and fat. Desserts and fruit are popular, and the average vegetable consumption is one or two servings a day.

Epidemiologists studied 150 cases of breast cancer that were diagnosed in 1984 and 1985 in women who had lived in La Plata for at least five years. Cases and controls were interviewed to obtain information about many personal characteristics and about diet. The dietary questionnaire covered an extensive list of food items, and allowed the scientists to estimate the calories consumed as well as the frequency of eating the different types of foods.

After controlling for such risk factors as age and body mass index, protective effects against risk of cancer were found for more frequent consumption of green leafy vegetables (cabbage, lettuce, broccoli, and cauliflower in this study), noncitrus fruits, whole milk, and preserved or freshwater fish. Higher risk for cancer was associated with more frequent consumption of eggs, animal fats (lard), desserts, legumes, grains, lean processed meats, stews, and fried meats. But when these food items were tested for risk while controlling for the other food items, only green vegetables and whole milk remained protective against breast cancer, and only eggs remained as a risk factor. High-fat foods and fats used for cooking were no longer risk factors. A significant risk factor was a high-calorie diet but, strangely enough, this characteristic was not related to body weight and so, remains to be explained. In terms of some specific nutrients that were calculated in the diets, fiber and beta-carotene were both associated with lower risk.

The risk reduction associated with more green leafy vegetables was considerable. The overall average frequency of having a green leafy vegetable was about three servings a week. Those women who were in the top quartile for these vegetables had a risk for breast cancer that was only 15% as high as those in the bottom quartile. This is a risk reduction of six- or seven-fold. It is interesting and perhaps important that the green leafy vegetables that were specified in the dietary questionnaire (at least the cruciferous vegetables—cabbage, broccoli, and cauliflower) are good sources of folic acid. The role of folic acid in preventing chromosome damage might lead to a cancer-preventing effect for this vitamin.

> Jose Mario Iscovich et al., "A Case-Control Study of Diet and Breast Cancer in Argentina," *Int. J. Cancer 44*, 770 (1989).

Colon cancer is another disease that varies greatly in occurrence in different countries. Like breast cancer, it is more common in the more affluent countries where meat and fat make up a large part of the diet. Colon cancer is not as common in the United States as is breast cancer, but still, about 4% of the U.S. population will develop cancer of the colon or rectum during their lifetime.

International studies in the 1960s led to strong suspicions that meat or fat in the diet was a partial cause of the disease. When the per capita meat or fat intake in many countries was compared with the mortality rate from colon cancer in these countries, there was a very strong correlation between these two statistics. But since the affluent countries have many differences in their culture, environment, occupations, and diagnostic capabilities compared to less developed countries, it was necessary to study individuals as subjects in order to control for differences in ethnic backgrounds, life style, area of residence, and other important factors. The disadvantage of studying individuals from the same area has already been mentioned—their dietary customs may be so similar that many large and careful studies are needed in order to find statistically significant differences related to risk.

The results of case-control retrospective studies on fat and colon cancer have not been consistent. Many studies have found a higher risk associated with a high fat or meat diet, but quite a few studies have found no excess risk associated with meat or fat. In contrast, case-control studies have consistently found lower risk of colon cancer associated with higher vegetable intake.

It is difficult to estimate the proportion of risk that is due to diet and the amount due to other factors. The two expert epidemiologists from

Oxford University, Doll and Peto, have estimated that 90% of colon cancer and 50% of breast cancer might be prevented by dietary changes. The trick is to find out exactly what changes are needed.

Current thinking on possible factors, in addition to meat and fat, that might be involved in the etiology of colon cancer include lack of fiber from vegetable sources, lack of fiber from cereal sources, and bile acids. Factors that might have anticancer effects include calcium, which has an antiproliferative effect on colon epithelium, and folic acid, which can help prevent mutations. This is a complicated set of factors to try to sort out and no doubt much new information will evolve slowly in the years to come. So far, the protective effects of large amounts of vegetables in the diet are being demonstrated consistently, from early studies up until the present.

As early as 1968 a study of life style factors and cancer of the gastrointestinal tract in Bombay, India showed a very low rate of colon cancer in one region among Hindus who are strict vegetarians and have plenty of dairy products in their diet. (They do have a high rate of cancer of the esophagus due to prevalent smoking and chewing habits.) Seventh-Day Adventists in California, about half of whom are vegetarians, have one-third lower mortality rate from colon cancer than the general population. We don't know exactly how much more vegetables either of these groups consumes compared to the general population, because these groups were studied before the vegetable hypothesis became widely known and tested.

At Roswell Park Memorial Institute they did ask about specific vegetables, and a reduced risk of colon cancer was found for increased consumption of raw vegetables or cruciferous vegetables. More than five hundred men with cancer of the colon or rectum were interviewed between 1959 and 1965, and these were compared with fourteen hundred controls. There were no statistically significant differences between cases and controls in frequency of eating meats of any kind or beef, specifically. Likewise, the use of various types of fats for cooking or seasoning was not associated with risk of colon cancer. Nor were smoking and drinking.

Eating raw vegetables appeared to provide a protective effect. The scientists found a statistically significant higher risk (almost twice as high) for colon or rectal cancer in those who seldom ate raw vegetables. Those who reported eating raw vegetables—coleslaw, tomatoes, red cabbage, lettuce, carrots and cucumbers—more than twenty times a month had the lower risk, compared to those who ate servings of these vegetables less than ten times a month.

Cruciferous vegetables—sauerkraut, coleslaw, Brussels sprouts, broccoli and cabbage—showed a strong association with reduced risk for colon cancer but not for rectal cancer. Those who ate cabbage at least once a week had one-third the risk for colon cancer as did those who ate cabbage only once a month. And for the whole list of vegetables questioned there was only half as much risk for colon cancer in those who ate a raw or cooked vegetable at least twice a day as there was in those who ate a vegetable less than once a day.

> Saxon Graham et al., "Diet in the Epidemiology of Cancer of the Colon and Rectum," *J. Natl. Cancer Inst. 61*, 709 (1978).

The same group of epidemiologists did a more recent large, detailed study of colon cancer patients in a wider area of western New York state. They wanted to try to unravel the apparent involvement of fat and total calories in the etiology of this disease. Some studies had previously found that total fat, total calories, and large body size were correlated with risk of colon cancer, but of course, these factors are closely interrelated with each other—a situation that makes statistical conclusions especially complicated.

The findings in the new study included higher risks for colon cancer in those people who consumed larger amounts of total fats in their diet. The effect showed up in both men and women and resulted in 2.5- to 4-fold higher risks for those in the highest quartile for fat con sumption. Higher amounts of fiber in the diet provided a small degree of risk reduction.

Cruciferous vegetables were not associated with risk in this study, done during 1975-1984, unlike the earlier study at Roswell Park. The scientists speculated that changes in the American diet during the intervening years might partly explain the failure to find an effect from cruciferous vegetables. The U.S. Department of Agriculture surveys confirm that Americans are not eating as much cruciferous vegetables as in earlier years.

Some vegetables, when studied separately, did show significant association with reduced risk for colon cancer. These were celery, carrots, green peppers, onions, and tomatoes. However, there was no indication that overall vitamin A, carotene, or vitamin C in the diet was associated with reduced risk for colon cancer.

> Saxon Graham et al., "Dietary Epidemiology of Cancer of the Colon in Western New York," *Amer. J. Epidem. 128*, 490 (1988).

The positive results for vegetables in protecting against colon cancer are totally in agreement with earlier epidemiological results on cancer in the gastrointestinal tract. Erik Bjelke, who discovered the lower rate of lung cancer in Norwegians who ate more carrots or milk, had earlier found low intake of several vegetables among colon cancer patients in Minnesota. This study had been done while he was completing doctoral studies at the University of Minnesota in the 1970s.

At about the same time at the University of Minnesota, Dr. Lee Wattenberg found that several cruciferous vegetables, when fed to rats, induced production of an enzyme in the liver and intestines that detoxifies many fat-soluble chemicals, including polycyclic aromatic hydrocarbons, some of which are known to be carcinogens. Later he found that a simple compound, indole, isolated from the vegetables, did the same thing when fed to the rats. Thus, there is at least one plausible explanation for cancer-preventing effect of cruciferous vegetables in man.

It had been known for several years that there are enzymes in man and other animals which are produced in larger amounts after exposure to foreign chemicals and which can convert undesirable chemicals from the environment to water-soluble compounds that can be flushed from the body. The enzyme induced by cruciferous vegetables is an example of the many detoxification mechanisms that exist in plant-eating animals that help protect against the natural toxins found in the plant world. (Plants and animals use many of the same chemicals for entirely different purposes. Plants have an important use for indole. They use it to make the auxin (plant growth hormone), indole-3-acetic acid. Beta-carotene is another plant product that has functions in the green plants that are entirely different from its uses in animals.)

As will be discussed in more detail in later chapters, the cruciferous vegetables have additional benefits for nutrition besides their ability to induce detoxifying enzymes. They are usually good sources of folic acid, which might help protect us against chromosome damage, and the dark green members of the group are good sources of beta-carotene.

A study on patients with gastrointestinal cancer had been done in Israel in 1967-1969 and had shown reduced risk if the diet was high in fiber. More recently, the epidemiologists in Tel Aviv reviewed the dietary questionnaires from this early study to see whether vitamin A was also related to risk. Their calculations showed no reduced risk for

milk. The highest level of vegetable intake was associated with about one-half as much risk for cancer as the lowest level, and the same was found for cooking oil. The risk reduction for the highest level of milk consumption was about one-third.

Food groups that were not associated with the risk of colorectal cancer were meat, fish, cheese, cured meats, eggs, butter, breads, bakery, sugar, alcohol and coffee, potatoes and fruit.

Unlike several other studies on colon cancer, the cases in the Marseilles study consumed slightly lower total calories than did the controls. The amounts of total vitamin A and vitamin C in the Marseilles study were well above the Recommended Dietary Allowance. The level of total vitamin A was not associated with differences in risk. An unusual result was a statistically significant doubling of risk associated with higher consumption of pasta and rice.

> Geneviève Macquart-Moulin et al., "Case-Control Study on Colorectal Cancer and Diet in Marseilles," *Int. J. Cancer 38*, 183 (1986).

In Italy, the mortality rate from cancer of the colon or rectum has increased about 40% since the mid-1950s, much like the situation with breast cancer. Part of the explanation for the breast cancer increase was the drop in birth rate in younger generations—many studies having shown lower incidence of breast cancer in women who have had more full-term pregnancies—but birth rate changes could not explain the entire rate increase, and have no bearing on the increase in colon cancer. Environmental factors of some sort are implicated by the geographical distribution of colon cancer cases in Italy—the northern part of the country having a three- or four-fold higher mortality rate than the southern provinces.

Epidemiologists in Milan in northern Italy conducted a case-control study on diet, smoking, drinking, medical history and socioeconomic factors, using as subjects 575 hospitalized cases and 778 hospitalized controls. Patients were interviewed and frequencies were recorded for the usual consumption of twenty-nine food items that provided most of the starch, protein, fat, fiber, vitamins A and C, nitrites and nitrates in the diet. The scientists hoped that the variety of the diet in Italy, along with differences in personal preferences, as well as recent migration from the south to the northern parts of Italy, which should provide a greater mix in the Milan population, would disclose whether dietary variation was related to colon cancer. The scientists found that frequent consumption of green vegetables was related to lower risk. The findings included higher incidence of colon cancer in those with higher socioeconomic status, a result found for several other types of cancer. Smoking and drinking were not related to risk. Foods that were not related to risk included bread, pastry, poultry, ham, canned and cured meats, milk, cheese, eggs, potatoes, fruit, cruciferous vegetables, carrots and lettuce.

Foods that were strongly related to increased risk of colorectal cancer were pasta, rice, beef and veal. (An increased risk associated with pasta and rice was also seen in the Marseilles study, and an increased risk from beef and veal was seen in the Athens study.) There was two- or three-fold higher risk associated with these foods in the top third of consumption frequency compared with the bottom third.

Foods that were significantly related to lower risk of both colon cancer and rectal cancer were green vegetables, tomatoes, melon, and coffee. (Coffee was also associated with lower risk in the Marseilles study but the lower risk was not statistically significant. In a recent study in Singapore, coffee drinking lowered the risk for colon cancer, and this was statistically significant.) Those subjects (cases and controls).who were in the highest third for frequency of eating green vegetables had one-half the risk of colorectal cancer as those in the bottom third. The risk reduction from tomatoes, melon, and coffee was a little less than that found for green vegetables. The results for green vegetables, etc., were independent of the results for pasta, rice, and beef.

> Carlo LaVecchia et al., "A Case-Control Study of Diet and Colo-Rectal Cancer in Northern Italy," *Int. J. Cancer 41*, 492 (1988).

A study on dietary habits in relation to colon cancer risk was carried out in Wisconsin by researchers at the University of Wisconsin. The researchers divided their patients with colon cancer into two groups—those with cancer in the upper part of the colon and those with cancer in the lower part—in order to find out more precisely whether fat and fiber in the diet were differentially associated with either of the two groups. This possibility had been suggested by some earlier studies.

The researchers found that more frequent consumption of vegetables greatly reduced the risk of both types of colon cancer, and more frequent consumption of processed lunchmeats and pan-fried foods was associated with higher risk for either type of colon cancer. They found no differences between different parts of the large intestine for risks associated with the dietary variables.

Several hundred surviving colon cancer patients from a two-year period in the early 1980s had been located through a state-wide cancer registry in Wisconsin. Appropriate controls, matched for age, sex, and area of residence, were located through state records of driver's license holders. Cases and controls were invited to fill out a questionnaire that asked about diet, occupations, previous residences, alcohol and tobacco use, medical history and other personal characteristics. Participants were not told that colon cancer was the focus of the study.

Medical scientists believe that the development of colon cancer is very slow. They think many years, perhaps decades, elapse between the initiation of precancerous changes in the lining of the gastrointestinal tract and the eventual development of a malignant tumor. For this reason, the researchers asked the participants in this study to describe their diets during three periods in their lives: under the age of eighteen, between eighteen and thirty-five, and over thirty-five years. From their answers, it could be seen that most people—both cases and controls—had changed their diets as they grew older. With increasing age, people ate fewer desserts, eggs, pan-fried foods, milk and gravy, and ate more salads, fruit, cheese, and broiled foods. This type of switch to a lower-fat, higher-fiber diet conforms to the recommendations for better diet that we have heard from nutritionists in recent years, although consuming less milk is not really recommended. In this study, the controls did a better job of switching to a lighter diet as they grew older than did the cases. But even after making changes in their diets, the controls averaged only about one and a half servings a day of vegetables.

The questionnaires from the six hundred participants were analyzed statistically for significant differences between cases and controls, adjusting for age and sex. Personal characteristics that were unrelated to risk for colon cancer included economic status, tobacco use, coffee and alcohol consumption, and body size. Foods that were unrelated to risk for colon cancer were ham, bacon, sausage, beef, chicken, pork, lamb, potatoes, fruit, desserts, cereals, and all types of fat added to foods. (Lard was the only type of fat that was associated with higher risk. Butter, oil, margarine, cream, and mayonnaise were not related to risk.)

Foods that were most strongly associated with risk for colon cancer were vegetables, processed lunchmeat, pan-fried foods, eggs, and cheese. Vegetables, including salads, miscellaneous vegetables, and cruciferous vegetables, reduced the risk for colon cancer by a factor of two to more than three between the bottom and top quartiles of consumption frequency. Frequent consumption of processed lunchmeats during the young-adult years and over-thirty-five years almost doubled the risk for colon cancer. Frequent consumption of pan-fried foods was associated with higher risk for colon cancer. Eating more cheese in early life was associated with lower risk. More frequent consumption of eggs in later life was associated with slightly higher risk. This observation about egg consumption might simply mean that these subjects had not tried as hard to adapt to modern diet recommendations.

Vitamin supplements had a cancer-preventing effect, but this was statistically significant only for men taking vitamins in later life.

Those people who had had an operation for gall bladder removal were at higher risk for developing colon cancer for a period of five years after their operation. Many other studies also have found higher risk for colon cancer in gall bladder patients. Some unknown personal characteristic, perhaps involving the bile acids, might predispose these people to both disorders.

To summarize, more vegetables in the diet were associated with lower risk for colon cancer. Most meats and fats were not related to risk, but this does not rule out some role for fat in contributing to the development of colon cancer. The higher risks associated with processed lunchmeats and pan-fried foods might mean that people who consume extra hidden fat in a more old-fashioned diet have a higher risk for this disease.

Theresa B. Young and Dennis A. Wolf, "Case Control Study of Proximal and Distal Colon Cancer and Diet in Wisconsin," *Int. J. Cancer 42*, 167 (1988).

Cancer of the pancreas is the fifth most common cause of cancer deaths in the United States. It is a disease that is difficult to diagnose, and it has been increasing gradually in the United States. Most cases are adenocarcinomas.

The pancreas has two important functions. The endocrine function is production and secretion of insulin, and the exocrine function is production of enzymes for digestion of starch, fats, and proteins. The enzymes are produced in epithelial cells of the pancreas and are secreted in a thick digestive juice into the small intestine as soon as food begins to enter.

The only known risk factor for pancreatic cancer is cigarette smoking. Other environmental agents have been suspected, but virtually nothing was known about other risk factors with certainty until epidemiologists in Sweden decided to conduct a case-control study in Stockholm and Uppsala. During 1982-1984, ninety-nine people in three hospitals were found to have adenocarcinoma of the exocrine pancreas. They were asked to complete a self-administered questionnaire for use in a health study. Two groups of controls were also asked to complete the questionnaire. The controls were a group of patients hospitalized for hernia and a group of residents from the same neighborhoods as the cases. The epidemiologists inquired about coffee drinking, alcohol, and tobacco use in addition to the dietary items.

The results of the comparison between cases and controls included several striking correlations with pancreatic cancer.

Smoking was a factor that increased the risk of pancreatic cancer. Smoking one pack a day increased the risk of pancreatic cancer by a factor of three compared to not smoking. Dietary factors that increased the risk were frequent consumption of grilled meats and high intake of some fats. Factors that reduced the risk were vegetables, especially carrots, and citrus fruit.

The finding of increased risk associated with frequent consumption of fried or grilled meat was striking, although the number of subjects who said they ate fried or grilled meat almost daily was small. For these people, there was a five- to ten-fold increased risk over those who seldom ate fried or grilled meat. At first the scientists thought their results also showed an increased risk for meat in general, but closer analysis showed that it was only the fried or grilled meats that produced the increased risk.

In some earlier surveys as well, meat and fat in the diet were suspected of being related to pancreatic cancer. For instance, in Japan the incidence of this disease has risen in recent years as the meat intake has gone up since World War II.

The comparison of cases and controls in Sweden showed increased risk associated with higher fat intake, with a strange contrast between butter and margarine. Those who preferred margarine on bread had an increased risk over those who preferred butter, with the risk increasing as the amount of margarine used went up. Such was not the case for using extra butter. (The Western Electric Study in Chicago had also shown increased risk of lung cancer associated with margarine use.)

The strong inverse relation between pancreatic cancer and vegetables and fruit in the diet, which was found in this study, is most welcome news. Pancreatic cancer is a mysterious and deadly disease, and the possibility of prevention by eating a better diet is our best hope for reducing the fatalities. The reduced risk from carrots that was found in the Swedish study was particularly striking, following a dose-dependent pattern, with those who ate carrots almost daily having only 30% as high a risk as those who ate carrots less than once a week, other things being equal. Citrus fruits provided the same degree of risk reduction as did the carrots, and for those who said they ate both carrots and citrus almost daily, the risk was even lower.

There was some slight elevation of risk from coffee drinking, and no increase in risk from artificial sweeteners or from alcohol. The scientists did not mention whether they had questioned the subjects about their use of milk or cooking oils.

> Staffan E. Norell et al., "Diet and Pancreatic Cancer: A Case-Control Study," *Amer. J. Epidem. 124*, 894 (1986).

The strikingly elevated risk of pancreatic cancer associated with frequently eating fried and grilled meats in the Swedish study is disturbing news for those who eat a lot of bacon and other fried meats, well-browned meat dishes, and grilled meats and fish. If this study is confirmed by more such studies, it offers an interesting possible explanation for the occasional studies which have shown an association between more frequent meat eating and various cancers. And it might be part of the explanation for the international studies showing positive correlation between per capita meat intake and cancer mortality around the world.

On plain chemical grounds it is difficult to imagine how meat could contribute to the development of cancer, but if the burned products of high temperature searing, browning, and charring of foods are considered, then it is quite easily imagined that toxic chemicals could be formed, and in fact, such products *are* formed and have been found to be mutagenic in laboratory tests. Now, the Swedish study provides strong evidence that these degradation products generated by frying and grilling meats can contribute to cancer of the pancreas in man.

The presence of carcinogenic benzpyrene in charcoal-broiled meat was first discovered in 1964. The benzpyrene was produced from the fat that dripped onto the hot coals and was carried in the smoke onto the meat. Since then, many experiments have shown the formation of mutagenic and carcinogenic (in laboratory tests) products from cooking protein foods, even at more moderate temperatures such as pan-frying of ground beef.

Mutagens are also formed by chemical reaction between amino acids and sugars when these are heated in boiling water for several hours. Amino acids are the building blocks of proteins, and sugars are present in the vegetables such as onions that are often cooked in the same dish. In the lab, aqueous solutions of amino acids and sugars turn brown during lengthy "cooking" and the resulting solutions test positive for the presence of mutagens.

When we brown pork chops with onions or make a well-browned pot roast or a grilled fish, we are adding some extra mutagenic chemicals to our diet. There are dozens of chemical reactions occurring between amino acids and sugars and the reactions produce many tasty new chemicals and, ultimately, brown polymerization products. Some of the new chemicals (benzpyrene, imidazoquinolines, and imidazoquinoxalines) have been shown to be carcinogenic or mutagenic in laboratory tests. These reactions between proteins and sugars are collectively known as "Maillard reactions," after the French physician and chemist who first studied the reactions in his Paris laboratory in the early 1900s. The same types of brown polymers form also in Nature during the breakdown of plant materials to form humus, the material we prize so highly for the garden.

I would not tell anyone to completely avoid all the tasty fried ham, hamburgers, steaks and grilled chicken and other foods we love—especially since our basic diet of edible plants is known to contain a considerable variety of toxic chemicals anyway that are a normal part of the plant world and which our bodies are equipped to detoxify—but the Swedish study is a clear warning that we should try to prepare most of our meats by methods other than frying and grilling. Baking, braising, stir-frying, and microwaving produce delicious dishes without including the burned crusty coating of carcinogens that may well increase the risk of cancer.

A large study on pancreatic cancer and life style factors in southern Louisiana was done in conjunction with a larger case-control study conducted by epidemiologists from the National Cancer Institute and Louisiana State University. As in Sweden, a powerful protective effect was found from high fruit intake and high vitamin C intake. Other positive and negative dietary factors were found, but some of the results were difficult to comprehend and seemed incomplete, perhaps due to lack of information on food preparation methods.

The southern Louisiana area is renowned for its Creole and Cajun styles of cooking and, unfortunately, it is one of the areas in the United States with a high incidence of cancer of the pancreas. By questioning 363 cases and more than twelve hundred hospitalized controls during 1979 to 1983, the epidemiologists sought to extract information that might provide clues to specific risk factors for this disease.

Questions were asked on coffee, alcohol, and tobacco use, on ethnic background (Cajun or non-Cajun) and cancer in close relatives, on residential area and occupation, as well as on customary diet.

When the results of the questionnaires were analyzed, the scientists found that cigarette smoking was a definite risk factor, producing twice as high a risk for those who smoked one pack a day as for non-smokers, like all other studies on pancreatic cancer. A family history of pancreatic cancer was also a strong risk factor. Dietary factors that were not related to risk included beef, seafood, vitamin A, coffee and alcohol.

Several findings of the survey were specifically related to Cajun life style. Being of Cajun ancestry was associated with a 40% higher risk for cancer of the pancreas than being non-Cajun. Vegetables and carotene were not associated with reduced risk, an unusual finding for carcinoma. Pork and rice in the diet were associated with elevated risk. At this point, the scientists decided to analyze the risks for Cajuns and non-Cajuns separately, since the study group was about evenly divided among Cajuns and non-Cajuns. Cajuns who lived in rural areas had twice as high a risk as urban Cajuns, but residence made no difference to non-Cajuns. The non-Cajuns did not show any significant increased risk from eating more pork or rice, but the Cajuns did. Cajuns who were in the highest quartile for amount of pork and ham in the diet had three times higher risk than Cajuns in the lowest quartile.

These unusual results for pork and pork products, rice, and vegetables made the authors of the study regret that they had not collected information on the food preparation methods that were used by the subjects in the study. The differences between Cajuns and non-Cajuns seemed to implicate something about food preparation methods as being an important factor. No information was collected on frequency of frying or grilling foods. The scientists could only speculate as to whether the characteristic cooking methods of southern Louisiana were partly to blame for the risks observed. In other words, some methods or ingredients used in preparing pork and rice dishes could have caused the increased risks. Or, large amounts of pork and rice in the diet could simply indicate a preference for the traditional Cajun cuisine. (It is not hard to imagine how carcinogens might creep into the Cajun diet. Cajun and Creole cooking includes hot red peppers, filé, and heavy use of roux as the basis of many dishes, and does not put much emphasis on vegetables.)

On the positive side, very significant risk reduction for pancreatic cancer was associated with fruit and with vitamin C in the diet. Cajuns who were in the top quartile for fruits and fruit juices had only 23% as high a risk of pancreatic cancer as Cajuns in the lowest quartile. Vitamin C intake was calculated from the fruit and vegetable frequencies, and for those Cajuns who consumed 150 milligrams per day or more, the risk was only 29% as high as for those who consumed less than 67 milligrams per day—a very remarkable effect for a rather small increase in vitamin C in the diet. Non-Cajuns who consumed a lot of fruit and vitamin C also had reduced risk of pancreatic cancer, but the magnitude of the effect was not as great as in Cajuns. Also, Cajuns who were heavy fruit eaters did not have any of the increased risk from pork and pork products that the other subjects did.

The scientists speculated that a possible explanation for the association between cancer of the pancreas and eating pork and pork products might be the presence of nitrite in cured pork products. Nitrite has the potential for being converted to carcinogenic N-nitroso compounds during digestion, a conversion that is inhibited by vitamin C. This might explain the striking protective effect of vitamin C in this study. N-nitroso compounds have also been found in cigarette smoke, and have been shown to induce pancreatic cancer in animals.

The scientists who conducted the study were hopeful that more research would be done to investigate further the possible relation between various Cajun dietary customs and cancer of the pancreas, and to pursue possible preventive measures.

Roni T. Falk et al., "Life-Style Risk Factors for Pancreatic Cancer in Louisiana: A Case-Control Study," *Amer. J. Epidem. 128,* 324 (1988).

I might here point out that again we see a protective effect from vitamin C for risk of cancers of the upper digestive tract. This has been seen in cancer of the esophagus (which is common in heavy smokers and drinkers and is also common in parts of China and other countries where salted and pickled foods are popular), cancer of the stomach, and cancer of the pancreas. Which raises the question of how much vitamin C should we consume? In Louisiana, cancer of the pancreas was much less common in people who consumed 150 milligrams per day from fruit—two and a half times the RDA. Scientists are still studying the question of how much vitamin C can be profitably used by the human body; so, no one really knows yet what the optimal intake might be.

Cajun cuisine is interesting for its history and its unusual, traditional dishes. Cajun cooking is said to have its roots in southern France, with adaptations from other cultures and the ingredients found in southern Louisiana.

Cajun cooking depends a lot on roux as the basis for many dishes such as gumbo, jambalaya, and fricassee. Roux is made from equal parts of fat and flour, cooked slowly in a heavy pan with constant stirring until the mixture has become a golden or deep red-brown paste. Different recipes specify the color that should be used. Roux takes time to make. The time required to make the roux might be half an hour to an hour, although *The Prudhomme Family Cookbook* (Wm. Morrow and Co., New York 1987) says making roux could take several hours in the more traditional country ways. (Making a white sauce starts out the same except that the flour and fat boil up together for only a few moments before continuing with the recipe.) Chopped onions, green pepper, etc., can be added to the roux to cook for a while, or liquid parts of the recipe can be blended into the roux next. If the roux winds up as a gumbo, it would probably have a pinch of filé added at the end. Filé is powdered sassafras leaves, an ingredient used originally by the Indians. Many Creole and Cajun sauces and soups and roast pork also include a Louisiana hot pepper for additional flavoring.

The results of the Cajun recipes are delicious, but the roux, the filé, and the hot peppers all add toxic chemicals to the stew. The lengthy cooking of the fat and flour mixture does more than just break open the flour granules to release the starch. The color change in the mixture from white to brown is visible evidence of charring and chemical reaction between the starch and protein in the flour. Mutagenic chemicals are no doubt being formed, just like in the Maillard reaction.

The Prudhomme Family Cookbook was written to capture the recipes for the traditional Cajun cooking as it was done on the farms in Louisiana. This wonderful book contains detailed instructions for some of the most mouth-watering, delicious-sounding recipes I've ever read. In addition to the roux and the very careful seasonings, the most noticeable characteristic of the cuisine is browning. Very thorough browning over high heat in oil was the rule for meats of all kinds. Meats, often with onions added, were browned in oil over high heat until a considerable amount of crusty residue formed in the heavy pan, which was scraped loose, stirred, and scraped some more. The browned crusty foods were essential for the proper flavor and color of the final dish.

The carcinogenic chemical in the filé (powdered sassafras leaves) that was often added to gumbo and jambalaya is safrole. The mutagenic chemical in hot red peppers is capsaicin. Filé is added to gumbo in rather small amounts and the hot peppers, obviously, are also used in small amounts. The amount of mutagens ingested from the filé and hot peppers is probably much smaller in quantity than the mutagens ingested from the roux and from the thorough high-temperature browning used for so many of the Cajun dishes. With a diet that contains extra doses of mutagenic chemicals, it is little wonder that southern Louisiana has higher incidence of several types of cancer than other regions. The dietary mutagens may add only a small extra risk to the population, but the risk for cancer is already high due to the common smoking and drinking habits in the area and the low popularity of vegetables in the Cajun cuisine. There is no other region in the country where the need is greater for people to acquire new enthusiasm for citrus fruit and green leafy vegetables in their daily diet.

The topic of mutagens and toxic chemicals that are present naturally in vegetables, herbs, and other edible plants such as the Louisiana hot peppers is a fascinating subject that has been much discussed in recent years since Bruce Ames of the University of California reviewed the topic in a 1983 article in *Science* magazine. The reason we survive without more damage from these natural toxins like the one in hot peppers is the evolution of enzyme systems in plant-eating animals (including man) which result in conversion of the toxins to water-soluble, non-toxic derivatives that can be flushed from the body.

The enzyme systems may not be a complete defense against carcinogens, since they may be deficient in some people, and they may be ineffective against some mutagens.

We can probably not avoid eating considerable quantities of the natural toxic chemicals from plant foods, but we *can* avoid over-indulging in charred foods. The most prudent path to take in our own diet planning would seem to be to go easy on the charred foods and to indulge in more fruits and vegetables.

Chapter 5

Significance of the Studies

In the last chapter, we saw many interesting studies on diet and the risk of cancer, with a considerable variety of findings depending on what specific dietary factors and what specific cancer sites were under investigation. For many of the cancer sites, a risk reduction was associated with more vegetables in the diet.

What are we supposed to think about the variation among the studies done so far, for instance, on diet and breast cancer? The studies have found a wide range of risk reductions. In Athens, they found ten times higher risk associated with low vegetable intake. At Roswell Park, they found 50% higher risk associated with low beta-carotene intake in women over fifty-five. In Milan, they found a risk reduction of more than half in women who had a high intake of green vegetables. In Australia, higher intake of beta-carotene was associated with 24% lower risk for breast cancer. And in Argentina, there was a risk reduction greater than six-fold for those in the top quartile for vegetable consumption compared to the lowest quartile.

Do the wide differences between the observed risk reductions mean the vegetable effect is untrue? I think not, and I am so impressed by the epidemiological studies done so far that I am thankful that I have been including the RDA amount of vitamin A and most other vitamins in my diet since the early 1970s when I first read about experiments that indicated that vitamin A-related compounds could prevent experimental cancer in animals. I wish I had known more about folic acid that long ago.

The differences in the magnitude of the vegetable effect across the various studies is not surprising considering the different environments in which the studies were done. In communities where vegetables are not very popular, there will be smaller risk reductions to be found than in communities where vegetables are popular among part of the population. Results will vary from one study to another depending on which vegetables are included in the dietary surveys. The difficulties in obtaining accurate recall about food frequencies from the subjects, as well as people's tendency to change their dietary habits occasionally, and the uncertainty about whether some periods in life are more important than others are all problems for the epidemiologists to deal with in designing their studies. The studies were not carried out under identical conditions. The results of any study depend on the ingenuity of the researchers in asking the right questions and using appropriate statistical methods.

When the most common kinds of errors that might occur from problems such as inaccurate recall are considered by statisticians, it can be calculated that the errors tend to reduce the magnitude of the true effect. In other words, likely errors from the dietary interviews tend to make differences in relative risks appear smaller than they really are. If we had truly accurate measures of people's diets, we would see differences in relative risks even greater than the differences that have been reported.

Another reason for differences in the magnitude of the vegetable effect derives from different methods for scoring the diets. Some studies counted vegetable servings from a long list of vegetables; other studies calculated vitamin intake using published tables of food composition. The inaccurate data in the tables of food composition for beta-carotene content of some vegetables has been mentioned. The use of total vegetable scores has the advantage of including any beta-carotene plus other possible cancer-preventing factors that might be in the vegetables.

What we as consumers of these studies should look for is consistency in the direction of the results rather than close agreement in the observed relative risks.

The studies on diet and risk for breast cancer, first published in the 1980s, offer the first possibility for prevention of this disease that has ever been suggested. Breast cancer has remained an unrelenting problem for many decades without much change in the incidence rate and without much reduction in mortality rate since the 1930s in the United States, in spite of many advances in treatment methods.

Many studies have been done to find the risk factors associated with breast cancer, but the risk factors that were found from medical histories do not offer any practical route to prevention. Having higher socioeconomic status or having no children or having a sister or mother who had breast cancer are associated with higher risk. Lower risk is associated with having a larger number of full-term pregnancies and especially with having the first child at an early age. The likelihood of breast cancer increases with age, and for older women, increases with obesity. In the United States, women who live in the North are more likely to have breast cancer than women in the South.

One risk factor that substantially increases a woman's risk is the combination of family history of breast cancer and a diagnosis of atypical hyperplasia in a breast lesion. This diagnosis can only be made from a biopsy. It is not the same as the very common diagnosis of cysts, which alone does not much increase a woman's risk for breast cancer. Since only about 3% of women who develop breast cancer had a previous biopsy done and, therefore, could have been warned if they had the dangerous atypical hyperplasia, it is important for all women to continue to make use of early detection methods conscientiously.

According to the American Cancer Society, 75% of women who develop breast cancer did not have any of the risk factors that have been associated with breast cancer. These are the risk factors mentioned above relating to family history and reproductive history.

I think this is one of the most interesting statistics in the cancer incidence story, but it has not received much discussion in the popular press. Rather, many women are aware that there are known risk factors, but they are not aware that the risk factors account for only 25% of the cases. I wonder about the 75% of cases who had none of the known risk factors. Did these breast cancer cases develop entirely at random without any risk factor that can be singled out, or might there be a risk factor that has yet to be identified such as deficiency of the important ingredients in green leafy vegetables and cruciferous vegetables?

Diet so far has not been widely recognized as a risk factor in breast cancer because not enough studies have identified specific dietary habits that are related. Many careful studies have been done to test for a link between dietary fat and human breast cancer, but the results of these studies have been inconsistent. The suggestion that fat in the diet causes breast cancer has not been substantiated. (From a biochemical point of view, the mechanisms that have been proposed for the involvement of fat in carcinogenesis are a bit farfetched anyway, compared to the direct involvement of vitamin A and folic acid in the normal functioning of the genome.)

The known risk factors from medical histories demonstrate that hormones have an influence on the development of breast cancer. But the quantity of vegetables in the diet also has an effect. In the vegetable studies, the statisticians in Athens, Milan, Adelaide, and La Plata used statistical methods to control for reproductive history, menopausal status, hormone use, and other variables before calculating the vegetable effect. So, the vegetable effect was independent of hormonal history and should be effective for all women. Let us hope that more studies will be done on dietary factors in breast cancer to find out more precisely the relative importance of diet and hormones.

Until the vegetable studies were done in the 1980s, there was little evidence for any specific effect of diet on breast cancer incidence. If the vegetable studies are confirmed by additional studies, we will have found a most welcome weapon against an all-too-common bane of women.

At the beginning of the last chapter we did not know whether we would find much evidence for a protective effect of vegetables or beta-carotene against the glandular types of carcinoma, called adenocarcinomas. Many early studies that showed protective effects of high vegetable or beta-carotene intake were studies on the respiratory tract, where squamous cell carcinomas are common. It was thought at first from some of the lung cancer studies that adenocarcinomas were not associated with vegetable intake. However, by delving into some of the recent studies on diet and cancer, we have found plenty of studies showing protective effects against adenocarcinomas such as cancer of the breast, ovary, and colon, and adenocarcinoma of the lung and of the pancreas.

Surely not all types of cancer will be found to be preventable by better diet. For instance, it is unlikely that we will find lower incidences of kidney cancer, brain tumors, lymphoma, bone cancer, or melanoma to be associated with better diet. The Seventh-Day Adventists do not smoke or drink, and they follow many specific recommendations aimed at conservative, healthful living. About half are vegetarians. The Seventh-Day Adventists have about one-half to two-thirds as many deaths from most types of cancer as the general population, but their mortality rates from cancer of the kidney, central nervous system, prostate, and from lymphoma are about the same as the general population. So it may not be possible to lower the incidence of these types of cancer through changes in life style or diet.

A few of the studies described in the previous chapter found that high consumption of green vegetables or fruit was associated with reduced risk of cancer, but when beta-carotene intake was estimated from the same data, the beta-carotene score was not correlated with reduced risk. Might there be other ingredients in vegetables with anticancer properties besides beta-carotene? This is a strong possibility that has been the subject of much speculation and some research for several years. I have already mentioned the indoles in cruciferous vegetables which can increase production in the body of an enzyme that detoxifies potential carcinogens before they can initiate cancer. This is only one example of the natural ingredients in food that have functions in metabolism that are very interesting puzzles to work out. There is continuing research on other vegetable factors such as vitamin C, folic acid, and selenium. It is very likely that some of these other vegetable ingredients will also be proven some day to have an anticancer function.

Indirect evidence for additional cancer-preventing ingredients in vegetables can be found in the study on breast cancer from Athens, Greece. In the 1986 study described in the previous chapter there was a ten-fold risk reduction, after adjusting for hormonal status and many other variables, for women in the highest quintile of frequency of eating a large variety of vegetables, compared to women in the lowest quintile. More recently, the same group of scientists calculated the nutrient content of the diet for these same subjects (Katsouyanni et al., *Cancer 61*, 181 (1988)).

After adjusting for calorie intake as well as for hormonal and other variables as before, they found that total vitamin A was inversely related to breast cancer risk, with a clear dose-dependent reduction in risk through quintiles of vitamin A intake. The risk for the group with highest vitamin A intake (which was more than twice the RDA) was about 40% as great as the risk for the group with lowest vitamin A intake.

This risk reduction associated with vitamin A was not as great as the risk reduction seen when total vegetable servings were counted, which could very well mean that vitamin A accounted for only part of the risk reduction and other uncalculated ingredients in the vegetables were exerting an additional cancer-preventing effect. A similar result was found in the study on lung cancer at the Hawthorne Works, where men who averaged three times more beta-carotene in the top quartile had only one-eighth as many cases of lung cancer as those in the lowest quartile.

These studies showing that vegetables or beta-carotene are related to lower risks for cancer offer intriguing possibilities for a new way to deal with the cancer problem. Being able to prevent many cases would be a welcome step toward the goal of reducing the damage caused by this disease. Finding out how beta-carotene and the other vegetable factors exert a cancer-preventing effect might someday lead to new forms of treatment. The reasons the medical community is currently so cautiously excited about the apparent value of beta-carotene come from the epidemiological studies described in the previous chapter (which was not an exhaustive listing by any means) and from a variety of laboratory studies on cells and on experimental cancer in animals.

In my opinion, the caution is understandable in view of the decades-long, frustrating search for the explanation for cancer in man, but I think the time has come for the scientists to be cheering wildly for their wonderful discoveries, and they ought to be shouting from the rooftops the good news about vegetables for cancer prevention.

Chapter 6

The Discovery of Vitamin A

Vitamin A was the first of the vitamins to be discovered. The feat was accomplished in masterly fashion by Elmer V. McCollum and Marguerite Davis at the University of Wisconsin, and was described in the *Journal of Biological Chemistry* in 1913. Their deliberate discovery, the landmark beginning of modern nutrition studies, came about after several years of elaborate feeding experiments on animals—experiments that were meant to enlighten the ancient and valuable business of animal husbandry; long, tedious experiments that required laborious preparation of purified foodstuffs, with careful record-keeping and observations of the animals for months on end and thoughtful planning of studies designed to test, four or five at a time, dozens of ideas about what might constitute the essential feed requirements of animals.

Very little was known at the beginning of this century about the nutritional requirements of animals. French and German chemists in the nineteenth century had ventured into completely uncharted territory when they began to inquire about the composition of animal tissues. These early chemists produced quite a stir when they proved that animals can convert starch into fat and sugar into glycogen (a polymerized form of sugar). Understanding of nutrition came slowly. The chemical composition of foods was a new and slowly developing science that was supported because it was expected to aid livestock production in time, but much work would have to be carried out before this goal would be reached. In order to find out which nutrients are needed by animals, actual feeding studies were done with livestock, giving foods in various combinations and proportions. It was hoped that chemical analysis of the foods would eventually show what were the nutrients needed for survival and growth.

The idea that there must be small amounts of unknown substances in food that are absolute requirements for animal nutrition was a brand new idea in the early years of the twentieth century. The idea had only been clearly enunciated in 1906. For more than thirty years before that, physiologists had seen that experimental animals could not live on an artificial diet of mixtures of purified proteins, fats, carbohydrate and minerals when these were isolated from natural foods, but the implications of this result had eluded them. The vitamins, being present in foods in only trace amounts, had not been isolated and their presence was not suspected until feeding studies on animals began to show the remarkable value of small amounts of whole, unrefined foods added to the artificial diet. The possible existence of vitamins was also hinted at by the discovery at the end of the nineteenth century that a fatal, human neurological disease, beriberi, could be cured and prevented by better diet.

During the nineteenth century, chemists had developed techniques for isolating the macronutrients—protein, fat, and carbohydrate—from foods and had begun measuring the amounts of these nutrients in various grains, animal feeds, milk and plant materials. When the amounts of protein, fat, minerals, and carbohydrate from a sample of dried foodstuff were added up, the result always came to very nearly 100%; so it was generally assumed that these nutrients were the only components of foods. Even the realization that foods contained these four different kinds of substances was a revelation. Until the early nineteenth century, the prevailing idea since the time of Hippocrates was that all foods provided a single nutrient, called aliment, which was thought to be extracted from food and absorbed by the body during digestion.

Also during the nineteenth century, chemists were beginning to learn about the composition of proteins, by hydrolyzing the proteins with acid and separating the amino acid building blocks. By the year 1900, sixteen different amino acids had been identified and chemists could state that the proportions of the amino acids were different in proteins from different sources. This work produced the first explanation of why some foods might be more nutritious than others. The livestock-feeding experiments that were being done in Europe had as their goal finding the optimal feeding methods for livestock. The fact that proteins from different feeds had different amino acid compositions gave some impetus to the further chemical analysis of foodstuffs. Livestock men knew that variation in feeds would give different gains in their animals and they thought more chemical knowledge of foods would provide a scientific basis for designing livestock-feeding methods.

Using the new methods for isolating and purifying the major components of foods, physiologists in Europe began feeding small animals (usually mice) defined diets consisting of mixtures of purified proteins, fats, starch and minerals, with the intention of finding out which minerals and which proteins, and in what proportions, would provide the best growth and physiological well-being for the animals. The problem was that the animals always died on these artificial diets!

A German scientist, N. Lunin, in 1881 fed purified milk sugar (lactose), milk protein (casein), minerals, and milk fat to mice and saw his mice die on this diet. When he added a small amount of whole milk to their diet, the mice survived. He concluded that his purification of the components of milk had removed some unknown indispensable substance found in milk. (His mice were in need of B vitamins, which were unknown at the time.)

A Dutch bacteriologist and professor by the name of Pekelharing did similar studies on mice and also found the value of whole milk. His mice died on an artificial diet of purified proteins, starch, lard and minerals unless he gave them a small amount of whole milk in addition. (His mice were lacking the B vitamins and vitamin A.) Pekelharing wrote in 1905 that there was an unknown substance in milk, and probably also in many other kinds of foods, that was absolutely essential for animal nutrition.

A German scientist, Wilhelm Stepp, came very close to the discovery of vitamin A in 1909 with his feeding experiments on mice. He found that if he extracted regular foods with hot alcohol and ether, thus removing fats and many other substances, the mice died when they were maintained on the extracted foods. He tried keeping them alive by adding back all of the known lipids to their diet (triglycerides, lecithin, cholesterol, and cerebroside), but the mice still died. The mice survived when he gave them the solid material from a cold alcohol extract of egg yolk. He concluded there was an unknown fatlike substance from egg yolk that benefited the mice. He did not know about several B vitamins in the egg yolk that would also have been present in the alcohol extract. If Stepp had extended his extraction work to several more kinds of fatty foods, he might have realized that not all fatty foods provided the unknown, essential fatlike substance.

These studies showing the failure of purified macronutrients to support animal life went on sporadically for more than thirty years with only an occasional conjecture from the scientists that there was something missing in the animals' rations. No systematic efforts were made to follow up on the results that were reported.

The full significance of these animal feeding studies was finally realized by a British physician and Cambridge professor, Frederick Gowland Hopkins, who saw a connection between the animal studies and several human illnesses where certain specific dietary improvements could produce a cure. Hopkins had started out as an analytical chemist, but he went into medicine because of his deep curiosity about the chemistry of living things. In his medical training he learned how to treat the common diseases, rickets and scurvy, which were prevalent in English babies and children at the time. Rickets could be cured with cod liver oil, and scurvy could be cured with lemon juice or a variety of other fresh fruits and vegetables. The curative properties of these foods had been known for many years, but nothing was known about the active principles in the foods—the foods were simply regarded as medicinal substances—and virtually nothing was known about the causes of the illnesses or the mechanisms of the cures. Also, at the end of the nineteenth century, Christian Eijkman and Gerrit Grijns, while working in the Dutch East Indies, had solved the mysterious disease, beriberi, by showing that it developed in men who were restricted to a limited diet of polished rice but not in men who were given whole rice (see chapter 13).

Hopkins considered together all of these partly solved medical mysteries, and in 1906 put forward the hypothesis that there must be many substances in foods other than the known proteins, fats, and carbohydrates that were just as essential for animal life as are the macronutrients. He called these unidentified substances the "accessory factors of the diet." Hopkins pointed out that cod liver oil might work by supplying some missing nutrient to the victims of rickets, and the curative agent in lemon juice, whatever it was, was neither a protein, a fat, nor a sugar. Some factor in rice polishings could cure beriberi, although the chemical nature of the factor was unknown. Hopkins' hypothesis that there were unidentified nutrients required by humans and animals was published in 1906 as a paper in a technical journal. His reasoning encouraged other scientists and physicians to begin thinking about the possibility that the absence of an essential substance could cause disease just as exposure to foreign substances or pathogens could cause disease. This concept of deficiency disease was a new idea in the medical sciences and it became accepted only very slowly over the next few years as detailed knowledge about the existence of vitamins was acquired.

Hopkins pursued experimental proof of his hypothesis by doing feeding studies on laboratory rats. He fed rats the same kind of artificial diets that others had used for mice and measured the rats' weight gain over time. The rats could gain weight at a normal rate only when some whole milk was added to the artificial diet. (Milk contains all of the known vitamins.) Without a small amount of milk (from 1 to 4% of the total diet) the animals could not metabolize the purified foods and use the foods for normal growth and survival, even though they consumed the purified food that was offered.

In addition to doing research in nutrition, Hopkins directed the biochemical research group at Cambridge University for many years. He became one of the great leaders of the new scientific efforts to define the chemical composition and metabolic requirements of living things. His generosity in helping struggling young scientists in England and from other countries to get a start in their careers was well known. Hopkins was awarded a Nobel Prize in 1929 for his vitamin hypothesis and for his contributions to the science of nutrition.

Meanwhile, at the Agricultural Experiment Station in Madison, Wisconsin, Elmer McCollum was also puzzling over the failure of artificial diets to keep animals alive. McCollum had grown up on a farm in Kansas and had studied chemistry at the University of Kansas. In 1906 he received a Ph.D. in chemistry from Yale, where he had the opportunity to listen to lectures on toxicology and nutrition given by some of the top experts of the day. After finishing his student years, McCollum had in mind to find a position teaching organic chemistry, but the first good job offer that came along was in the field of nutrition investigation at the University of Wisconsin.

McCollum took the job and, realizing he had no decent background in nutrition, he enthusiastically set about to educate himself in the field by reading the abstracts describing animal nutrition studies from the previous thirty-five years. The abstracts were compiled in the German publication, Maly's *Jahresbericht uber die Fortschritte der Thier-Chemie*. McCollum was astonished to read that none of the rations that were made from purified food components had been able to keep animals in a healthy condition. He realized that finding out the causes of these failures was the most important task to be undertaken in the field of nutrition.

McCollum was ambitious and was always determined to find out the answers to whatever problems he set out to study. McCollum had joined the College of Agriculture at Wisconsin while a feeding experiment was in progress using cows. His first stroke of genius was switching from cows for experimental study to rats. Rats lived out their life cycle in two or three years, and the amount of food needed for the rats was small compared to cows. Using cows you could not experiment with artificial diets, but with rats you could. His rat colony at Wisconsin was the first in the United States.

McCollum's first studies were designed to test the idea that lack of preformed phosphoproteins or other phosphorus-containing compounds in the artificial diets was the reason for animals' failure to survive. Two years of work with the rats told him that none of the known phosphorus-containing substances found in the animal body was essential in the diet, as these could all be synthesized as needed by the animals.

McCollum and his assistant, Marguerite Davis, continued working with the artificial diets. Much of their work revolved around efforts to optimize the mineral component of the diet. They realized early on that grains alone did not provide adequate nutrition for the animals. When certain minerals were added, a little better growth was seen, but the rats still could not grow normally. Thinking the malnourished animals might have poor appetites, they tried improving the taste of the rations by adding freshly cooked bacon or water that had been distilled from cheese for its aroma or proteins, starches, and fats from a variety of sources. Through these experiments, they finally saw that the rats could thrive on butterfat or egg yolk fat when these were part of the diet, but not on lard or olive oil. This was the first scientific evidence that certain fats were more beneficial than others, and this was the key observation that produced the discovery of vitamin A.

Young rats that had used up their stored vitamin A stopped growing and only resumed growth when a vitamin A-containing food, such as butter or egg yolk, was included in their rations. This was the explanation for the rats' failure to grow that would eventually become clear to the chemists as they continued their work.

McCollum and Davis showed that the beneficial substance was not the butterfat itself, but was, rather, a fat-soluble substance that remained active and could be extracted with ether after the butterfat was destroyed by alkaline hydrolysis. They called this substance "fat-soluble A." (The term, vitamin, would be adopted a few years later.)

McCollum had kept some of his former professors at Yale informed about his research program and they had started similar work. One of their findings was that "fat-soluble A" could also be supplied in the diet of rats by giving cod liver oil.

This raised the next obvious question of where do animals normally obtain "fat-soluble A" in their diet? Not many animals consume butter, eggs, or cod liver oil, but many animals obtain most of their nutrients from pasture grasses. Were the good pasture grasses that normally sustain many kinds of livestock a source of the "fat-soluble A"? After another two years of work, McCollum was able to show that his rats could obtain the nutritional equivalent of butter from clover, alfalfa, cabbage or yellow corn.

McCollum and Davis conducted a large number of feeding studies on the rats during these years and made several more discoveries about essential factors in the diet. They tackled the partly solved beriberi problem by studying diets based on polished rice. The devastating neurological disease, beriberi, had been shown to be caused by a diet heavy in polished rice, which had become a staple grain in the Far East in the last part of the nineteenth century. McCollum and Davis used the same type of experimental strategy to study the deficiency in polished rice that they had used for the "fat-soluble A" discovery. A basic ration of purified food components was supplemented with additional nutrients to find out the nature of the deficiency. In 1915 they published their feeding studies based on polished rice and showed that the dietary deficiency in polished rice was not a mineral or a protein or "fat-soluble A" and it was not a toxin, but it was a water-soluble substance that could be extracted from rice polishings, or from wheat germ, milk, skim milk, or egg yolk. They concluded that there were two accessory substances of the diet: one of them soluble in fats and one soluble in water, which they called "water-soluble B."

Although the rats in the original experiments had been fed a basic diet of purified protein, carbohydrate, lard, and minerals, they had also been fed B vitamins inadvertently as a contaminant in the lactose (milk sugar), and this had contributed to their ability to survive.

McCollum and Davis realized this during the following years of work and learned how to purify lactose to the degree that B vitamins could be removed if desired.

By this time McCollum really knew quite a bit about how to keep rats healthy on an artificial diet. Whole grains alone did not supply complete nutrition. Grain with the addition of minerals, especially calcium, iron, magnesium, sodium, potassium and phosphorus, gave a slightly improved weight gain. This had been clearly shown also in the cow-feeding studies. Grain plus minerals plus a little extra protein gave some further improvement. And complete nutrition, as proven by normal growth and normal reproduction, was obtained from the four-way combination of grain plus extra protein plus minerals plus "fat-soluble A." McCollum used the rat bioassay to figure out what was missing from the various deficient types of diets. He found that the animals could not thrive on grains alone, even combinations of several grains, due to lack of minerals and lack of the fat-soluble vitamin in grains. Only a few grains such as corn contained any of the fat-soluble vitamin and even in these, there was only a small amount present. (The grains did provide sufficient amounts of the "water-soluble B.") Animals fared one hundred per cent better on a combination of grain and green plants, and, in fact, could thrive on a diet of wheat or corn and sun-dried alfalfa and nothing else. Alfalfa was a rich source of minerals, especially calcium, and also provided the fat-soluble vitamin, some protein, and we know now that it also provided some vitamin D which would have been useful for the rats as they were kept indoors and did not get any sun.

McCollum also did the first experiments that showed some protein combinations were better than others for growth of the animals. For instance, wheat plus peas provided a good source of protein but oats plus peas did not support growth. Oats plus navy beans were much more beneficial for growth and reproduction. The concept of the supplementary relationships between foods became clear from McCollum's dietary studies and was one of the constant themes of his later efforts to educate the public.

McCollum received much recognition for his early successes and soon was offered the post of head of the chemistry department at the new Johns Hopkins School of Public Health. This position he accepted eagerly because it offered the chance to learn about medical research problems from leading specialists. At Johns Hopkins he continued making discoveries in the field of nutrition and, in addition, took up the task of promoting better understanding of nutrition by the American public. His nutrition work with animals and reading about the dietary customs of peoples in different parts of the world led him to value most highly a diet based on combinations of whole grains with some additional protein, additional minerals (especially calcium), and the green leaves of plants.

He was concerned that the high level of white flour, cornmeal, potatoes and sugar in the American diet was far from the ideal diet, which he thought should contain generous amounts of green leafy vegetables and milk. As early as 1918 he called milk and leafy vegetables "protective foods" because their high nutritional value helped compensate for the deficiencies of many other foods. These principles of good diet were the theme of his lectures throughout the country in 1918, which were part of his contribution to Herbert Hoover's U.S. Food Administration campaign against hunger and malnutrition. His enthusiastic lectures were always well received, including as they did explanations of the dietary studies on rats and translations of the experimental findings into useful information for human diets. He was often told by people in the audience that they had never before heard that the choice of foods could have an impact on health.

McCollum accepted a responsibility to help educate the public as well as other scientists, and the responsibility to help government agencies. He served on many advisory committees throughout his long career. McCollum wrote and lectured for agricultural groups and for professional groups, and became well known from his popular writing on nutrition. Between 1922 and 1946 he contributed 169 articles to *McCall's* magazine, explaining better nutrition for American families.

Looking back in later years over the work done at Wisconsin, McCollum remembered some of the flaws in the research work as well as the notable discoveries. The famous cow-feeding experiment that was in progress when he arrived contained a flaw in the method of preparation of those animals' feed, which may have influenced the results somewhat, and the work with the rats could have proceeded more efficiently if pathologists or other medical scientists had been recruited to help evaluate the condition of the animals. McCollum's realization that his work needed the advice of medical specialists was a big reason for his elation at being offered the post at Johns Hopkins. At Johns Hopkins, he was to benefit from collaboration with medical specialists in his 1922 discovery of the existence of vitamin D in cod liver oil, a substance so valuable for its ability to cure rickets.

When McCollum left Wisconsin, vitamin D had not been discovered and neither had vitamin C. The concept of deficiency disease was a new idea. Casimir Funk had suggested from human studies that there were at least four deficiency diseases—beriberi, scurvy, pellagra, and rickets—and that each would be found to be caused by deficiency of a separate vitamin. McCollum did not agree with this suggestion in 1917 because his rats thrived on diets that contained only 3% wheat germ as a source of the B vitamin and 5% butterfat for the A vitamin. He thought it unlikely that such small amounts of wheat germ and butterfat would be supplying any other vitamins simultaneously. In this, McCollum was in error we know now, because the butter and egg yolk contained small amounts of vitamin D. The sun-dried alfalfa also contained a small amount of vitamin D from conversion of ergosterol to vitamin D. McCollum's rats thrived without vitamin C in their diets because rats do not require vitamin C—they make their own supply of ascorbic acid from glucose. For a short while, McCollum thought that some of the deficiency diseases would turn out to be caused by unbalanced diet rather than by vitamin deficiencies.

When McCollum left Wisconsin in 1918, he left unfinished the investigation of the "fat-soluble A" nutrient in the green leafy plants like alfalfa and clover. No one knew anything about the chemical nature of this nutrient. Some work was beginning to show its wide distribution in foods and its usefulness to the animal body in allowing normal growth, in curing an eye disease that developed in deficient animals, and in preventing lung infections. But the only way to assay for the substance was by means of the rat growth-promoting test.

Harry Steenbock was another chemist at the Agricultural Experiment Station, a former student of McCollum and a coworker, who took over the work with the rat colony when McCollum left. Steenbock set out to investigate a variety of plant foods to find out their relative values as sources of the fat-soluble vitamin. He knew this type of information could have economic value. He hoped also to be able to find out something about the chemical nature of the substance.

These chemists, McCollum and Steenbock, cared much about the details and quantitative aspects of their work. They were able to extract much new information about nutrition from their studies, but this was only because of the thoroughness with which they set up the research programs and thought about the possibilities. The rats were fed rations that had been carefully mixed up from precisely weighed amounts of certain grains or purified proteins with carbohydrates and fats added in exact proportions, with precise amounts of sodium chloride, potassium phosphate, magnesium sulfate, calcium lactate, ferrous lactate, calcium phosphate and other salts all added in certain quantities. Variation in the proportions of the minerals, grains, starches and fats and variation in the plant sources of the grains and proteins made possible a large number of different diets. Over three thousand different rations were formulated and tested at Wisconsin during these years. The chemists were motivated in their labors by a powerful curiosity about the workings of the still-unknown nutrients and by the obvious implication that their discoveries might have important bearings on human health as well as on animal production. Their early success in drawing out new knowledge from the feeding studies gave them the confidence to continue. The new knowledge—always accompanied by new, unanswered questions—fueled their curiosity about the nutrients.

It was especially important to Harry Steenbock to find out exactly how much of the fat-soluble vitamin was present in different foods. McCollum had shown that green leaves could supply the vitamin—would other parts of food plants also contain it? Steenbock tested a series of root vegetables in 1918-1919. He found the growth-promoting, eye-saving vitamin in the yellow roots like carrots and sweet potatoes, but none at all in other roots like Irish potatoes, taro, and beets.

Then Steenbock remembered from two years earlier one of the feeding studies on rats that had not turned out right. The rats had been on corn rations with some other nutrients added, but they were not successful in rearing their young as rats usually did on this diet. He did not pay much attention at the time because of other work, but after the studies of carrots and sweet potatoes, the two year-old problem came back to mind. He remembered that yellow corn had been unavailable on the local market two years earlier, so the lab had substituted white corn instead. It was a diet of white corn that had caused failure of reproduction, as well as eye disease, in the rats.

The feeding studies with corn were repeated, using four varieties of white corn and four varieties of yellow corn that were all grown in the Midwest, and the results were clear. The yellow corn was far more nutritious than the white. On white corn the rats died in three months and on yellow corn they could grow and rear their young.

Steenbock wrote a short article for *Science* magazine to make these studies known and to explain why he thought there was a good possibility that the fat-soluble vitamin was a yellow pigment in plants, or a compound closely related to a yellow pigment. At the time, several yellow pigments called carotenoids had already been isolated from plants and it was known that carotene was one of the common carotenoids. Carotene had been discovered in carrots in 1831, and in 1907 Willstatter and Mieg had shown that carotene could be isolated from either carrots or green leaves. It was also known by this time that animals could not synthesize carotene. Steenbock thought that the fat-soluble vitamin might very well turn out to be carotene itself.

Steenbock's suggestion of 1919 turned out to be correct, but the proof remained ten years in the future, when it would finally be shown, after years of contradictory and confusing experiments, that the fat-soluble vitamin exists in foods in two forms: an almost colorless form in milk, butter, eggs, and liver (retinol), and a bright orange form in plants (carotene).

Steenbock set out in 1919 to try to extract the fat-soluble vitamin from plant materials. Preliminary work had given the impression that the vitamin was unstable; so gentle methods of extraction were tried first. These methods did not work very well. Steenbock found that cold alcohol did not extract much vitamin from ground, dried carrots. McCollum had found that ether did not extract much vitamin from cornmeal.

When he switched to lengthy extractions using alcohol, Steenbock had greater success. Using alcohol, he was able to extract active vitamin from carrots, alfalfa, and yellow corn. Alfalfa was an especially good source of the vitamin for further study—the rat bioassay showed seventeen times more vitamin in alfalfa than in yellow corn. The purified carotene had an intense deep red color. When present as a minor component of plants, carotene imparts some shade of yellow to the plant. (In green leaves the yellow color is masked by the strong green of the chlorophyll.) If carotene were the fat-soluble vitamin, one would expect that foods that had a stronger yellow color would be richer in the vitamin than pale-colored foods. This had been true in the root vegetables, but was not true in all other foods.

Steenbock's idea that vitamin A was a yellow pigment from plants was put to a test by Leroy Palmer and Harry Kempster from the University of Missouri. They thought to find out whether chickens could be maintained on a diet completely lacking in yellow-pigmented foods. In this they were successful. They raised chickens to maturity on a completely white diet consisting of white corn, skim milk, bone meal, and some pork liver which contained no carotenoids or other yellow pigments. The mature chickens had white legs, beaks, and ear-lobes instead of the normal yellow and laid eggs that had white yolks, but the eggs could be hatched to produce healthy chicks. These work-ers realized that the pork liver contained the fat-soluble vitamin in a non-yellow form, and, since yellow foods were not necessary for the chickens, they concluded yellow pigments were not necessary for vi-tamin A activity.

Another puzzle was connected with the variation in color of butter samples. Steenbock obtained from the university creamery butter sam-ples that had been produced at different times of the year and had dif-ferent intensities of yellow color. When tested in the rats, the vitamin activity of the different butters did not correlate with the yellowness of the samples. Cod liver oil was another puzzle. It was known to be about 250 times more concentrated in the vitamin than butter even though it had only a very light yellow color.

So Steenbock's idea that the vitamin and carotene might be one and the same could not be accepted after all. There were too many food sources of the vitamin where color and vitamin activity did not go together.

During the next few years, highly purified carotene was tested for vitamin A activity in several laboratories with variation in the results. Carotene did not always produce good growth-promoting effects in A-deficient rats. This may have been because vitamin D was also needed for good growth, a point that was not properly understood until 1928, when the von Eulers in Stockholm provided vitamin D along with car-otene in their assays, and proved the vitamin activity of carotene; or, some of the carotene samples may have been inactivated by air oxi-dation. Chemists in England, Sweden, and Switzerland were studying the problem of how a substance from plants and a different substance from cod liver oil could have identical effects in the growth-promoting bioassay. Carotene and vitamin A had both been purified from several materials and the two substances had some very different chemical properties such as their solubilities in various solvents, yet they seemed to have the same beneficial effects on nutrition in test animals. The chemical structures were not yet known. The carotene structure had been partly figured out, and the structures of both substances would be completely determined by 1931. Some other carotenoids be-sides carotene were tested and at least one was found to have vitamin activity. In the meantime, the dissimilarities between the spectro-scopic properties of carotene and the pale-colored vitamin in cod liver oil brought about the suggestion that there might be several substances with similar chemical structures that all have vitamin activity.

The carotene puzzle was finally solved in 1929 through a series of careful and clever studies that were devised by Thomas Moore at Cambridge University in England. Moore decided to purify carotene from carrots and from red palm oil and test the material in rats at various stages in the purification procedure. This approach to the problem, he knew, would show whether or not the vitamin activity increased as carotene became more highly purified. Moore used rats on a diet of purified protein, starch, vegetable oil containing added vitamin D, salts, and a source of B vitamins. Without a source of vitamin A, rats could live only about two months on this diet before developing eye disease, lung infections, weight loss, and dying.

Moore's careful testing of carrots and extracted and purified carotene proved again that carotene was a very potent fat-soluble vitamin in the rat bioassay. The higher potency of the more purified carotene compared to the less pure material made it unlikely that some contaminant was producing the vitamin effect.

Another laboratory had claimed that dietary carotene was stored in the liver of test animals. Moore looked into this assertion and found a different result. He examined the livers of rats that had been fed high doses of carotene and did not see the bright yellow color of carotene. He extracted the fats from the livers and tested the solutions with a chemical reagent that produces a bright blue color when mixed with vitamin A from cod liver oil or butter. The color test had been devised a few years earlier and was known to produce a very weak blue-green color with carotene, also. By clever use of this color test, which could distinguish between carotene and vitamin A, and the distinctive yellow color of carotene, Moore could estimate the amounts of the two substances when both were present together. The livers from carotene-fed rats produced a bright blue color identical to that of cod liver oil in spectroscopic tests.

This was the experiment that solved the puzzle. Large amounts of carotene had been fed to the rats and large amounts of vitamin A were deposited in the animals' livers. Moore realized that dietary carotene had been converted into vitamin A in the animals. This discovery could explain all the confusing results from the previous ten years and showed that carotene was indeed equivalent to vitamin A after all. Moore went one step further and proved that it was really vitamin A itself and not some similar compound that was deposited in the livers of carotene-fed rats by showing that the deposited vitamin A was effective as the growth-promoting vitamin in a bioassay for the vitamin.

Moore continued to study carotene and vitamin A. He noted in 1930 that preformed vitamin A, such as that found in cod liver oil, was effective in much smaller doses than carotene in the form of carrots or greens. He realized that this might be explained by inefficient conversion of carotene to vitamin A.

Moore did further studies with carotene-fed rats to find out something about how and where carotene is converted into vitamin A in the animal body. He found that in rats fed lavish amounts of carotene, carotene was still present throughout the length of the digestive tract and appeared also in the feces. This experiment told him that carotene was not being converted while it was in the contents of the digestive tract; it must be converted instead after it was absorbed from the small intestine. Since liver contained a larger amount of stored vitamin A compared to any other tissue, as well as small amounts of carotene, Moore thought the site of conversion would most likely turn out to be the liver. Even in animals that developed very high concentrations of vitamin A in their livers, the level of vitamin A in other organs and tissues remained at a limited level; so it appeared that the liver also performed some function in controlling the amount of vitamin A distributed to the tissues.

During these same years, the detailed chemical structures of beta-carotene and vitamin A were being worked out by chemists in England and Switzerland. Beta-carotene contained two ring systems separated by a hydrocarbon chain that included eleven conjugated double bonds, which accounted for its intense color, and vitamin A contained only one ring and a shorter hydrocarbon chain containing five double bonds, being the result of oxidative cleavage of a symmetrical carotene molecule in the middle.

So, in the case of plants, Steenbock's suggestion that the yellow versus white color of the vegetables is a good indicator of their vitamin A content was right all along. But in the case of animal products such as butter, eggs, and fats, one could not tell the vitamin A content from the color because in the animal body the carotene had been converted to the very pale-colored product, retinol, which was the form of vitamin A that was useful for the animal's needs.

Chapter 7

Night Blindness and Other Ills

Everyone knows that vitamin A is good for the eyes. This has been understood in a practical way since at least the time of Hippocrates, who wrote in the fourth century B.C. that eating liver would cure night blindness. This traditional remedy has been passed along by seafaring people through the centuries. For instance, fishermen in Newfoundland have long known that consuming cod liver or seagull liver would cure their night blindness when it developed after long days in the sun with the glare of the sea falling all day on the retina of the eye. The sunlight used up part of the vitamin A in their retinas to the point where the eyes no longer functioned properly. Eating liver to cure the condition was the practical solution to the problem long before anything was known about the vitamins or their functions.

During the 1920s and 1930s medical investigations into the effects of vitamin deficiencies gradually produced some explanations for some of the old-time home remedies and called attention to specific conditions that could occur when the diet does not contain sufficient quantities of the vitamins. Night blindness is one of these conditions.

Night blindness—difficulty seeing when going from a brightly lit area into a dark area—is sometimes an early sign of vitamin A deficiency. (Some people have a congenital type of night blindness that may not be more than an occasional inconvenience for them, and is not due to vitamin deficiency.) In cases where the night blindness is due to a simple lack of vitamin A, it is easily corrected by including liver or cod liver oil or some other good source of vitamin A in the diet. Difficulty in adjusting to bright daylight is another early symptom of vitamin A deficiency. These symptoms often go together and can persist for many years without leading to any further eye problems, but they are known to be caused by the vitamin deficiency. Night blindness was discovered to be a consequence of vitamin A deficiency in 1925 from work with rats that were kept on a diet that lacked vitamin A. The A-deficient rats could not find their usual hiding places just after they were subjected to large changes in the level of the room lighting. Their ability to adapt to sudden darkness or to bright light was impaired.

Vision in dimly lit areas, called twilight vision, depends on the rod cells of the retina which contain the pigment, rhodopsin, which has also been called "visual purple." The biochemistry of vision is an extremely complicated process with some parts of the process still a bit of a mystery. One of the unanswered questions about vision involves dark adaptation, which is impaired in people suffering from vitamin A deficiency. It is not known why rod cells are less able to respond to low levels of light just after entering a dark theater than they are after a few moments. This process of dark adaptation is normal. In individuals deficient in vitamin A, the length of time they must spend in the dark before being able to use their rod cells for twilight vision is noticeably longer and the amount of light they need to see anything at all is greater. It is this condition that is called night blindness.

The ability to see in a low level of light after a brief period of darkness was made into a test and used in surveys among school children in the 1930s in attempts to find out whether vitamin A deficiency was very common and to find out what dose of vitamin A was needed to restore good dark adaptation. The test was somewhat crude and gave different results for different investigators, but it was common to find symptoms of night blindness in twenty to eighty per cent of the children in some areas of the United States.

The ability to see in twilight or in daylight is an ability we naturally take for granted. Occasionally we pause to wonder at the miraculous delicacy of a flower, or the glow of a piece of finely polished wood or stone, or the different types of flight patterns of the birds. We should also wonder at the miracle of sight that enables us to observe such things. Biologists who study the visual process have found a complex system of highly specialized cells and structures in the eye that make use of complicated physics and chemistry to convert photons of light into nerve impulses that result in vision.

The retina is the inner layer of the eyeball where vitamin A functions in the visual process. The retina consists of several fine layers of membranes and nerve cells and a layer that contains the specialized nerve cells called the rods and the cones. The rods and cones are the cells in the retina that respond to light in the visual process. Using the electron microscope, rod cells can be seen as close-packed cylinders in one layer of the retina all standing perpendicular to the light source, interspersed with the smaller cone cells. One blunt end of the cells is in contact with the next layer of the retina, the pigment epithelium layer. Some internal structures of the rods and cones, the disk membranes, are constantly being renewed in the cells, and parts of the old disk membranes are shed from the ends of the cells and are phagocytized by the pigment epithelium.

The form of vitamin A that is used by the rod cells for vision is 11-cis-retinaldehyde which combines with the protein, opsin, to form the visual pigment, rhodopsin. Even in the dark, the rod cells are functioning. Sodium and calcium ions diffuse into the cell at one end and are pumped out the other end in an energy-requiring process that moves one billion electronic charges per second in each cell. This dark current is drastically reduced when light impinges on the retina and some of the ion channels in the cell membrane close. Light converts the 11-cis-retinaldehyde to the all-trans isomeric form in a very fast reaction that initiates a cascade of chemical changes in the rod cell that result in production of a signal in the optic nerve. As part of this cascade of changes following the light-induced isomerization of the retinaldehyde, the conformation of rhodopsin is altered and several enzymes closely associated with rhodopsin become activated. A cascade of enzymic changes in the cell amplifies the effect of light on a molecule of rhodopsin. (There are about thirty million rhodopsin molecules in each rod cell.) The exact mechanisms whereby the dark current in the cell is reduced after a flash of light are still being worked out; biochemists have shown that cyclic guanosine monophosphate and calcium ions are involved as signal transducers. The all-trans isomer of retinaldehyde produced by the photon of light separates from the rhodopsin and is reduced enzymatically to retinol (vitamin A), which moves out of the rod cell and into the pigment epithelium layer of the retina where the vitamin A is stored, mostly as retinyl ester.

Restoration of light sensitivity in the rod cell after exposure to large quantities of light is not yet completely understood, but this is a field of active investigation in vision biochemistry, and many of the enzyme reactions have been worked out. All of the molecules must be restored to their original condition. The ion channels must reopen, cyclic guanosine monophosphate must be resynthesized, and 11-cis-retinaldehyde must be resynthesized and transported from storage back to the rod cell where it recombines spontaneously with the protein, opsin, to form rhodopsin.

Most of the vitamin A in the retina is reused, so that dietary deficiency does not produce deficiency symptoms for some time. However, the fact that deficiency symptoms can develop, as in the Newfoundland fishermen after much exposure to the sun and the sea, demonstrates that part of the vitamin A is lost to the retina during the chemical changes and is excreted. A fresh supply of vitamin A is required to make up for the fraction that is lost.

If you have followed all of this chemistry carefully, you may be wondering what happened to the explanation for night blindness. The details of how vitamin A deficiency results in impaired dark adaptation have not been completely worked out. It is known that during dark adaptation more vitamin A moves from the storage site in the retina to the rhodopsin in the rod cells. Also, recent studies are beginning to explain how calcium ions in the rods and cones are involved in the adaptation to varying light levels. Further understanding of the role of calcium ions will no doubt add more to the explanation of the processes involved in normal vision.

Night blindness is a symptom of mild vitamin A deficiency. It is also the first symptom of a much more serious eye disease that results from severe vitamin A deficiency and is a major public health problem in many parts of the world, especially for children. Xerophthalmia is a major cause of blindness in third world countries in areas where malnutrition is chronic and medical attention is lacking. Xerophthalmia results from deterioration of the tear glands and keratinization of the conjunctiva, resulting in ulceration of the cornea and total blindness. It has been estimated recently that a quarter million children go blind every year from this disease in Asia, and the situation in some other parts of the world is probably just as shocking.[1]

Xerophthalmia develops through a series of stages of increasing deterioration of the eye, and the early stages can be diagnosed upon close inspection by a physician. In the earlier stages the disease can be arrested by giving vitamin A. In India, successful field trials were started in the late 1960s to combat eye disease in young children by giving large doses of vitamin A twice a year.[2] Children can be given 200,000 International Units of retinyl palmitate dissolved in corn oil twice a year by the oral route without producing toxic effects. Several months' supply of vitamin A can be taken up from this dose and stored in the liver. If the children have adequate amounts of protein in the diet, they can use the stored vitamin A as needed by the eyes and other tissues.

Surveys have been done in many countries to try to ascertain just how widespread is the problem of vitamin A deficiency.[3] Malnutrition, vitamin A deficiency, and xerophthalmia are often found together in poor regions of less-developed countries. Giving large doses of vitamin A in the early stages rescues the eyes but only works over the long term if there is enough protein in the diet to make the necessary, specific retinol-binding protein that transports the vitamin A out of the liver and into the circulation.

Babies come into the world with very little vitamin A stored in the liver. This is why xerophthalmia is seen most often in young children who have not built up a reserve supply of the vitamin. In many cultures where nutrition information has been lacking, it has been widely thought that green vegetables and fruits are difficult to digest, and these foods are not given to small children or to sickly older people in the belief that they would cause illness or aggravate existing conditions. Yet these less healthy people are the ones who have the greatest need for the vitamins and other nutrients in vegetables.

Malnourished children are especially susceptible to exacerbation of their hypovitaminosis A when they become ill. Diarrhea (common in regions with poor sanitation) can interfere with absorption of vitamins from food, and infectious diseases that produce fever cause the tissues to take up vitamins from the circulation at an increased rate. The result is worsening of the eye condition. This is noticed especially as an aftermath of measles, which has inflammation of the cornea as one of the symptoms. Measles is an especially serious disease in some parts of the world, causing eye disease and death in children, even in areas where the population is not generally deficient in vitamin A. Children admitted to the hospital with severe measles benefited from large doses of vitamin A when this was tested in Tanzania. This is one of the countries in East Africa where measles is an especially virulent disease in small children, and measles is the cause of most cases of childhood blindness. Those children in the hospital who received the vitamin A treatment had only half the mortality rate due to measles or complications as did the cases who were not treated with the vitamin.[1] As a result of this work by Dr. Alfred Sommer and his colleagues during the 1980s, the World Health Organization and UNICEF now recommend that a large dose of vitamin A be given routinely to children who live in vitamin A-deficient communities when they come down with measles.

Doctors in South Africa have also demonstrated the dramatic effects of a high dose of vitamin A in small children who were hospitalized with measles.[4] Children who were given the vitamin A treatment recovered from pneumonia, diarrhea, and croup in less time than untreated children, and only half as many died. In this population, vitamin A deficiency is rare; so it seems that the sudden requirement by the tissues for extra vitamin A in children with severe measles cannot be met properly by the child's normal stores of vitamin A. In any event, the vitamin A treatment provided great improvement.

High mortality rate in young children is a major public health problem for the less-developed countries. A lack of vitamin A seems to be associated with lowered resistance to infectious diseases common in children such as diarrhea and lower respiratory infections. Trials have been carried out in several countries which showed that giving vitamin A supplements to deficient children resulted in less illness. Reduced rates of lower respiratory infections were seen in Australian children (who were well-nourished except for their vitamin A deficiency), and reduced rates of respiratory disease and diarrhea were seen in children in Thailand.

In controlled intervention trials in Indonesia, mortality rates in preschool-age children were one-third less in villages that were supplied with vitamin A compared to villages where the vitamin was not given out. This was a conclusion from a large project to find out whether giving extra vitamin A to children in areas where mild vitamin A deficiency exists would improve the statistics on childhood disease and death. An area at the northern end of the island of Sumatra in Indonesia, where xerophthalmia is common, was studied by a group from Johns Hopkins University, the government of Indonesia, and Helen Keller International. Two medical teams visited 450 villages to examine all children under six years of age, except infants. In half the villages, volunteers then gave out a large dose of vitamin A (and made sure the child swallowed it) and returned about six months later to give a second dose. In the other half of the villages, vitamin A was not given until after the end of the study a year later (unless a child was seen to have active xerophthalmia at the initial examination—these children were given vitamin A immediately and were excluded from the rest of the study).

The medical teams returned a year later to do a second examination of all the children. They found four times as many cases of active xerophthalmia in villages that had not received the vitamin A doses as they found in the vitamin A-treated villages, and there were 50% more deaths in children in the untreated villages during the elapsed year. The differences between the two sets of villages would have been even greater if all the children in the treatment villages had been dosed, as planned, but ten to twenty per cent of the twelve thousand children escaped from the treatment. (Try to imagine rounding up twelve thousand one-to-six year-olds and having them hold still to take their medicine.)

The prevalence of xerophthalmia in Indonesia has been declining due to government efforts in education and in provision of vitamin A supplements or fortified foods to the population, but further efforts are needed to wipe out this disastrous disease. The intervention trials of the type done in Indonesia and Tanzania serve to prove the benefits of providing vitamin A to deficient children and encourage governments to increase their efforts to overcome this deficiency.

There are several possible ways to improve the dilemma of children in poor regions who are deficient in vitamin A. The best solution to the problem is the educational approach, where the necessity of including green leafy vegetables and carotene-containing fruits in the diet is emphasized to the point where it becomes a normal part of the traditional diet. However, this is a slow method. A faster method that has been tried and found to produce good results is fortification of a commonly used food item with vitamin A. In the Philippines and in Indonesia, addition of vitamin A to monosodium glutamate has been found to be an efficient, cheap way to provide vitamin A to most of the population in the areas where this has been tested. The MSG is produced and packaged in only a few factories in these countries and is used by practically the whole population, rich and poor.[5] So, strategies for aiding the malnourished children who are so susceptible to serious diseases in third world countries have been thought out, tested, and found to be effective, but a great deal of government effort is still required to see to it that these programs are implemented wherever they are needed.

There are several reasons why vitamin A helps improve disease resistance in children. Experiments in animals and in humans show that vitamin A helps the functioning of the immune system, and the important vitamin A effect of maintaining normal, healthy epithelial linings of the respiratory tract probably helps to reduce the severity and frequency of respiratory diseases.

In humans the first signs of vitamin A deficiency, besides night blindness, are changes in the epithelial tissues. Internal epithelial structures in glands, ducts, and mucous membranes lose their normal appearance and functions and become atrophied, stratified, and keratinized. Keratin is a type of protein that can be easily identified in microscopic examinations by means of staining with a dye. Keratin formation is normal for the outer layer of the skin, the nails, and the hair, but is not normal for epithelial tissues in the internal organs.

In severe vitamin A deficiency in animals, the basal cells of the epithelial tissues in glands, ducts, and mucous membranes respond to the deficiency by proliferating, but the new cells are deficient in normal functions such as secretory activity and pile up in layers of excess cells that are sloughed off into the ducts of the lungs and trachea, parts of the kidney, the conjunctiva, the nasal sinuses, and ducts of the pancreas. In the kidney, the deterioration of the mucosal linings produces conditions that make infections and calcium phosphate stone formation more common. In glandular organs, in the lungs, and at the base of the tongue cysts form filled with yellow, cheesy masses of keratinized cells. In the lining of the gastrointestinal tract there are fewer of the mucus-secreting cells and less mucus to protect the GI tract from abrasion and contact with toxins. In animals there are changes in the bone marrow.

In experimental animals, these changes in the epithelial tissues of the body that develop from a vitamin A-deficient diet are reversible. When vitamin A is supplied, the layers of excess keratinized cells that clogged the ducts are sloughed off or disintegrate, and normal functions are restored. Scientists have known about the changes in epithelial tissues that accompany vitamin A deficiency since the 1920s, but they still do not understand in detail why so many normal tissues convert to stratified, keratinized tissues from lack of vitamin A.

The failure of proliferating A-deficient epithelial tissues to produce cells with the expected normal functions is called a failure of normal differentiation. In 1925, Wolbach and Howe, of Boston, described in great detail the effects of vitamin A deficiency on rats that were fed an artificial diet lacking vitamin A.[6] Young rats on an A-deficient diet stopped growing, developed bad posture and a rough coat, emaciation, the eye disease, and lost their stored fat. Many of the glands in the body became atrophied and cysts developed filled with keratinized cells. Wolbach and Howe summarized their extensive observations on the effects of "fat-soluble A" deficiency as being mainly an alteration of epithelial tissues, which began to proliferate but without producing normal epithelium. They described the main tissue change as being the substitution of normal epithelium by stratified keratinizing epithelium, arising by focal proliferation of basal cells from the original epithelium rather than by changes in preexisting cells, with some characteristics of augmented growth that suggested the acquisition of neoplastic properties.

A few years later Wolbach and Howe described how rats in this terrible condition could recover normal epithelial tissues by sloughing off the abnormally keratinized cells after vitamin A was restored to their diet.

McCollum had also seen his rats recover their normal appearance and growth and recover from the eye disease if the "fat-soluble A" was restored to their artificial diets soon enough. McCollum was a chemist, not a physician; so he was not knowledgeable in the techniques of microscopic examination of tissues and investigation of gross pathology at the beginning of his work with nutrition around 1910. His chief laboratory measurement was the failure of young rats to continue to gain weight when vitamin A was lacking in the diet. McCollum and his coworkers had noticed eye disease in their rats, but for several years they thought this was due to infection or irritation. Eventually he read further in the reports of the nineteenth century chemists who had experimented with artificial diets and found that they, too, had seen eye disease in small animals that were deficient in vitamins. The eye disease in people living on poor diets had been described in the nineteenth century also, as had been the night blindness condition.

A Japanese physician, M. Mori, published a report in 1904 describing the serious eye disease, xerophthalmia, in fourteen hundred small children. He said the disease was common in people who ate mostly rice, grains, and beans, but was not common in fishing villages. Mori discovered that he could cure the eye disease in the children by giving them cod liver oil (a good source of vitamin A), chicken livers, or eel fat. He thought the eye disease was caused by dietary deficiency of fat.

In Denmark during the First World War, xerophthalmia afflicted malnourished children, usually those who were already sick with measles, scarlet fever, or diarrhea. Dr. C.E. Bloch, a professor of pediatrics, studied the problem and he also thought it was due to a deficiency of fat in the diet. Poor people were living on skim milk, potatoes and bread, and never got eggs, butter or whole milk. Even those who lived in the country drank skim milk, unless they owned a cow, because the whole milk and the milk fat were being sent to the dairies and only skim milk remained cheap. (In the United States today skim milk and low-fat milk have vitamin A added to replace the natural vitamin A removed when fat is removed from the milk, but in Denmark years ago the skim milk did not contain vitamin A.) In 1917, Dr. Bloch discovered that giving cod liver oil cured the eye disease in children. He gave them two teaspoonsful of cod liver oil twice a day (which they relished) and in a week the eyes looked better. Bloch did not learn of McCollum's discovery of "fat-soluble A" until a couple of years later, after the War, but McCollum did read about Dr. Bloch's work with the malnourished children who had eye disease.

McCollum was always one to keep abreast of the scientific literature. When he read about Mori and Bloch using cod liver oil to cure the serious eye disease, xerophthalmia, he realized this was the same disease he had been observing in the rats that were deprived of the substance, "fat-soluble A." In the rats, the disease was definitely caused by deficiency of the specific substance, "fat-soluble A," that was present in egg yolk, butterfat, and cod liver oil, and was not caused by deficiency of total fat in the diet. Rats could develop deficiency symptoms even if they had plenty of fat; for instance, A-deficient diets that included lard or vegetable oil, which lack vitamin A, could cause the eye disease. McCollum published his conclusions about xerophthalmia in children being caused by a dietary deficiency of "fat-soluble A" in 1917.[7] McCollum's efforts to understand all the relations between dietary variables and deficiency diseases were sometimes temporarily off the mark, but eventually his research efforts led to greater understanding.

The devastating eye disease that has caused so much misery and blindness in children around the world occurs in those whose diets are extremely low in vitamin A. When an infectious disease puts extra demands for nutrients on the metabolic system of an undernourished child who has no liver stores of vitamin A, the eyes deteriorate rather quickly due to the near total absence of vitamin A in the circulation. Some of the studies on children showed that the eyes could be improved by giving small amounts of whole milk, which contains natural vitamin A in both of its forms, retinol and beta-carotene. As long as small amounts of vitamin A are included in the diet, and major infectious diseases are avoided, there are no cases of blindness due to xerophthalmia.

In better-nourished populations, like we have in the United States, the blinding eye disease is extremely rare. But milder forms of eye disease such as night blindness and dryness of the conjunctiva are common in people who do not have much vitamin A in their diets. A government nutrition survey in 1971 found that children of American migrant farm workers commonly had eye symptoms caused by vitamin A deficiency. These were physical changes that could be seen by a physician upon inspection of the eyes, not night blindness.

In the early 1970s, scientists from the University of Iowa and the U.S. Army Medical Research and Nutrition Laboratory collaborated on a study using eight healthy adult volunteers who agreed to live on a vitamin A-deficient diet in a hospital metabolic ward.[8] The scientists wanted to observe their symptoms as the stored vitamin A in the liver was used up, and then calculate the amount of vitamin A needed to restore the level in the circulation to normal at the end of the experiment. Deficiency symptoms appeared in the volunteers after their vitamin A stores were reduced. One of the symptoms was a bumpy skin condition called follicular hyperkeratosis. Small raised, solid bumps developed at the hair follicles due to hypertrophy of the outer layer of the skin. Other symptoms that developed were changes in the senses of smell, taste and hearing, and changes in the cerebrospinal fluid pressure. Of course, impairment in dark adaptation also developed in the volunteers as they became depleted of vitamin A.

The night blindness condition is not unusual in the United States, at least in its milder forms, and occurs most often in younger people. Young people who have not paid much attention to their diets and who have not built up a reserve supply of vitamin A in the liver can have some deficiency symptoms.

Dr. Harold Jeghers studied night blindness in medical students at Boston University in 1937. The entire freshman class and some of the upperclass students (except for a few who had taken vitamin supplements) were tested for their ability to use their rod cells for twilight vision after going from bright light to near darkness.[9] A photometer that had been designed for the purpose of testing for the ability to see in low light levels was employed for the test.

About 35% of those tested had low scores in the test. Many of these fifty-five students already knew they had problems seeing at night, but never knew what to do about it. They complained about difficulties with driving a car at night, recognizing friends on the street at night, or trying to play golf at dusk. Another common symptom was difficulty in adjusting to bright light outdoors, or suffering from temporary blindness while driving at night from the glare of oncoming headlights.

One poor fellow had developed severe night blindness as a college student. After having an accident at night, he had his eyes examined, but nothing was found to be wrong. After another accident in which he injured a pedestrian, he gave up driving at night and had his eyes examined two more times. After dark he could barely see the edge of the road, signs or pedestrians, and upon entering a darkened theater, he could not walk down the aisle alone for ten or fifteen minutes. His general health was fair, except for dry skin, enlarged hair follicles (follicular hyperkeratosis), some dryness of the conjunctivae which caused him to complain of burning of the eyes, and inflammation of the eyelids. His diet was the explanation. Jeghers had done elaborate dietary interviews with the students—they participated in the testing and interviews as an educational exercise in biochemistry and physiology. This student had lived away from home for seven years and had adopted a poor diet simply out of habit. For breakfast he had black coffee and doughnuts. For lunch he had two sandwiches, coffee, and dessert. Dinner was meat, white potatoes, white bread, one pat of butter, one vegetable, coffee and dessert. The vegetable was either green beans, lima beans, beets, peas or corn—all are very low in vitamin A. His vitamin A intake was calculated to be only one-fifth the level that is now recommended. For years he had not eaten any fruit, spinach, carrots, liver, milk, ice cream or cheese.

When Jeghers compared the fifty students who had the worst photometer scores with the fifty who had the best scores, he found striking differences in their eating habits and their vitamin A intakes. Those on the bottom averaged only half as much vitamin A in their diets as the top group. The top group had more students who lived and ate with their families; those on the bottom were more likely to be eating in restaurants or cooking for themselves. Those in the top group all ate at least two well-balanced, complete meals every day, in contrast to the low group where 60% ate only one complete meal a day. (Coffee and doughnuts or a sandwich and soda were considered to be not complete meals.) There was no difference in the frequency of head colds in the two groups, but the low group reported that their colds lasted longer and they reported having had more serious infectious diseases that kept them home in bed for more days during the previous year. Skin problems due to vitamin A deficiency occurred in the low group, but this was not as common as the night blindness.

The students with the low scores in the dark adaptation test were given vitamin A supplements and then were retested. All of those who suffered from night blindness were cured of this condition. Jeghers experimented with different dosages and generally gave large doses for two weeks followed by more moderate doses. The cures required from one week to five months. The student with the bad case of night blindness saw an improvement in his handicap after ten days of vitamin A supplements and tested normal in the dark adaptation test after he had included vitamin A supplements, milk, butter, and fresh fruits and vegetables in his diet for two months.

Jeghers was very concerned that the rather high percentage of the students who had night blindness might be representative of the general population. Other small studies on dark adaptation had also found impairment to be rather common. The difficulties of people with this condition driving on unlighted roads at night are just one of the potentially serious consequences of low vitamin A intake in the diet.

Chapter 8

Metabolism and Toxicity of Vitamin A

A deficiency of vitamin A leads to eye disease, but vitamin A must surely have beneficial effects for the whole of the animal body, not only for the eyes. McCollum's rats developed eye disease if they were on rations that lacked vitamin A, it's true, but the eye disease did not cause their death. The rats succumbed to a mysterious general failure that involved slowed weight gain in the half-grown rats, followed by some weight loss and then sudden death. They sometimes developed lung infections, but not always. Mature rats stopped producing any offspring.

The failure to grow if vitamin A is lacking in the diet is only one of the many consequences of a deficiency of vitamin A. Animals that are deficient suffer from a decline in the number of secretory cells lining the intestine, suffer from thickened and scaly skin and from changes in the epithelial linings of the respiratory, urinary, and genital tracts. Bone development in growing animals is not normal. There is atrophy of the spleen and bone marrow with the development of anemia. Disturbances of the reproductive system occur in mature animals that become deficient in vitamin A.

Such a variety of effects from a lack of vitamin A tells us this is a nutrient that is involved in basic development of tissues throughout the body in ways that are fundamental to the health and functioning of the animal system. Just how much is really known about the details of the vitamin A story? How much information have the scientists gleaned from their continual quest for understanding of nature's ways? How does beta-carotene pass through the complicated system of absorption and conversion mechanisms in the body? What happens to the conversion product, retinol, that is the linchpin in our precious eyesight, as it is transported to the retina of the eye and to all other parts of the body? Where else is the retinol used, and are there any clues in the scheme of transport and conversion mechanisms and cellular functions that might explain why carotene in the diet is associated with lower incidence of carcinomas, according to so many of the epidemiological studies that have been done in recent years?

Retinol from animal foods such as milk and eggs and beta-carotene from fruits and vegetables have identical effects for preventing and curing the known deficiency symptoms in animals, except for the remarkable association of beta-carotene in the diet with lower rates of many types of carcinomas. Why is it that beta-carotene is so often associated with less cancer but retinol is not? What could be so special about beta-carotene? Rather, is there truly anything at all special about beta-carotene in comparison with retinol, or is the apparent beta-carotene effect on cancer incidence merely a coincidence, with some other vegetable ingredients having the true cancer-preventing properties? As carotene from fruits and vegetables passes into the bloodstream by way of the lymph circulation, partly in the form of carotene and partly converted to retinol; as it is deposited in fat cells as carotene or stored in the liver as an ester of retinol; as retinol is metered out from the liver in regulated quantities and taken up by the retina of the eye or by other tissues; as retinol is used by the cells for their own purposes and then is converted to metabolites, some of them water-soluble, and used again or excreted, does the vitamin A have any functions that could explain its apparent role in preventing cancer?

In this chapter I will describe how beta-carotene is converted into other necessary chemicals in the animal body, and how they are stored and passed through the metabolic system. I will also explain the important cautions against the consumption of excessive amounts of vitamin A from animal foods or supplements, especially during pregnancy, and why there are no such cautions needed against consuming beta-carotene in fruits and vegetables. The popular suggestion that beta-carotene might function through an antioxidant mechanism will be discussed later, in chapter 14.

During the 1930s, '40s, and '50s, scientists studied the chemistry of vitamin A and its precursors, the carotenoids, and learned how to isolate, purify, and measure the quantities of vitamin A-related chemicals in plant and animal tissues. Chemists devised methods for making synthetic vitamin A and synthetic beta-carotene. Biochemists learned how the carotenoids such as beta-carotene are synthesized by plants starting with two-carbon fragments from sugar metabolism. George Wald at Harvard University studied the chemistry of vision for many years and discovered that a form of vitamin A is involved in the capture of photons of light by rhodopsin in the rod cells of the retina.[1] Physiologists studied the symptoms of vitamin A deficiency and vitamin A overdose in humans and in animals.

By the late 1930s it was known that both carotene and vitamin A are absorbed from the digestive tract into the lymphatic system, but to different degrees. Preformed vitamin A (retinyl ester) is well absorbed, but carotene absorption is incomplete when large amounts of it are ingested, especially if the meal is low in fat. It was also known that the liver could store enough vitamin A to last many weeks should the dietary supply be cut off.

At this time scientists thought that the conversion of carotene into retinol took place in the liver. This had been suggested by Thomas Moore in 1931 when he proved that animals convert carotene into vitamin A. Animals had been fed large amounts of carotene, and vitamin A (retinol) was found deposited in the liver; so it was natural to assume that the liver was the site of the conversion.

The liver was known to be the site of many kinds of enzymatic reactions in metabolism, but it was not the site of the carotene conversion into retinol. During the 1930s and until 1946, many researchers assumed it was and attempted to study the carotene-converting enzyme by incubating carotene solutions with liver slices from many kinds of experimental animals, but no substantial amounts of vitamin A could be detected in these experiments.[2] Another puzzle was the wide differences among different animal species as to the amount of carotene present in their livers or circulating in the blood. In a study of sixty different species of animals, two Danish researchers, H.B. Jensen and T.K. With, found many species where carotene could not be detected in blood or liver. Many groups of scientists found that carotene could not cure the symptoms of vitamin A deficiency if the carotene was injected, although injections of vitamin A could cure the symptoms quite well. For several years the answer to these puzzles about carotene conversion eluded the scientists.

Harry J. Deuel, Jr., a biochemist at the University of Southern California, was studying carotene absorption and the levels of carotene in cows' milk and hens' eggs in the early 1940s. He, too, assumed that carotene was converted into retinol in the liver. In studies designed to find out more about the liver's capacity for converting carotene, he and his students decided to compare the fate in animals of injected carotene with the fate of orally fed carotene.

For the experiments they used rats fed or injected with carotene that had been solubilized in blood plasma, cottonseed oil, or a lecithin-glycol solution. Carotene is not at all soluble in water, being a hydrocarbon; so special methods must be used to put it into solution.

When rats were injected with carotene and sacrificed twenty-four hours later, carotene was found in the liver according to how much had been injected, but no retinol was found. In contrast, when carotene was fed orally, there was no carotene deposited in the liver, but retinol was found instead.

Deuel and his associates did extensive analyses to check the accuracy and validity of their experiments. They showed, as several other groups had also shown without understanding the meaning, that injected carotene could not cure the symptoms of vitamin A deficiency in rats that had been on vitamin A-deficient rations. When they reported on their studies in 1946, they explained their results as being consistent with a new idea, namely, that carotene is converted into retinol before it reaches the liver and before it even reaches the bloodstream, possibly in the intestinal wall.[3] Their further experiments in the following years and studies in several laboratories in England where vitamin A metabolism was under study proved this conclusion to be correct.

The reason there was great variation in animals as to the amount of carotene that circulates in the bloodstream was due to different abilities to absorb unconverted carotene from the intestinal tract in different species. The reason that injected carotene could not cure symptoms of vitamin A deficiency was that the injected material did not have the chance to be converted to retinol in the cells of the small intestine.

Additional details about the animals' method of converting carotene to retinol became known from enzyme studies by two medical laboratories in 1965. James A. Olson and DeWitt S. Goodman studied the carotene-converting activity of partly purified enzyme from rat liver and from the mucosal cells lining the small intestine. They both showed that the conversion is accomplished by an enzyme in the cytoplasm of cells.[4] The enzyme uses molecular oxygen to split a beta-carotene molecule in the middle and produces retinaldehyde, a form of vitamin A closely related to the form used for vision. Using their test tube method for studying the enzyme, chemists could now find out which of the carotenoids from plants can be converted into vitamin A by animals.

The green plants synthesize more than five hundred different carotenoids. These pigments usually contain forty carbon atoms and a system of conjugated double bonds that is responsible for their strong yellow and orange-red color; some of the carotenoids also contain oxygen atoms and are called xanthophylls. The carotenoids are present in all higher plants and in algae and some fungi. They serve several useful purposes in the plants, from providing color in flowers to serving an essential role in photosynthesis. The carotenoids contribute the yellow and orange coloration in flowers and fruits and vegetables, and also the orange color of the goldfish and some other animals. (Another class of pigments, called anthocyanins, is responsible for the pinks, reds, and purples of the flowers.) Plants also use carotenoids as the starting material to make some additional chemicals useful for their own survival. An example is sporopollenin, the degradation-resistant, probably cross-linked polymer in the walls of pollen grains that is made from carotenoids. Another chemical made from carotenoids is abscisic acid, the plant hormone that regulates dormancy and leaf drop.

The animals have taken advantage of the plants' ability to synthesize these complicated molecules and have converted some carotenoids to their own purpose—a purpose never dreamt of by the plant that manufactured the carotenoid. Thus, the members of the animal kingdom, most of which must be able to see to locate their food, have adopted as the linchpin of their visual apparatus a chemical ubiquitous in the plant kingdom, plentiful in plants that are useful as food, from the algae of the streams and seas to the green leaves of the eucalyptus tree.

Only about fifty of the five hundred known carotenoids are useful to the animal system, because of the strict requirements for the molecular structure needed for the visual process. Beta-carotene is the most important carotenoid for human nutrition because its chemical structure is such that it can be split in the middle to yield two identical molecules of retinaldehyde. We can produce more retinaldehyde from beta-carotene than we can from other carotenoids such as alpha-carotene or cryptoxanthin, both of which can be split in the middle but yield only one molecule of retinaldehyde. (The other half of these carotenoids has a slightly different structure which destroys its usefulness for vision.) Most of the five hundred or so carotenoids in nature have small variations in their chemical structure which make them of no use for the visual process in animals.

Beta-carotene is an essential molecule in photosynthesis in green plants. During photosynthesis plants use energy from the sun to convert carbon dioxide from the atmosphere and water from the soil into sugars. A by-product is gaseous oxygen, which is released to the environment. Carotene has two important functions in photosynthesis. The first is as an absorber of sunlight. Carotene or similar carotenoids absorb photons of light and efficiently transfer the sun energy to chlorophyll, which is also an absorber but not at the same wavelength. The chloroplasts in the cells of green leaves contain the chlorophyll and carotenoids, and also contain quinones, alpha-tocopherol (vitamin E), vitamin K, and several kinds of lipids. In the chloroplasts a complicated series of reactions converts sunlight into electrochemical energy which is used to split water and to synthesize chemicals needed by the plant to produce carbohydrates from the carbon of carbon dioxide and from part of the oxygen in carbon dioxide. During the complicated process of splitting apart water molecules, a strong oxidant is produced which could damage the plant cells. This is where carotene finds its second vital function in photosynthesis. The strong oxidant is deactivated by carotene to eliminate potential toxic effects. We should probably assume that many of the other carotenoids in plants have functions that are entirely similar to the functions of beta-carotene.

The animals' use of beta-carotene begins with the enzymatic splitting of the molecule in half. Carotene in the diet of an animal was shown to be converted into retinaldehyde in the wall of the small intestine. Other enzymes in the same cells lining the small intestine can make further conversion products from the retinaldehyde.[5,6] The retinaldehyde can be converted into retinol and then esterified to form the retinyl esters that circulate in the lymph and bloodstream before reaching their destination, the liver. Or the retinaldehyde can be converted to retinoic acid. The retinyl esters and some absorbed but unconverted beta-carotene pass through the intestinal cells where they are packaged in chylomicrons along with all the other fatty nutrients absorbed from the diet, to be transported first by the lymph and then by the general circulation.

The retinyl esters are taken up by the liver within a few hours, and the carotene and any other carotenoids that were absorbed are stored in many different tissues, including fat cells, the skin and liver, and glands. It is fortunate that the retinyl esters are removed from the circulation and stored in the liver because the retinyl esters are the form of vitamin A that is toxic in high doses.

Before I go on with the explanation of how retinyl esters are stored in the liver, this would be a good place to digress to relate some research on retinoic acid, a natural anticancer compound. I mentioned above that retinaldehyde can be converted into retinol or into retinoic acid in the wall of the small intestine. The whole story is not yet known, but the ability of carotene to produce retinoic acid might turn out to be the explanation for the apparent association of dietary carotene with lower rates of cancer.

When vitamin A-containing foods of animal origin (milk, eggs, liver, cod liver oil, and also vitamin supplements) are consumed, the vitamin A, which is in the form of retinol and retinyl esters, is easily absorbed by the small intestine and is efficiently repackaged into chylomicrons for shipment to the liver storage site.

Beta-carotene from fruits and vegetables takes a longer route to formation of retinyl esters and there is a fork in the road. Beta-carotene is first split by the converting enzyme in the wall of the intestine, as discussed above, to produce retinaldehyde. Retinaldehyde can then be converted to retinol and retinyl ester for shipment to the liver, or the retinaldehyde can take the other fork in the road and be oxidized enzymatically to retinoic acid.

The two routes can be shown diagrammatically.

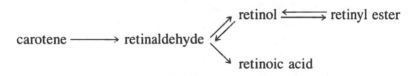

An arrow in the diagram denotes an enzymatic conversion.

The importance of all this is that retinoic acid is a normal form of vitamin A found in the tissues and circulation, and it is one of the most potent anticancer compounds known in laboratory studies of cancer cells growing in culture. Many drugs (chemotherapy) can stop tumor cells from dividing, but retinoic acid does this in laboratory experiments and goes one step further, causing differentiation of many tumor cells, meaning an alteration from uncontrolled proliferation to the acquisition of normal cell characteristics.

The cancer-preventing and reversing effects of retinoic acid that are seen in laboratory studies were first observed in 1971 by Werner Bollag at Hoffmann-LaRoche Co. in Switzerland. Because high doses of retinoic acid are toxic, synthetic chemicals related to retinoic acid are being much studied as potential anticancer agents in human patients.

It is known that the lining of the intestine has an efficient system for absorbing vitamin A from animal foods and then shipping the retinyl esters off to the liver. This system might make it unlikely that the vitamin A from animal foods remains long enough in the intestinal cells to be much converted to retinoic acid. There is a possibility that beta-carotene absorbed from foods is a more important source of retinoic acid in the circulation than is retinol. (Retinoic acid is also produced within the cells of various tissues. This retinoic acid is made from retinol that has been delivered to the cells from the liver storage site.)

The natural production of retinoic acid from carotene and from retinol has been known since the early 1960s.[7] Two Dutch chemists, J.F. Arens and D.A. van Dorp, made some synthetic retinoic acid in 1946, before retinoic acid had been found in animals, and demonstrated that it had potent vitamin A activity when fed to rats. In 1949 and in following years, retinoic acid was retested in animals by several groups of scientists and was shown to have most of the curative powers of vitamin A in animals that had deficiency symptoms. (However, the retinoic acid did not function in the retina of the eye or in the reproductive system.) In 1961 the biosynthesis of natural retinoic acid from retinaldehyde was detected in the intestinal wall of animals by biochemists in Russia and at the NIH. Other biochemists began to study the production of retinoic acid from retinaldehyde. They soon found out that retinoic acid could be made in other animal tissues besides the intestine, that its formation is an irreversible enzymatic conversion, and that it has considerable vitamin A activity when given to deficient animals. They also found that retinoic acid could be made from retinol by way of retinaldehyde as intermediate, as can be seen in the diagram. The idea began to evolve that retinoic acid might be the active form of vitamin A in many tissues. This idea had been first suggested cautiously by Thomas Moore in 1951 at a symposium on nutrition honoring Elmer McCollum. At the time, retinoic acid was known to be functional when given to animals but was not known to be synthesized by animals. The idea remains today a completely viable hypothesis. The active form of vitamin A and the function of vitamin A at the cellular level remain uncertain, other than for the vitamin function in the retina. The problem is that there seems to be more than one fundamental active form and function for vitamin A at the cellular level. In the general scheme that is envisioned, vitamin A (retinol) is delivered to the tissues from the storage site in the liver and many tissues convert the retinol to retinoic acid if need be for use by the cells.

In 1967, F.D. Crain and associates demonstrated that the rat can produce retinoic acid from carotene as starting material in the wall of the intestine.[8] (The earlier work had used retinaldehyde as starting material.) And they made an enzyme preparation from the cells that could produce retinoic acid from carotene. The major products of dietary carotene were already known to be retinol and retinyl ester, and now another product was detected from the retinaldehyde that had taken the other fork in the road. So dietary carotene can be converted in the intestine to two forms of vitamin A: a larger amount of retinol and a smaller amount of retinoic acid.

A small amount of retinoic acid is found in normal human serum and a small amount is found in the tissues. A great deal of research has been done on the metabolism of retinoic acid since its discovery as a normal form of vitamin A. Much of the research has been directed at finding out what happens chemically to retinoic acid in the body and whether any conversion products have much vitamin A activity.[7] Retinoic acid is rapidly converted to several types of water-soluble derivatives which can be excreted in urine or bile, but none of these derivatives has been proven to have an indispensable function in the tissues. The derivatives are most likely one of the body's methods for excreting vitamin A after it has served its purpose in the body.

Much of the early research work on retinoic acid—its production from vitamin A (retinol), its biological activity, and its conversion in animals to a variety of metabolites—was carried out in the laboratory of Hector F. DeLuca at the University of Wisconsin. During the 1960s and 1970s, biochemists there proved that retinol could be converted *in vivo* to retinoic acid.[9] In order to study this conversion they were forced to use the most sensitive analytical techniques that were then available because retinoic acid is present in only minuscule amounts at any one time in animal tissues. DeLuca's laboratory produced many new procedures for the study of metabolism of the fat-soluble vitamins during these years, and many new scientists—diligent biochemists, some of whom have continued to work on various aspects of vitamin A research during recent decades.

Research on retinoic acid has been stepped up in the last few years as laboratory methods for analyzing small amounts of physiological products have become more sensitive and also because drugs that are related to retinoic acid have been studied for possible use in preventing recurrences of skin cancer and for treatment of skin diseases.

Joseph L. Napoli at the State University of New York at Buffalo has reopened the study of retinoic acid production in animal tissues because of the apparent anticancer effects of carotene in the diet. His recent studies have shown that several animal tissues other than intestine can convert carotene into both retinol and retinoic acid.[10] At low concentrations of carotene, the two products were made in equal amounts. Napoli raises the question of whether carotene in the diet might produce a slightly higher level of retinoic acid in the tissues, which might account for the lower risk of cancer in people whose diets are high in carotene.

Whether or not this is the explanation remains to be seen. Until recently, scientists did not know whether carotene that is stored in human fat cells and other tissues had any function at all in these tissues. A few older studies on animals (not humans) had shown that carotene can be converted into retinaldehyde in tissues other than the wall of the small intestine.[6] In 1991, a study at Tufts University in Boston showed that beta-carotene can indeed be converted to other forms of vitamin A in human adipose tissue as well as in the small intestine.[11] The products of the beta-carotene conversion included retinoic acid, the form of vitamin A that has powerful anticancer effects in animal and cell studies. Other human tissues were not tested because the reason for the study was a question about the mechanism of carotene conversion.

If it is shown in future studies that beta-carotene is a better source of retinoic acid in man than preformed vitamin A is, either in the intestinal mucosa or in some other tissues, this might explain why dietary carotene from fruits and vegetables is so often associated with lower rates of cancer in epidemiological studies while dietary retinyl ester from animal foods or vitamin supplements usually is not. If it is shown in future studies that beta-carotene stored in various tissues can be converted to retinoic acid, this might explain how beta-carotene could have a cancer-inhibiting effect independent of the level of circulating retinol in the bloodstream.

The interesting questions surrounding the possible functions of beta-carotene in the body are producing new research work and new speculations. But a real-life problem associated with vitamin A intake remains to be discussed and that is the problem of toxicity from overdoses of retinyl ester.

The retinyl esters that are transported out from the small intestine are packaged into fat-filled, protein-coated droplets called chylomicrons while they are still in the cells of the intestine. The droplets are transferred to the lymphatic system, and soon enter the blood circulation. (Many of the details surrounding the route taken by newly absorbed vitamin A were figured out during the 1960s using radiolabeled versions of the vitamin.)

When the chylomicrons reach the liver, the retinyl esters are taken out and transferred to liver cells and the esters are hydrolyzed to produce retinol. The retinol can either be put in storage in the liver (after re-esterification) or be shipped out to the tissues complexed with a specific protein (retinol-binding protein) that is made within the liver.[6]

The complex between retinol-binding protein and retinol is the package that is used by the liver to send vitamin A (retinol) to the eyes, mucous membranes, skin, reproductive organs, growing bones in the young, and all the other tissues that require vitamin A. Retinol cannot leave the liver storage site unless it is complexed with a molecule of the retinol-binding protein, and the amount of retinol-binding protein that is produced by the liver is kept within controlled limits. So, consuming large amounts of vitamin A, as from liver or vitamin supplements, does not help deliver much extra vitamin A in its useful form to the tissues. In fact, eating very large amounts of retinyl ester will cause toxicity if the liver storage space is already filled. (Beta-carotene from fruits and vegetables, on the other hand, never causes toxicity—see below.) The amount of dietary retinyl ester that can cause toxicity is about five times the RDA level, or higher, if this amount is consumed for some time. (The RDA is about 5000 IUs per day; intakes of 25,000 IUs per day have produced toxic effects in humans.) The tissue damage caused by high levels of vitamin A was discovered by Honor B. Fell at Cambridge University. She and her coworkers studied chick embryo tissues in the 1950s and 1960s.[12] They noticed that excess vitamin A caused the cells to release enzymes which broke down extracellular material, including cartilage, and the cells themselves were damaged. This was a definite toxic effect from high levels of vitamin A.

The vitamin A package from the liver, containing a molecule of retinol complexed with the small protein molecule called retinol-binding protein, travels by way of the bloodstream to the cells where it is needed.[13] The retinol-binding protein remains outside of the cells as retinol is taken up by the cells. After delivering vitamin A, part of the free retinol-binding protein is lost through the kidneys, so that more retinol-binding protein must be produced by the liver each day. The newly synthesized molecules of retinol-binding protein are then secreted from the liver already complexed with another retinol molecule from the liver storage site to deliver more vitamin A to the tissues. As long as vitamin A is complexed with retinol-binding protein in the circulation it is never toxic, but various forms of vitamin A (but not beta-carotene) can cause damage to tissues if they circulate at high levels without the normal retinol-binding protein accompaniment—in other words, if the vitamin A did not come from the liver storage site.[13] Situations where this potentially toxic condition could happen include chronic consumption of large amounts of vitamin A-rich foods (liver, cod liver oil, vitamin A supplements), or a single massive dose of one of these, or the medical use of drugs related to vitamin A to treat diseases.

In the case of chronic overconsumption of vitamin A, retinyl ester circulates without the protective benefits of retinol-binding protein. In the case of medical uses of retinoic acid or similar compounds, these forms of vitamin A circulate in combination with serum albumin rather than with retinol-binding protein.

In cases of chronic overdose of vitamin A, the storage capacity of the liver becomes filled, and retinyl esters can no longer be removed from the circulation as they normally are within a few hours of consuming a meal high in vitamin A. This produces toxicity from high levels of circulating retinyl esters, with possibly damaging results.

This possibility of toxic overdose is one of the major concerns of health professionals whenever the subject of vitamin supplements is brought up in popular books and magazines. However, it is easy to maintain completely safe intakes of vitamin-rich foods if you know which foods have the potential to cause overdose. The especially rich sources of preformed vitamin A (retinyl esters) that must be used in moderation are: liver (including beef liver, chicken liver, liverwurst, and braunschweiger), cod liver oil, and vitamin supplements. These are the vitamin A sources that are fine in their recommended amounts but which should not be overindulged in. The beta-carotene in fruits and vegetables has never caused toxicity in humans, probably due to our limited ability to absorb carotene and convert it to retinol; so there are no restrictions on using fruits and vegetables for their vitamins and minerals. The wonderful variety of beneficial nutrients we can obtain from fruits and vegetables, which includes carotene, vitamin C, folic acid, indoles, fiber, and minerals, makes the vegetable part of our diet the part we should continue to emphasize and enjoy, guilt-free and fearlessly.

The medical literature contains several hundred case reports of incidences of toxicity from overdose of vitamin A from liver or vitamin supplements. Overconsumption of halibut liver oil was the culprit in the earliest documented case of toxicity in a child, which happened in Baltimore in the late 1930s. Birth defects are another possible result of overdose of vitamin A. New drugs closely related to vitamin A are causing serious birth defects when a woman does not heed the warning against taking the drugs during pregnancy.

The most important advice that should be emphasized in any discussion of the dangers of overdoses of vitamin A is the warning against overindulging in vitamin A when pregnant, or even when considering pregnancy.[14] This warning does not apply to beta-carotene from fruits and vegetables, which has never caused birth defects.

Vitamin A is needed for proper development of the fetus in animals and in humans. The fetus obtains retinol (vitamin A) from the mother's circulation by a transfer mechanism across the placenta that is not completely understood.[15] In normal, good nutrition the amount of retinol that is passed to the fetus is kept within the proper limits by the normal control mechanisms for the level of retinol in the circulation, namely, the amount of retinol-binding protein circulating in the mother and also in the fetus.

Birth defects occur in animals if very high doses of vitamin A are given to the mother.[16] This was first demonstrated by Sidney Cohlan in 1954. Cohlan was studying the effects of vitamin A on bone development in rats when he noticed that birth defects resulted if he gave either a single large dose or several large doses of retinyl ester to pregnant rats.[17] The doses he used were many times larger than the dose required by the animals. Many more experiments on animals have also shown that birth defects result from high doses of vitamin A.[14]

It is always prudent when a woman is contemplating having a child to check with a doctor about what type of vitamin supplements, if any, should be taken. The World Health Organization considers that supplements of vitamin A are not needed during pregnancy if the mother has normal, good nutritional status. But many people do not get the RDA levels of all the necessary vitamins in their usual diet; so doctors these days usually recommend multivitamin supplements during pregnancy. The wise thing to do is to get specific medical instructions on the brands and dose that are acceptable. The doses of multivitamin supplements that are recommended during pregnancy are not mega-doses—the doses prescribed are practically the same as the RDA level. Another reason to get medical advice early is to take advantage of new epidemiological findings that show that the B vitamin, folic acid, may prevent a serious birth defect, spina bifida. Doctors think that to be effective for this purpose, folic acid in the diet or in supplements must be adequate during the first six weeks of pregnancy.[18]

Birth defects have occurred in humans as well as in animals from excessive doses of vitamin A. A woman in Stockholm was treated for acne with large doses of vitamin A. She was given 150,000 IUs of vitamin A daily (about thirty times more than the RDA) for only three weeks, but, unfortunately, she was pregnant at the same time. The baby was born with microcephaly and did not survive.[19] A new drug for severe acne, Accutane (TM), has also caused birth defects in cases where a woman neglected to heed the strong warning against becoming pregnant while taking the drug.[14] The drug is 13-cis-retinoic acid, which is now known to be present at a low level in normal human plasma; but when used as a drug, the dose taken is several hundred times higher than physiological levels of such compounds.

In the case of Accutane (TM), the minimum dose that can cause birth defects in animals has been determined, but in the case of vitamin A from vitamin supplements or cod liver oil, this information is not available. The only thing that can be stated with confidence is that women who are considering pregnancy should consult a physician and avoid supplements containing vitamin A in doses that are higher than the RDA. For drugs and for vitamins, as for all the useful chemicals in our foods and in our environment, it is the dose that makes the poison.

Birth defects have not been the only toxic outcome from overdoses of vitamin A. Overdoses have caused brief severe illnesses, chronic mysterious illnesses, and even a few deaths. Overdoses have occurred in situations where well-meaning but uninformed people have fed large amounts of the vitamin to children or to themselves in the mistaken belief that the vitamin could cure some disease if large amounts were taken.

The symptoms of toxic overdose from taking too much vitamin A in the foods mentioned above (liver, cod liver oil, vitamin A supplements) are: bulging of the "soft spots" in a baby's skull or headache in adults, nausea, vomiting, vertigo, visual disturbance, bone and joint pain.[15] Other symptoms are cracking of the lips, dry skin and deep peeling of the skin, intense itch without any eruption, and hair loss. (Retinoic acid causes the same toxic symptoms as vitamin A, but, of course, retinoic acid is used only in laboratory experiments or under medical supervision.)

In Seattle in 1980, twin baby girls aged seven months were admitted to the hospital with alarming symptoms. At least, their mother was undoubtedly alarmed, but the physicians quickly found out the diagnosis. Each of the infants had suddenly developed irritability, vomiting, and bulging of the "soft spot" on top of the head. Several dozen cases of vitamin A poisoning in children had already been reported in the medical literature. Most cases resulted from excessive dosing with vitamin supplements. The doctors considered the symptoms along with a blood test for vitamin A and the dietary history to make the diagnosis.[20]

The twins had been getting fruit and vegetables since two months of age and daily feeding of chicken liver since three months. Their mother prepared her own baby foods, and found it convenient to cook, puree, and freeze chicken liver for a nutritious meat dish. Chicken liver is one of the foods that is very rich in vitamin A (retinyl ester). The infants had been eating about four ounces a day of the liver, which gave them 3600 micrograms of vitamin A. Along with the vitamin A they were getting from milk and vitamin supplements, they were eating over ten times more vitamin A each day than their RDA, and this had been going on for four months.

The bulging of the "soft spot" disappeared two weeks after vitamin A-containing foods were stopped. Their other symptoms also disappeared within a few weeks and the twins had no aftereffects from their bout with poisoning. The bulging was caused by an increase in the cerebrospinal fluid pressure, which causes some of the symptoms associated with overdoses of vitamin A.

If you like liver, chicken livers, or liverwurst, how much of these foods could you eat before you would need to worry about overdose of vitamin A? The amount of vitamin A in these foods can be found in the U.S. Department of Agriculture tables of food composition (see chapter 11). Using these tables you can calculate that a quarter pound serving of beef liver contains enough vitamin A to last an adult female for fifteen days. The RDA for women is 800 RE; for men it is 1000 RE because of larger body size, so the vitamin in a quarter pound serving of liver is thought to be used up faster by men. If an adult were to eat a quarter pound of beef liver every three days (five times more frequently than the vitamin A could be used up) on a regular basis, it might be possible to produce symptoms of vitamin A poisoning. Chicken liver and liverwurst contain a little less vitamin A than beef liver; so they would have to be eaten almost every day, in quarter pound servings, to cause overdose.

A more common cause of vitamin A poisoning than liver is vitamin supplements. Vitamin supplements are freely available in drugstores and health food stores, and megadoses of vitamins have been recommended by some medical and some nonmedical practitioners for chronic ailments that are difficult or impossible to cure. If the ailment was a result of vitamin deficiency, then a temporary course of vitamin therapy would be called for. But megavitamins have been claimed to bring beneficial results on the basis of studies that were not properly controlled or designed, and the results of which are not to be trusted. Megavitamins can be dangerous, and the poisoning that results from overdoses of vitamin A is the most common example. We can tell the difference between vitamin supplements that are acceptable and those that are potentially dangerous by inspecting the fine print on the label. The label lists the dose in one capsule in terms of the RDA (Recommended Dietary Allowance). Daily doses of vitamins that are close to 100% of the RDA are never toxic for adults if only one capsule is taken each day. It is only after taking five or ten times this amount for some period of time that vitamin A (retinyl ester) becomes toxic.

In Connecticut, a four year-old boy was brought to the hospital with symptoms of vitamin A overdose. He had fever, irritability, cracked lips, enlarged liver, abnormal liver function tests, pain in the leg bones, and an abnormal bone scan. The doctors suspected vitamin A poisoning from part of his medical history, and a blood test for vitamin A confirmed this diagnosis.[21] The child suffered from minimal brain dysfunction (hyperactivity) and, apparently, a physician had suggested the megavitamins as a therapy. The boy's family had given him vitamin tablets, which he gobbled up like candy. He was kept in the hospital for four weeks, during which time the symptoms of vitamin A poisoning subsided.

Some of the most bizarre tales of vitamin A poisoning have come from the polar regions of the world where desperate situations and tragic outcomes are part of the human adventure of exploration and risk-taking. When European explorers ventured into the distant reaches of the Arctic and the Antarctic, they had to learn some of the things the Eskimos and the Samoyeds already knew about survival in frigid lands—they had to learn about the toxicity of polar bear liver, bearded seal liver, and husky dog liver. The liver of certain animals is so rich in vitamin A that it cannot be used as food by humans without immediate danger of poisoning.

Vitamin A poisoning caused the death of one explorer in Antarctica in 1913 and extreme illness in a companion. The two explorers were forced into the desperate situation of killing their sled dogs for food after they lost their food supply. The dogs were completely consumed by the survivors. The animals' livers being softer than other parts of the carcasses, these were consumed eagerly with disastrous results.[22] Sir Douglas Mawson and Dr. Xavier Mertz were Australian scientists on a surveying expedition in Antarctica. Thirty-three days into the trip, a fatal accident occurred as they neared their turn-around point. One of their two sleds had been loaded with most of the food in preparation for the return journey when it fell without a sound, along with a third man, Ninnis, into an eleven foot-wide crevasse, gone forever. Mawson had crossed the unseen crevasse safely while riding on his sled, but Ninnis, who was on foot next to the other sled, put more pressure on the snow lid and it gave way. Mawson and Mertz were left with one and a half weeks of man food, no dog food, six dogs, their cooker and kerosene. They decided the only thing to do was slaughter the remaining dogs as necessary on the return trip. Mawson made it back to base camp in fifty-four days but Mertz died from vitamin A poisoning after twenty-three days.

Mawson's diary and a book he wrote two years later described the terrible symptoms of acute vitamin A poisoning.[23] "The skin was peeling off our bodies and a very poor substitute remained which burst readily and rubbed raw in many places." Mawson used bandages to keep loosened skin in place on the bottoms of his feet. Mertz became sicker than Mawson from the vitamin A poisoning. Both men had definite symptoms of toxicity. We can only speculate as to why Mertz died and Mawson survived. This could have been due to individual variation in resistance or unequal consumption of liver. Mertz became weakened and sick with stomach pains, which lasted for a week. He then began having fits and became delirious, and died within the day. Mawson was also sick and weak and briefly considered giving up the struggle to return, but the habit of "plugging away" won out. He decided if he could not reach base camp, at least he would try "to reach some prominent point likely to catch the eye of a search party, where a cairn might be erected and our diaries cached."

Ten days after Mertz died, Mawson suffered another accident. While pulling the sled by a rope harness, he fell into a six foot-wide crevasse and, as he related, "found myself dangling fourteen feet below on end of rope in crevasse—sledge creeping to mouth—had time to say to myself, 'so this is the end,' expecting the sledge every moment to crash on my head and all to go to the unseen bottom . . . " The sled held fast at the top, stuck in the snow. With great effort, Mawson drew himself back up to the top, only to fall again to the full length of the rope when the edge gave way again. Tempted briefly to release the rope and end "all the pain and toil," he made another decision to postpone eternity and hauled himself out a second time. Two weeks later he reached base camp and found five men waiting. He had lost nearly half his weight, and suffered from boils and swollen legs and what he thought was a deranged mental condition. He recovered his health slowly during the next several months, and survived to old age.

In the Arctic regions, a common source of dangerous amounts of vitamin A has been polar bear liver. The toxic effects of eating polar bear liver became known to European explorers as early as the sixteenth century. In the sixteenth century, sailors from Norway, Holland, and England began exploring the Arctic Ocean in search of a Northeast Passage to China by way of a northern route past Scandinavia and Russia. Although they did not reach China, they managed to start up international trade in the fish, furs, and game resources of the coastal region of northwest Russia. The great Dutch navigator, Willem Barents, reached the northern part of the island of Novaya Zemlya off the northern coast of Russia in 1596 and spent the winter on shore. The crew suffered great hardships during the winter with two deaths and much illness. It has been reported that all those who ate bear liver became ill, some losing all their skin from head to foot.[24]

A group of nineteen men exploring Greenland in 1913 all became ill after killing a bear and preparing a stew that contained the liver. They developed severe headache, irritability and vomiting, and half the men suffered from peeling skin. Several other instances of similar illness during polar expeditions were reported in the nineteenth century.

In 1935, three young men fishing near the city of Adelaide on the south coast of Australia got sick from eating seal liver. They were admitted to the hospital with a variety of symptoms—headache, vomiting, convulsive seizure, abdominal pain, and peeling of the skin. At the time, poisoning from high doses of vitamin A was not yet recognized as a medical problem, so the correct diagnosis was not made. The victims suspected that their sickness might have been caused by the seal liver, and this information went down in the hospital records, to be remembered and discussed years later in an article by two Australian physicians on the history of acute vitamin A toxicity.[25]

In 1940, a Norwegian phsiologist, Kaare Rodahl, collected samples of polar bear liver and seal liver in Greenland with a view to identifying the toxic substance.[24] The samples were analyzed for vitamin A content in the laboratory of Thomas Moore at Cambridge University. Rodahl and Moore found a level of vitamin A in bear liver that was about 18,000 IUs per gram of wet sample, which is about fifty times more concentrated than beef liver. Feeding the bear liver to rats gave the same toxic symptoms as feeding high doses of vitamin A.[26]

These tales of toxicity, miserable symptoms and, occasionally, death explain why health professionals are so often opposed to the idea of people self-medicating themselves with vitamin supplements. They fear some people will overdo it. Only a few hundred cases are known where overdoses of vitamin A have caused symptoms, but the symptoms can be frightening and painful. The discomfort of losing large amounts of the outer layer of the skin seems to occur only in acute vitamin A poisoning, which can be caused by a single meal extremely high in vitamin A, such as a meal of bear liver or seal liver. The more common occurrence of poisoning from chronic ingestion of overdoses of vitamin A, as in the case of the infants who were fed chicken liver daily or the four year-old boy who ate vitamin tablets like candy, usually causes bone pain and changes in the bone density and symptoms that result from excess pressure in the cerebrospinal fluid, with effects on the brain. Nausea, vomiting, delirium, irritability, headache and lethargy are brain symptoms of vitamin A poisoning.

So, vitamin A in animal foods like liver and fish liver oil, as well as the vitamin A in supplements, must be used in moderation because of the real potential for toxic effects and birth defects that can occur from excessively high levels of retinyl ester in the circulation.

In complete contrast with the well-known toxicity from retinyl ester is the total lack of toxicity from beta-carotene, the precursor of vitamin A that is supplied by the fruit and vegetable part of our diet. The absence of toxicity from beta-carotene can be accounted for by the limitations in the animal system for converting beta-carotene to vitamin A. The carotene-converting enzyme in the cells of the intestinal wall can produce only a limited amount of vitamin A at any one time. When large amounts of beta-carotene are consumed, part of the excess is absorbed unconverted and stored in several different tissues, as discussed earlier, and part of the excess is excreted in the feces.

James A. Olson has calculated the maximum amount of vitamin A that could be produced in a day's time from dietary beta-carotene, at least in the rabbit making maximal use of the enzyme in his intestinal wall.[27] The calculation showed that a rabbit could theoretically make 230 times more retinaldehyde in a day than he needs. But even this amount of vitamin A is less than half the amount that would be needed to produce toxic overdose in a rabbit. Of course, the rabbit's intestinal converting enzyme is not working anywhere near top speed full time in real life because he is not likely to get a diet that is so rich in beta-carotene; so, the probability is remote that he would ever come close to a toxic overdose.

This situation, where the amount of vitamin A that can be produced from beta-carotene is limited, is part of the explanation why there have never been any cases of human toxicity from the beta-carotene in fruits and vegetables. Another safety factor operating in our favor to avoid toxicity is a lower proportion that is absorbed and converted to vitamin A when foods especially rich in beta-carotene, such as carrots or mangoes, are consumed.

Scientists at Hoffmann-LaRoche Company in Switzerland demonstrated this effect using pure beta-carotene. They compared the curative powers of vitamin A acetate (retinyl ester) and beta-carotene over a wide range of doses to find out how much of these two forms of vitamin A is absorbed.[28] Two species of animals were used—chicks and rats—and three different kinds of bioassay for vitamin A efficacy were used. They found that when low doses were fed, one molecule of beta-carotene had the same efficacy as one molecule of retinyl ester, but as larger doses were fed to the animals, beta-carotene was not absorbed, converted, and stored in the liver nearly as efficiently as was retinyl ester. The point was reached where doubling the dose of retinyl ester resulted in a doubling of the amount of retinyl ester stored in the liver two days later, but doubling the dose of beta-carotene produced only a small increase in the amount of retinyl ester that was stored.

No one knows whether the limitations on absorption and conversion of beta-carotene are entirely similar in man to the situation in the animals that have been studied. Humans can absorb unconverted beta-carotene (and other carotenoids) and store carotene in several tissues. Beta-carotene can be found in human skin, in liver, in fat cells, and in many glandular tissues. As mentioned earlier, little is known as of 1991 about whether the stored beta-carotene in human tissues is converted to retinol or retinoic acid.

In people who consume large amounts of beta-carotene, higher than average amounts of carotene can be found in the blood, but the blood level of retinol, which is released from the liver storage site, is normal. In Ghana in West Africa, the traditional diet is rich in beta-carotene. One of the oils used for cooking in Ghana is red palm oil, which is loaded with beta-carotene, the only cooking oil that does contain this vitamin. The diet also includes green leafy vegetables, mangoes, and pawpaw (papaya). Scientists in Ghana measured the blood levels of retinol and carotene in several dozen individuals and found retinol levels that were similar to those in the United States and western Europe, but carotene levels that were several times higher than those in the United States.[29]

When small amounts of beta-carotene are consumed, as in a normal food serving, much of the beta-carotene in the food is absorbed, although there is variation among different individuals. In a small study on human volunteers in India in 1970, nutritionists studied the absorption of beta-carotene from several foods.[30] The absorption from cooked carrot or from raw papaya ranged from 73% to 98% in the four people studied. Absorption from a cooked green leafy vegetable (amaranth) ranged from 52% to 100%, and absorption from a serving of mixed vegetables ranged from 16% to 60%. The unabsorbed carotene was lost in the feces.

More studies are being done on carotene absorption in recent years because of the growing medical interest in using beta-carotene for clinical trials to see whether it can reduce cancer incidence. Scientists want to know more about how well it is absorbed and what, if any, symptoms of toxicity could be expected. A recent study on thirty men was done at the Human Nutrition Research Center, part of the U.S. Department of Agriculture. The study showed considerable variation among individuals as to how much carotene shows up in the blood plasma following a large dose of carotene. There appeared to be a three- to four-fold variation in absorption either from pure carotene or from carrots, even though all the subjects were on the same basic diet while their blood levels were being checked.[31] It was not determined whether the variation was due to individual differences in absorption from the intestine, or individual differences in conversion to retinyl ester.

When carotene is consumed regularly in large amounts, it can cause yellowing of the skin. The same group of scientists mentioned above found this to be true when they gave volunteers thirty milligrams a day of pure beta-carotene for several weeks. The yellowing occurred mostly on the hands and face, and disappeared slowly after stopping the beta-carotene capsules. Several other studies have shown the same type of temporary, innocuous yellowing of the skin from beta-carotene.

In another recent study, volunteers were given forty-five milligrams a day of pure beta-carotene for eight weeks.[32] None of the fifteen volunteers developed toxic symptoms. Some yellowing of the skin was reported in another group after three weeks. Plasma carotene levels became higher if the volunteers were given a high-fat diet than when they were given a low-fat diet.

These studies where very high doses of beta-carotene were given to volunteers were carried out to study the time course of elevated carotene levels in the blood plasma and to find out whether adverse reactions would develop from the pure beta-carotene. The absence of toxic reactions confirms long-term studies in animals. The safety of beta-carotene has been tested in animals by feeding large amounts for up to two years at a stretch and by feeding large amounts to two generations of rats.[33] No signs of birth defects were found from the high doses of beta-carotene, in contrast to the situation where high doses of retinyl ester are fed, with resulting birth defects in animals.

We know from long experience that beta-carotene has never caused toxicity problems in man.[28] Foods that are especially rich in beta-carotene have not caused toxicity, and the administration of high doses of beta-carotene prescribed for certain photosensitivity diseases has not caused toxicity and has not caused excessively high levels of retinol in the circulation.[34]

The lack of toxicity from beta-carotene allows us plenty of freedom to indulge in the especially rich carotene-containing foods such as carrots, sweet potatoes, apricots, papayas, and cantaloupe, and the green leafy vegetables that are so important in our daily diet. The high doses of carotene that have been given to human volunteers or to certain patients are much higher than the amount we consume in a normal diet. Normal intakes of carotene from fruits and vegetables range up to ten milligrams a day. A person who consumes 1000 Retinol Equivalents a day (RDA for vitamin A) solely from fruits and vegetables would be consuming six milligrams a day of beta-carotene. However, government surveys show that Americans on the average consume less than one-third of their vitamin A as carotene; so the usual carotene consumption in the U.S. is only two or three milligrams a day.[35] How much improvement in the cancer incidence rates might we see if we all increased our average carotene intake to ten milligrams a day? This would be so easy to do. Approximately fifteen milligrams of beta-carotene could be obtained in a day by having three dried apricots with breakfast (6 mg), a quarter cup of cooked fresh carrot with lunch (6 mg), and half a cup of cooked kale with dinner (2.7 mg).

This discussion about the lack of toxicity associated with beta-carotene is meant to be part of the explanation of the differences between vitamin A from animal foods and supplements (retinyl ester), which can cause toxicity, and beta-carotene from fruits and vegetables. It is not meant to be a recommendation for consuming pure beta-carotene in capsules. So far, we have no proof, as of 1990, that consuming beta-carotene supplements can reduce the incidence of cancer, although we do have dozens of dietary studies from around the world that show that people who consume more vegetables have fewer cases of cancer than their neighbors who eat fewer vegetables. It may turn out that consuming beta-carotene Hunza style, in frequent small servings, is the best route to human health. It may be that the production of retinoic acid in the cells of the small intestine during the process of absorption is more beneficial than large amounts of beta-carotene stored in the tissues. And it may turn out that a certain other component of green leafy vegetables, namely, folic acid, is also necessary for cancer prevention.

More than seventy years have passed since Harry Steenbock made the suggestion that the "fat-soluble vitamine" we need for normal growth, vision, and reproduction might be obtained from the plant pigment, carotene, as well as from butter and eggs. These years have been filled with an abundance of discoveries by chemists and medical researchers seeking to understand all the details of vitamin A conversions and functions in the animal body. A prodigious number of details are known, but important parts of the story remain to be puzzled out. In this chapter I have described only a few of the highlights of the steps involved in the process of converting carotene to more useful forms of vitamin A—my chief concern being to explain how and why to avoid toxic overdoses of vitamin A in the coming public appreciation that carotene and the retinoids are important for cancer prevention.

The student of vitamin A metabolism will find in the scientific journals many more details on all parts of the story. The lifelong labors of diligent scientists using whatever was the most up-to-date technology they had at their disposal in these years have elucidated the details about the absorption of carotene and preformed vitamin A from foods into the cells of the small intestine. They have described the properties and capabilities of the cellular enzymes that convert the vitamin into several chemical forms. They have described the details of the liver function in storage of vitamin A and in mobilizing stored vitamin into the circulation. They have described specific retinoid-binding proteins in many tissues which might have important roles in the cells that make use of vitamin A. They have described a variety of degradation pathways and conversion products that the cells employ to remove and excrete vitamin A after it has served its purpose.

The vitamin A story continues to unfold. During the late 1980s, scientists discovered specific receptors—proteins in the cell nucleus whose sequence in this case shows them to be related to an oncogene—that bind to retinoic acid and then bind to DNA to influence gene expression. So far, four of these receptors have been identified in human cells and they each have their own pattern of tissue localization; so the variety of effects of vitamin A in different parts of the body begins to see some explanation. The genes that are regulated by the retinoic acid receptors are beginning to be identified.[36] This is accomplished through studies of DNA binding by the receptors. The studies done so far show that retinoic acid is involved, with thyroid hormone, in production of growth hormone in the pituitary gland and is involved in helping vitamin D to maintain strong bones. Another finding of the studies on retinoic acid receptors is their involvement with production of laminin, an extracellular glycoprotein that may be important in preventing metastasis of tumor cells. (Laminin is a sticky adhesive-like material that is part of the basement membrane that separates epithelial tissues from the general circulation.)

In laboratory studies that go back to the 1950s, it has been demonstrated that vitamin A has a controlling function in differentiation as well as a role in controlling cell proliferation, but how these roles are played out in normal cells is not yet completely understood. Laboratory studies are only now beginning to produce some understanding of these processes at the molecular level. These are complicated fields of study, and require the ability to isolate genes and monitor the interactions of many regulatory factors. Eventually we might learn how the axolotl uses vitamin A to control the regeneration of a lost limb, or how vitamin A accomplishes a variety of different effects, depending on the tissue. One hope expressed with the laboratory studies is that we might eventually be able to take better advantage of vitamin A-related compounds to counteract the mistakes in the growth control process that lead to cancer.

Other recent work on vitamin A seeks to find out whether beta-carotene functions as an antioxidant in animal tissues, somewhat like it does in the photosynthetic process of green plants. Beta carotene can be demonstrated to work like an antioxidant in artificial mixtures of chemicals and artificial membranes, but whether or not this property of carotene would have any effect in prevention of cancer is completely unknown at the present time. There is no doubt, however, about the important effects of vitamin A in gene regulation. The gene regulator and antiproliferation effects of vitamin A may be the entire explanation for the anticancer effect of vitamin A.

While we wait for the rest of the vitamin A story, we owe it to ourselves and our families to do the best we can in maintaining good health. We cannot ignore the dietary studies that show that people who consume more vegetables are less likely to develop cancer. The dietary studies on cancer incidence are a large part of the basis for the recommendation to have at least five servings a day of fruits and vegetables, emphasizing the dark yellow and leafy green vegetables and citrus fruit. This 1989 recommendation from the Committee on Diet and Health of the National Research Council (see chapter 11) is the most important thing we need to remember about vitamin A metabolism.

Chapter 9

RDA and Vitamin A — How to Measure?

We can greatly improve our diets by one of the most simple and enjoyable means imaginable. Frequent servings of the beta-carotene-containing fruits and vegetables will benefit us individually and as a society from now on as we return to our basic nutritional requirements of whole grains, vegetables, fruits, milk, meat and fish. The best sources of the beta-carotene that we seem to require in frequent small doses in order to reduce the risk of cancer can usually be identified simply by color—fruits that contain beta-carotene always have some degree of orange color and vegetables are either orange in color or dark green because of the chlorophyll. Specialists in nutrition and those individuals who desire to know more exactly how much beta-carotene is present in a particular food will want to consult the food composition tables published by the U.S. Department of Agriculture. These tables provide the best information generally available on the vitamin A content of all of our dietary items, as well as information on a host of other nutrients.

Foods have been analyzed for their vitamin A value ever since McCollum and Steenbock began testing edible plants for "fat-soluble A" using the growth-promoting effect that could be measured in the rat. In modern times, the rat bioassays have been replaced by chemical and microbiological methods of analysis for the various nutrients; but in the case of beta-carotene, technical problems remain in the chemical analytical methods of analysis. The chemical analysis of beta-carotene in foods can be surprisingly complicated because of the presence of numerous carotenoids that are similar to beta-carotene. As mentioned in chapter 4, the Department of Agriculture has become aware of potential errors in older analyses of beta-carotene, and is currently working to improve the data on the beta-carotene content of fruits and vegetables. This will result in further updating and revising of Department of Agriculture Handbook No. 8 "Composition of Foods."

The vitamin A value of foods has been expressed in two systems of measurement. The original system, dating from the 1930s when many foods were first evaluated for vitamin A content, gave vitamin A value in International Units (IUs). More recently, a new system has been adopted and the vitamin A value is given in Retinol Equivalents (REs). The switch to a new system of measurement was desired in order to use the quantity of retinol in a sample, measured in micrograms, as the basis for comparison with other forms of vitamin A, rather than continuing to use 0.3 micrograms of retinol as the basic unit of measurement. Also, studies on absorption efficiency of carotene have led to the realization that carotene in food is not completely absorbed and converted to vitamin A in man. Newer understanding of the limited absorption of carotene in man required some changes in the assessment of vitamin A value of carotene-containing foods. Chemical analysis of foods for the carotene content does not tell the whole story about the vitamin A value of foods because of this limited and variable intestinal absorption.

The newer system of measurement uses a simple definition of Retinol Equivalents for the amount of preformed vitamin A (retinol) found in foods of animal origin. One microgram of retinol in these foods equals one Retinol Equivalent. Calculation of Retinol Equivalents for carotene-containing foods (fruits and vegetables) is a little more complicated and rather uncertain. The intention is to estimate the amount of retinol that can be obtained from the vitamin A precursors in fruits and vegetables.

This leads to the question, then, of how do they determine the vitamin A value of fruits and vegetables, and how do they determine how much vitamin A is needed for good health in man? One might expect that these two questions would be straightforward problems for the nutritionists to solve, but both problems involve considerable difficulties in their solution. In fact, the best information we have is often but a very rough estimate. It is relatively easy to study the dietary vitamin requirements of experimental animals by feeding artificial diets, but the results cannot be directly related to human needs because the species are so different. There have been only a few small scientific studies, carried out on volunteers, that were designed to study the human requirement for vitamin A. Additional information on human requirements, which has usually been in general agreement with the scientific studies, has come from clinical observations where the dietary habits of people who appeared to be healthy were compared with diets of people who had symptoms of vitamin A deficiency such as night blindness.

The first attempt to standardize the measurement of vitamin A value of foods took place at a conference of nutrition experts sponsored by the League of Nations in 1931. The conference set up standard units of measurement for the most important vitamins known at that time. Vitamin A activity was to be measured in International Units based on the biological activity of a sample of pure beta-carotene that had been prepared through collaboration of seven laboratories. Samples of carotene from the seven laboratories were sent to the Institute for Medical Research in London where they were pooled, recrystallized, and tested for growth-promoting activity. One microgram of the sample would equal one International Unit. The growth-promoting activity of food samples would then be tested in rats and the IUs in food samples would be calculated from comparison with the standard.

As laboratory work on the chemistry of carotene continued, chemists soon realized that the original standard sample was not pure beta-carotene, as had been thought, but was actually a mixture of alpha- and beta-carotene. So, in 1934 Paul Karrer, the Nobel prize-winning chemist from Switzerland, supplied a pure sample of crystalline beta-carotene to be used as the new reference standard. Karrer and his colleagues at the University of Zurich had accomplished the final elucidation of the chemical structure of beta-carotene in 1930 and also proved the structure of retinol in 1931. After they provided a genuine sample of pure beta-carotene, it was necessary to make a new definition of the International Unit of vitamin A activity; so now this was set as the activity of 0.6 micrograms of pure beta-carotene.[1,2]

In 1949 the International Unit was further defined as the activity of 0.3 micrograms of retinol. When small amounts of pure retinol and carotene were fed to rats, it was always found that twice as much carotene was needed to produce the same curative or growth-promoting effect as a certain amount of retinol. Theoretically, the two forms of the vitamin should have the same effect based on the weight of the sample that was fed because a molecule of carotene is converted into two molecules of retinaldehyde in the wall of the small intestine, but conversion inefficiency in the rat always causes the loss of about half of the small dose of carotene that is fed.[3]

By now it should be clear that "vitamin A" is a general term that is used for any version of the fat-soluble vitamin that promotes growth in the young and prevents eye disease. Several variations of vitamin A are known. Included are retinol, retinyl ester, retinaldehyde, beta-carotene, and a few other carotenoids. Some of these exist in more than one stereoisomeric form. All of the variations have a part of their molecular structure in common, namely, a beta-ionone ring with a polyene side chain containing conjugated double bonds. (See the structural formulas in the appendix.) Beta-carotene has two beta-ionone rings linked by a polyene hydrocarbon chain with a central point of symmetry. Plants make beta-carotene from a precursor carotenoid that has the same forty carbon atoms but no rings.

The growth-promoting activity of vitamin A in young rats was the original method used for comparing the vitamin A value of standards and food samples. Even though standard conditions were used for raising the animals and monitoring their weight gain, the results of the bioassay were not very reliable. Chemical analyses for vitamin A content of foods were much to be preferred, but in the early days, bioassays were the only methods that were sufficiently sensitive to detect the trace amounts of the vitamins present in foods. In the late 1920s, a color reaction was invented for chemical analysis of vitamin A in food extracts, enabling easier routine testing of some samples. The retinol in milk, eggs, and fish liver oil, or in vitamin A-fortified foods, could now be analyzed by the intensity of the blue color produced from treatment with antimony trichloride, but many similar compounds such as carotene and cholesterol also produced bluish colors; so careful spectrophotometry was required for the analysis. Chemical methods of analysis for vitamin A became more accurate in the following decades when chromatographic methods for separating closely related compounds came into general use.[4] The chemical extraction of carotenes from food samples with determination of the amount of carotene in the sample is the method that has been used for most modern estimates of the vitamin A value of carotene-containing foods.

Chemical analysis of plant and animal materials can be extremely complicated. Any material from the world of living things contains about ten thousand different kinds of molecules in the smallest sample—thus, a humble blade of grass rivals a redwood in chemical complexity. The five hundred or so different kinds of carotenoid pigments that have been identified in plants testify to nature's prolific inventiveness, and make our efforts to quantify the one carotenoid we like best sometimes a difficult task. Most of the carotene analyses that have been done for the food composition tables used a simple chromatographic method that had the potential for inaccurate results.[5,6] The "carotene" fraction from plant materials that is obtained with this simple procedure often contains a few of the other carotenoids that are chemically similar to beta-carotene but which have little or no vitamin A value for man. Examples of such carotenoids are alpha-carotene, cryptoxanthin and lycopene. These carotenoids are so similar to beta-carotene that they are not separated from beta-carotene in the old-fashioned analysis and, if they were present, they contributed to the "beta-carotene" fraction, giving false high results for the vitamin A value. The false high results for oranges and tomatoes and peaches were good examples. This difficulty with the older analytical procedure is part of the reason why older tables showing vitamin A content of foods may differ from the tables found in recent publications. There is now available a more powerful analytical method that can provide accurate information on the quantity of beta-carotene in food samples, and it is being used by the Department of Agriculture to revise the food composition tables. The 1984 edition of the USDA vegetable handbook (Handbook No. 8-11) and the 1982 edition of the fruits handbook (Handbook No. 8-9) contain some corrected values for vitamin A content. Additional corrections in the vitamin A values of fruits and vegetables can be expected as the chemical analytical work continues.

Even if the analysis gives an accurate result for beta-carotene, the laboratory extraction method does not predict how much of the carotene will be extracted by the human digestive system. The conversion of carotene into vitamin A by the rat was noted to be about 50% efficient for small doses of carotene, but absorption efficiency goes down as the amount of carotene in a meal goes up, and in humans, other factors such as whether a little fat is present in the meal and whether the vegetables are raw or cooked, can affect carotene absorption and often result in poor carotene utilization.

In 1967, an expert committee of the Food and Agriculture Organization of the United Nations and the World Health Organization recommended a new system for expressing the vitamin A value of foods. The committee met to review and evaluate studies from around the world that have attempted to define the vitamin A requirement of man or that have described vitamin A intake in different populations, and to consider the problems that are evident in many parts of the less-developed world in obtaining sufficient vitamin A, especially by young children.[7] On the basis of one small human study that seemed to show that humans, like rats, have a 50% efficiency in converting carotene to retinol and on the basis of many studies in different countries that showed that carotene is not well absorbed by man, the committee suggested a new system for calculating the vitamin A value of carotene-containing foods. The new system would compensate for the inefficient absorption of carotene in man by counting only a fractional amount of the beta-carotene found to be present in fruits and vegetables.

In the new system, one Retinol Equivalent would be defined as one microgram of retinol or six micrograms of beta-carotene. Retinol (preformed vitamin A) in foods like milk, eggs, and liver is thought to be completely absorbed and, of course, does not require conversion, but carotene is estimated to be approximately only one-third absorbed from a variety of vegetables and then is only 50% converted to retinaldehyde or retinol. So the new system assumes that only one-sixth of the carotene in foods will be converted to vitamin A in man.

The 1967 recommendation has been adopted by British and American government committees on dietary allowances.[2] The newer tables of food composition published by the U.S. Department of Agriculture contain vitamin A data in Retinol Equivalents (REs) as well as in the former International Units (IUs).

The estimate that carotene is only one-third absorbed from foods is a rough approximation. We saw in chapter 8 that carotene absorption from several foods in a small study in India ranged from 16% to 100%. The 1967 FAO/WHO committee reviewed many other such studies. In these studies, known amounts of carotene-containing foods—carrots and spinach were usually tested—which were prepared by different methods, were fed to a few volunteers. (Adults, children, and infants have been studied.) The foods were analyzed for carotene content and feces were collected for several days and analyzed to find out how much carotene was not absorbed. The amount of carotene that was absorbed ranged from 1% to 98% in different studies and there were many instances where the same food was utilized to widely different extent by different individuals in a study. The FAO/WHO committee concluded that it is not possible to predict accurately from these studies how much carotene is absorbed, and the best approximation of carotene availability is about 33%. The one-third estimate for absorption of carotene might some day be revised, but in the meantime, it will be used for all carotene-containing foods to simplify the evaluation of diets for vitamin A content. Consuming a variety of carotene-containing foods if possible will help compensate for errors in the one-third estimate for any particular food.

Although the new system of evaluating diets in terms of Retinol Equivalents was adopted by the U.S. Food and Nutrition Board in 1974, we are still in a transition period in converting over to the new system. Some nutritional information that is available to consumers still makes use of the IU system. The equivalencies listed below can be used by consumers to convert from one measurement system to another:[8]

$$
\begin{aligned}
1 \text{ RE} &= 1 \text{ microgram of retinol} \\
&= 6 \text{ micrograms of beta-carotene} \\
&= 3.33 \text{ IU of retinol} \\
&= 10 \text{ IU of beta-carotene}
\end{aligned}
$$

The switch to the new system of evaluating diets for vitamin A content can cause some confusion. Under the new system, carotene is assumed to be only one-third absorbed from food, an assumption that was not used in the IU system. If you were accustomed to using the older food composition tables published by the U.S. Department of Agriculture in 1963, you would have thought that half a cup of mustard greens or half a cup of winter squash or one cup of broccoli provided enough vitamin A to reach the RDA level of 4000 to 5000 IU. But according to the new tables using REs, you must triple these quantities of the same foods in order to reach the RDA level of 800 to 1000 RE.

Not all of the vegetables must be eaten in greater amounts to overcome the one-third absorbability consensus that is incorporated into the Retinol Equivalent calculation. Newer analyses of carrots show that more carotene is present in modern carrots, because of richer cultivars now being grown or because of later harvesting when the carotene content is higher. The 1963 USDA vitamin A rating for cooked carrots showed that half a cup provided about 9000 IU, or about twice the RDA, and the 1984 value is about 2000 RE—still twice the RDA.

Sweet potatoes are another vegetable for which the vitamin A value did not decline with use of the one-third absorbability calculation. A medium sweet potato still provides vitamin A at twice the RDA level.

There are doubtless quite a few more sources of confusion to be found in our ordinary dietary evaluations. Vitamin supplements still list the vitamin A value of one tablet in terms of IUs, even though many brands acknowledge the newer emphasis on carotene by including some carotene in their formulations. One major brand contains 5000 IUs as retinyl acetate (retinyl ester) plus 1250 IUs of beta-carotene. One wonders how much beta-carotene this represents: since they use the older system of measurement where 1 IU = 0.6 microgram beta-carotene, this means the tablet contains 0.75 milligram beta-carotene—a very stingy amount of a most valuable nutrient. For comparison, one carrot contains about 12 milligrams carotene. (The 5000 IUs of retinyl acetate equals 1500 REs.) Food processors provide nutritional information on the labels of packaged foods, but they use the percentage of RDAs as their method of scoring their products for each nutrient for which an RDA has been established. (Actually, food processors are required to calculate the percentages for vitamins not from the average vitamin content of their food items, but from a value that is a little less than the average vitamin content.) As of 1992 the food processors and vitamin manufacturers still use the 1968 RDAs as their basis for calculation of percentages, by order of the Food and Drug Administration, even though RDAs for a few nutrients have been changed since 1968. The Food and Drug Administration has plans to update this rule in conjunction with new regulations for nutrient labeling, and will set new values called Reference Daily Intakes (RDIs) for use in listing nutrition information on food labels.

The Retinol Equivalent system will eventually be more widely employed and understood. It should be kept in mind that REs are approximate and the vitamin A value of a fruit or vegetable can vary with the cultivar, with the ripeness, with the length of time it was held in storage and the growing conditions, as well as with the conditions of chopping and cooking, to say nothing of how close to the one-third estimate for absorption that might apply to the particular vegetable and the particular individual.

The Department of Agriculture publishes revised editions of the handbooks "Composition of Foods" every few years. Some of the reasons for updating the handbooks are: new analyses are performed as the requirements for nutritional labeling increase, new analyses are done on foods that are prepared by different methods, new products come on the market or new strains of a vegetable are developed with different amounts of nutrients, and new analytical methods are devised that yield more accurate results.

As mentioned in chapter 4, the U.S. Department of Agriculture, in conjunction with the National Cancer Institute, is in the process of analyzing many carotene-containing foods by a new analytical method that gives accurate results for beta-carotene (or any other compound of interest) even in the presence of many similar chemicals.[9] More accurate data on the beta-carotene content of foods will help epidemiologists who are studying the correlations between diet and cancer and will help the many other specialists who use the food composition tables. The new analyses of fruits and vegetables may also provide details about the content of other nonvitamin A-generating carotenoids, which is a subject that interests some cancer researchers. More accurate knowledge of the beta-carotene content of fruits and vegetables may also help the educational efforts in less-developed countries where consuming adequate amounts of beta-carotene is a major nutritional problem in some areas.

The approximate amount of vitamin A needed by healthy people has been fairly well known for many decades in spite of the obvious difficulty of doing experimental studies on humans. The first estimates of human requirements for vitamin A were published in the 1930s.[1] By 1937 many foods had been assayed for their vitamin A content using chemical analysis, and the Department of Agriculture had published the results with IUs as the measuring system. The estimates of human needs were based on clinical observations such as the amount of dietary vitamin A needed to avoid or cure night blindness, and various estimates were made that between 4000 IUs and 5600 IUs per day was the amount needed.

One of the usual methods for estimating human requirements for a nutrient is the observation of deficiency symptoms combined with analysis of dietary intakes. This can be a complicated and lengthy undertaking. Vitamin deficiencies usually cause symptoms that have a gradual onset in adults, and malnourished people often suffer from multiple deficiencies that make diagnosis of a particular deficiency a matter for skilled judgment. In the case of vitamin A, it is the eye symptoms that have been most often used to decide whether a certain population is deficient. If the vitamin is lacking, night blindness will be common as well as dryness of the conjunctiva and ulceration of the cornea. Vitamin A can be measured in blood samples, and surveys in many countries have been done to correlate the average blood level with the frequency of occurrence of eye symptoms. When blood levels of retinol are below twenty micrograms per deciliter in a population, it is common to find eye symptoms.

The first RDAs (Recommended Dietary Allowances) were published by the government in 1943 and were meant to serve as a guide for nutrition planning in connection with national defense and the procurement of appropriate food supplies for the armed forces. Over the years, the RDAs have found wider usage in nutrition education, in planning food supplies for groups and institutions, and in evaluating food consumption patterns that are developed from dietary surveys. The RDAs are based on the best available scientific knowledge and are updated from time to time by a Committee on Dietary Allowances of the Food and Nutrition Board, under the auspices of the National Research Council.[10]

The Recommended Dietary Allowances were never meant to be a set of dietary rules for individuals to follow. They are meant, rather, to describe the average dietary requirement over a period of time of a healthy population, with an extra allowance included so as to encompass most of the variation in requirements that might be expected in a group of individuals.[8] So, the RDA of any nutrient (other than calories) is higher than the requirement of the average healthy person. The RDA is also not meant to be used as a reason for cutting down on the habitual consumption of any nutrient. Most nutrients other than calories can be tolerated at dietary levels that are higher than the RDA and if the habitual intake is higher than the RDA, this may be perfectly acceptable. An example is dietary protein, which is consumed in quantities greater than the RDA level by most people in the developed countries without any deleterious effects.

The Committee on Dietary Allowances establishes an RDA for a nutrient only after sufficient information has been collected about the requirements of healthy people in various stages of life. There are a number of problems involved in estimating RDAs and differences of opinion sometimes arise on the criteria to be used for particular nutrients. The RDA might be set at the amount needed to avoid development of deficiency symptoms, or it might be set at the amount needed to avoid loss of body stores. When information is lacking about a nutrient that is known to be essential, the Committee on Dietary Allowances might recommend an intake level that is "safe and adequate" as a preliminary recommendation until enough information is available to establish an RDA. This has been done for some of the essential trace minerals. The Committee assumes that a wide variety of foods will be used to obtain the nutrients for which RDAs have been established. When this assumption is followed, essential nutrients for which RDAs have not yet been established will also likely be included in the diet.

This is a word of advice from the nutrition experts that should be taken greater note of by health-conscious consumers. A variety of foods is important. Nutrition is a rather new science, and new discoveries about our dietary requirements for vitamins, minerals, and fiber are being made every year with no let up in sight. The truth is that we do not know enough yet to devise an artificial food, such as a fortified cereal or a multivitamin tablet, that can guarantee all our vitamin needs, no matter what advertising may claim. Even if vitamin supplements are used, we still need to make every effort to have a variety of foods from the four major food groups—whole grains, vegetables and fruits, milk, and meats—to better guarantee our own good health.

Two scientific studies have been done on volunteers to determine how much vitamin A is required by man. One study was done in England in the 1940s and one was a collaboration between the University of Iowa and the U.S. Army Medical Research and Nutrition Laboratory in the early 1970s. In both studies the volunteers were put on a vitamin A-deficient diet for one to two years until symptoms appeared and then they were given retinol or beta-carotene in an attempt to estimate what dose would cure the symptoms and restore the circulating blood level of retinol to normal. These studies were extremely complicated to perform and analyze. The studies have been of considerable interest to nutritionists; they are discussed and summarized by the Committee on Dietary Allowances in the tenth edition of *Recommended Dietary Allowances.*[10]

Using these two studies as well as earlier studies on the amount of vitamin A needed to prevent night blindness, the RDA is estimated to be 1000 Retinol Equivalents for men and 800 Retinol Equivalents for women. This is unchanged from the older system of measuring vitamin A in International Units. In IUs the RDA was 5000 IUs, and vitamin A was thought to be obtained in American diets approximately half from retinol and half from beta-carotene.[8] The 2500 IUs of retinol and the 2500 IUs of carotene must be converted to Retinol Equivalents separately because of the one-sixth utilization rule for carotene. The 2500 IUs of retinol equals 750 Retinol Equivalents, and the 2500 IUs of carotene equals 250 Retinol Equivalents for a total of 1000 REs.

There will continue to be some uncertainty about the exact amount of beta-carotene in anyone's diet for a few more years, until we have the results of the newer analyses of the carotene content of fruits and vegetables. The new analytical method, high performance liquid chromatography, is being used by the U.S. Department of Agriculture to determine more accurately the carotene content of the popular fruits and vegetables. When these results are available, we will be better able to analyze people's diets for the carotene content.

The uncertainty in present knowledge about the true amount of beta-carotene in some vegetables and fruits is another good reason for keeping a variety of these foods in our diets. Tomatoes were formerly rated as good sources of beta-carotene (two tomatoes were thought to supply 5000 IUs vitamin A), but it is now known from the more accurate chemical analysis that there is very little beta-carotene in tomatoes; the "total carotene" fraction of tomatoes as analyzed by the traditional method is largely composed of another carotenoid, lycopene, which is responsible for the bright orange-red color of tomatoes but which has no known function in animal metabolism.[5] And yet, tomatoes might still turn out to have some specific benefits in the diet; in dietary surveys that show less cancer in people who consume more vegetables, tomatoes are often among the vegetables preferred by these people.

Carrots are a different situation—the major carotenoid in carrots is actually beta-carotene according to modern chemical analysis, in agreement with the older analyses.[6] Carrots are still one of the best sources of carotene in the diet. Apricots are also an excellent source of beta-carotene according to the latest analysis, apparently even richer than they were thought to be by the old-fashioned method. One fresh apricot contains more than 2 milligrams of beta-carotene according to a recent analysis by the Department of Agriculture, and dried apricots do not appear to suffer any loss of carotene upon drying.[11] The same workers also showed that cantaloupe is an especially rich source of carotene. A quarter of a cantaloupe (150 to 200 grams of edible fruit) contains from 32 to 43 milligrams of carotene, according to my interpretation of their analysis.

Some other good sources according to recent tests are kale and spinach. Kale has about twice as much carotene as spinach,[12] but spinach has ten times more folic acid than kale according to the 1984 edition of USDA Handbook No. 8-11.

Other laboratories are also publishing the results of carotene determinations in fruits and vegetables using the modern methods of chromatography. Many of the new results are in line with the vitamin A values listed in the 1984 edition of Handbook No. 8, but some results are different and they can be either higher or lower than the old results. Lower results will be found for some foods like tomatoes and peaches where the old-fashioned method counted other carotenoids as "carotene," and low results will also be found if the chemists fail to completely extract the beta-carotene. This seems to be happening in some laboratories. Differing results for a certain food are expected when the variety or ripeness is different, but different extraction procedures can also yield big discrepancies in the results. The chemists would do well to review the difficulty that Harry Steenbock had in extracting the "fat-soluble vitamine" from alfalfa when he was trying to prove that beta-carotene was responsible for the vitamin A activity of green plants.

We cannot yet rely on the food composition tables to give us a completely accurate reading on the amount of vitamin A precursors in all of the fruits and vegetables because the new analytical work is still continuing. But the 1989 report from the National Research Council has made it easy for us to calculate how much fruit and vegetables we need. Their recommendation to have at least five servings a day, taking care to emphasize the yellow and green vegetables and citrus fruit, is a dietary standard we can all follow together to battle the cancer problem.

Chapter 10

The Folic Acid Connection

There is another vitamin in vegetables that might play an important role in cancer prevention. Folic acid is best known as a B vitamin that is required to prevent a type of anemia, but its role in maintaining normal chromosomes and genes during cell division has much broader significance for human health and is the explanation for its possible cancer-preventing effects. Folic acid guards against chromosome aberrations similar to those that are usually seen in cancer cells and which become more numerous as cancer becomes more advanced. Folic acid may also help to maintain the normal activity of genes through its indirect role in the transfer of methyl groups to the genes—this is a mechanism used by higher organisms for switching genes on and off. The functions of folic acid in normal metabolism have been studied for more than forty years and the biochemistry of folic acid has been explained fairly well. The potential mechanisms whereby a deficiency of folic acid could lead to the gene damage that is thought to be involved in the earliest events that lead to cancer are much better understood than are the potential mechanisms of vitamin A involvement in cancer. And yet, the importance of folic acid in the diet is not widely appreciated—in the cancer-prevention field folic acid is the sleeper.

Folic acid is obtained from a wide variety of vegetables and legumes and is especially rich in the green leafy vegetables such as spinach. Liver, yeast, and wheat germ are also good sources. The name derives from the Latin word, folium, meaning leaf.

Folic acid was first isolated from natural sources in the 1940s by several groups of scientists who were tracking down unknown growth factors that were required by different organisms. University scientists who were studying the nutritional requirements of chicks on the one hand and of a bacterium on the other hand found that there was a missing nutrient. Neither of these species could be grown properly on artificial diets that included the full array of vitamins that were known at the time. This meant that unknown factors remained to be discovered. The unknown growth factors were water-soluble—they could be obtained from water extracts of natural foods—so they fell into the class of vitamins called B vitamins. As it happened, the growth factor needed by the chick and the factor needed by the bacterium were the same vitamin. The story of the discovery of folic acid has been told by nutrition specialists at the University of Alabama[1] and by other scientists who were involved in the early experiments.[2]

Chemists who were studying the nutritional requirements of chicks at the University of Missouri in the 1930s had observed and characterized a type of anemia which they traced to some bad batches of commercial liver extract. Their studies led them to believe that the anemia was a deficiency disease, but the vitamin that was lacking was not one of the previously known chick vitamins. A similar type of anemia in humans had been described by a British scientist a few years earlier. Lucy Wills had discovered that a type of macrocytic anemia that was common in pregnant women in India could be cured by giving liver or yeast extracts. Wills and her associates tried to isolate the unknown factor but they had difficulty with this because they did not have a convenient bioassay method for testing their extracts.[3]

At the University of Wisconsin, also in the 1930s, biochemists were studying the vitamin requirements of one of the lactic acid bacteria, *Lactobacillus casei*. This organism required several B vitamins in order to thrive in an artificial culture medium, but unknown factors were also required. Good growth of the bacterium was not achieved unless additional natural foods such as yeast extract were added to the culture medium. Curious about the identity of the unknown factor, the biochemists sought to isolate the growth factor from yeast and succeeded in making a partly purified vitamin. They employed activated charcoal to adsorb the unknown compound from the yeast extract in their purification procedure. A bioassay based on the growth rate of *L. casei* was used to great advantage subsequently by them and by other groups of chemists who finally isolated the pure vitamin. (The *L. casei* growth test is used to this day as a method for estimating the amount of folic acid in foods.)

In 1941, chemists at the University of Wisconsin who had tackled a project to purify the vitamin described how they made a concentrated preparation of the vitamin from liver extract. They repeatedly used the activated charcoal method to adsorb the vitamin from solution and eluted the vitamin from the charcoal with aqueous ethanol containing ammonia. This procedure produced a vitamin solution that was two hundred times more concentrated than the original extract. The chemical structure of the vitamin was not yet known, but these workers wondered whether their concentrated vitamin, which allowed *L. casei* to thrive, might be the same factor required by chicks. They tested their preparation in chicks and found some evidence that the two growth factors might be identical.

Meanwhile, at the University of Texas, another group of chemists had been busy testing a variety of foods as sources of the unknown B vitamin that was required by some bacteria. They found that the vitamin was present in liver and in many plants, especially in green leaves. Also in 1941, they reported having made a highly concentrated form of the vitamin by starting with four tons of spinach (using large-scale equipment at the Eli Lilly Company) and making use of the activated charcoal method for purification. They showed that the nutrient was useful for the proper growth of rats as well as for bacteria, and they suggested the name "folic acid" because of the relative abundance of the nutrient in many kinds of green leaves.

The Texas chemists made an estimate of the molecular weight of folic acid from diffusion tests, and they determined its UV absorption spectrum and tested the compound for its chemical reactivity. At this point the detailed chemical nature of the vitamin was still not known. Preparation of pure folic acid and determination of its chemical structure were soon accomplished by chemists at two drug companies.

Preparation of pure, crystalline vitamin from liver was announced by chemists at Parke, Davis and Company in 1943. With pure material to work with, it would now be possible to determine the chemical structure of the vitamin. The Parke, Davis group confirmed that the vitamin was able to prevent anemia in chicks and also served as a growth factor for the *Lactobacillus*. They continued the work on the chemical nature of the vitamin by finding out something about the different forms of folic acid as it exists in different natural sources, showing that the vitamin in yeast is attached to a peptide containing several glutamic acid residues.

Meanwhile, at another pharmaceutical company, Lederle Laboratories, chemists were working out the detailed chemical structure of the complicated folic acid molecule. Former students from the Wisconsin group had joined Lederle and continued to work on folic acid chemistry. The Lederle group discovered the entire chemical structure and devised methods for synthesizing the vitamin from simpler molecules. They did further investigations into the nature of the polyglutamate chain attached to the folic acid molecule in natural sources, and published the description of their work on the structure of folic acid from 1946 to 1948.

Folic acid has a complicated structure and it is converted into different chemical forms during its metabolic functions. (See appendix for a drawing of one of its forms.) Folic acid can have different states of oxidation or reduction of the heterocyclic pteridine ring, different length chains of glutamate residues, and different forms of a one-carbon unit attached to the nitrogen atoms.[1] Folic acid goes by several names today, depending on its chemical form. In food composition tables it is called folacin. Other names for folic acid compounds are folate, pteroylglutamic acid, PGA, THFA, citrovorum factor, leucovorin, and folinic acid.

We all know vitamins are important, having heard this refrain all our lives, but we may not have a very clear idea of why this is so. A complete understanding of the importance of vitamins would require a rather sophisticated knowledge of biochemistry, but it may be possible to appreciate the importance of vitamins well enough by realizing that they are essential participants in many of the thousands of chemical reactions that occur daily in living cells.

The B vitamins, including folic acid, are used as coenzymes in enzymatic reactions. These reactions convert nutrients into the structural elements and essential molecules of the cells and help provide the chemical energy needed to keep everything going. The enzymes of metabolism break down some chemical components of the body and build up others in order to meet the lifelong needs of living things for growth and continued activity, and many of these enzymes require a coenzyme. If a B vitamin is lacking, then a coenzyme is lacking, and the particular enzyme that required the coenzyme in order to carry out its reaction simply doesn't work and some needed job doesn't get done. The type of job done by folic acid enzymes is the transfer of single-carbon groups like methyl groups from one chemical constituent to another in the cells of plants and animals. This is one of the critical jobs necessary for growth and normal metabolism. It is especially important in the production of DNA. Folic acid enzymes play a direct role in providing single-carbon groups that are used in the biosynthesis of the bases needed to make new DNA—specifically, the bases adenine, guanine, and thymine—and they play an indirect role in providing methyl groups that are added to finished DNA as part of the system for switching genes on and off. (The term "base" as used for DNA refers to the alkaline, rather than acid, nature of the four nitrogen-containing compounds—A, T, G, and C—that are found in DNA.)

The methyl groups that are found on finished DNA in normal cells of higher plants and animals originated on the amino acid, methionine. Methionine acquires its methyl group with the help of enzymes that make use of folic acid and vitamin B12. So, both folic acid and vitamin B12 are needed for synthesis of methionine from its precursor. Methionine is also obtained from dietary protein; it is one of the essential amino acids. Even though methionine is obtained from proteins, the body needs to synthesize more of this amino acid using folic acid, vitamin B12, and homocysteine. Methionine is constantly being reworked in a metabolic cycle that uses folic acid and the amino acids, homocysteine and serine. Part of the methionine is drawn off for use in protein synthesis and part of the methionine is converted to S-adenosylmethionine, which is the immediate source of the methyl groups that are added to DNA to help control the activity of the genes. S-adenosylmethionine also provides the methyl groups needed for synthesizing the choline component of the phospholipid, lecithin, and it provides the methyl groups for several other chemical reactions in metabolism.

Folic acid in the circulating blood contains a methyl group that must be removed by transfer to homocysteine, producing methionine, before folic acid can be used in the synthesis of the bases of DNA. So, the metabolic cycles for folic acid and for methionine are interrelated—if one cycle is disrupted, the other also suffers some damage. Knowledge of this interrelationship helps in the understanding of folic acid-related laboratory studies.

Both vitamin A and folic acid play roles in human metabolism that can help prevent cancer. Vitamin A in its retinoic acid form is involved in suppressing cell proliferation. It works at the level of the

DNA-binding proteins (transcription factors) that control gene expression. A deficiency of vitamin A results in increased proliferation by stem cells in the basal layer of epithelial tissues (see Night Blindness). Folic acid, on the other hand, is required for efficient cell division. It is required for production of the purine and pyrimidine bases that are needed for DNA replication during cell division. All of the bases that are needed for new DNA are assembled from scratch by the biosynthetic enzymes of the cells, and folic acid enzymes are involved in this process. A deficiency of folic acid results in visibly defective chromosomes, and this is how folic acid deficiency might be involved in the initiation of cancer. Such a deficiency is quite possibly the most common enabling condition that leads to the genome abnormalities that eventually cause cancer.

The evidence for a connection between folic acid nutrition and the incidence of cancer is circumstantial only at the present time. In this chapter I will describe some of the research that touches on the probable anticancer role of folic acid. The evidence for a connection between folic acid and cancer incidence comes from the following areas of cancer research:

1. A lack of folic acid is associated with chromosome aberrations and chromosome fragile sites and breaks. Chromosome aberrations are observed under the microscope in cancer cells and become more numerous as cancer cells progress. Chromosome aberrations are seen at characteristic locations in many types of cancer.

2. Animals that are fed a diet that is deficient in methyl groups develop cancer of the liver and other tissues. Animals that are fed a diet deficient in folic acid show an increase in chromosome breaks.

3. Folic acid is involved indirectly in DNA methylation. The normal pattern of DNA methylation in the genes is altered in cancer cells and also in benign tumors and in some other disorders. One of the earliest alterations in the progression of human colon mucosa to colon cancer is a decrease in the amount of methyl groups on the DNA.

4. The consumption of more green leafy vegetables—a good source of folic acid—is associated with lower incidences of cancer in human populations.

Chromosome aberrations

A severe deficiency of folic acid in the diet is well known to cause a type of anemia called megaloblastic anemia. One of the characteristics of the disease is damaged chromosomes. Deficiencies of folic acid that last five months or more can produce this anemia. Other conditions that interfere with absorption of folate from foods or that cause an increase in the body's requirement for folate, such as pregnancy, can also cause the anemia. Occasionally, the same symptoms are caused by vitamin B12 deficiency because, without vitamin B12, folic acid does not carry through its normal metabolic functions. The two vitamins work together to transfer methyl groups during one step in one-carbon metabolism. (This is the transfer of methyl from folate to homocysteine to produce methionine.)

In megaloblastic anemia, the red blood cells are enlarged because of abnormal DNA synthesis in the bone marrow cells that are precursors of red blood cells. The precursor cells are unable to multiply efficiently because they lack adequate supplies of the purine and pyrimidine bases that make up the DNA and which cannot be synthesized without folic acid. The cells are larger than normal because they are in the growth part of the cell cycle, but the slow, abnormal DNA synthesis delays their progression into the cell division stage. Characteristics of the disease are increased cell size and slowed DNA synthesis in many of the proliferating cells of the body, not only in the bone marrow.[4]

In 1966, researchers in Boston and New Zealand described in detail the damaged chromosomes that are found in people suffering from megaloblastic anemia. The Boston group studied specimens of bone marrow taken from their anemia patients. The chromosomes in the bone marrow cells showed three types of abnormalities: chromosome breaks, chromosomes that were elongated when they should have been compacted, and centromere spreading. The treatment that was required was determined from blood tests for folic acid and vitamin B12, and the appropriate treatment was given. Within a few days, the patients began to improve. When bone marrow was tested in a few patients after treatment, there were no longer any chromosome breaks observed in the developing blood cells. So it seemed likely that the vitamin deficiency was solely responsible for the chromosome breakage.[5]

A group of scientists in Christchurch, New Zealand made an even more careful study of the chromosome abnormalities in megaloblastic anemia patients. They also studied cells taken from bone marrow and found numerous abnormalities in the chromosomes. The abnormalities were of the same types as were described in the Boston study, with the addition of some chromosomes that had pronounced degeneration.

They noticed that the chromosome breaks occurred in one but not both of the chromatids of replicated chromosomes. The type of damage to the chromosomes was different than the type of damage that is caused by high-dose radiation, and the damage was of a more random nature than the chromosome damage that is observed in cancer cells. (In cancer, clones of cells arise that all appear to have the same chromosome abnormality.) The damage in the anemia patients resembled the damage that is caused by DNA-inhibiting nucleoside drugs. But even the sickest patients in the study had plenty of bone marrow cells that appeared normal in addition to their abnormal cells.[6]

These studies published in 1966 brought together the biochemical work on folic acid function, which had shown by this time how folic acid was needed for synthesis of the purine and pyrimidine bases of DNA, and the microscopic studies of abnormal blood cells that are found in megaloblastic anemia patients. The abnormal cells could now be understood in terms of disruptions in DNA synthesis that seemed to throw a monkey wrench into the fine machinery of cell replication if folic acid was deficient for some reason.

The chromosomes that can be seen in the cell nucleus during part of the cell cycle are complicated structures. A chromosome appears to be coiled up like a telephone cord when seen from a certain distance, but on closer inspection each turn of the coil is seen to consist of a close-packed series of smaller coils of the DNA polymer and associated proteins.

The most important part of a chromosome is the DNA double helix, the high molecular weight, two-stranded polymer of nucleotides containing the four bases whose sequences ultimately determine the structure of all proteins in an organism through transcription of the sequences and translation of the genetic code. The two strands of DNA are held together by hydrogen bonding between pairs of bases on either strand. The hydrogen-bonded base pairs have been likened to the rungs of a ladder for the purpose of describing the double helix. The DNA polymer backbones made up of alternating sugar and phosphate groups, two strands of which would be the side rails of the ladder, twist continuously from one end of the ladder to the other.

A gene consists of a section of the DNA that may contain several thousand pairs of bases. There is a nearby section in the DNA called a promoter region that controls whether or not the gene is transcribed (activated). The promoter region may work by binding to specific proteins called DNA-binding proteins, nuclear receptor proteins, or transcription factors. The mechanisms whereby promoter regions control the activation of their associated genes are subjects of great interest in present-day biological research.

In addition to the DNA double helix, chromosomes contain proteins in amounts that are roughly equal to the amount of DNA, and they contain a small amount of RNA.[7] The proteins of the chromosomes contribute to their three-dimensional structure. The DNA double helix and the chromosomal proteins are held together in a complex arrangement of sections of the DNA helix wrapped around globules of protein to form beadlike nucleosomes. A nucleosome consists of a spherical octet of protein molecules with DNA wrapped around the outside; the DNA molecule continues and wraps around more spheres of proteins. The result might look like beads on a string except that the string of nucleosomes is further wound into several higher levels of coiling, like a miniature solenoid that is folded into looped domains and then coiled some more to make the chromosome that is visible under the microscope.[8] The resulting structure is much wider and more condensed and organized than a stretched-out DNA polymer would be. The configuration of the chromosome structure can change somewhat as a cell passes through various stages such as activation of genes, or cell division, or differentiation into a specialized cell type.

Microscopic examination is one of the methods used to study the chromosomes. During some parts of the cell cycle, it is easy to inspect the chromosomes in the nuclei of cells after first staining the chromosomes with a dye. This method has been used to study abnormal chromosomes in cancer cells and in other diseases. Human cells contain 23 pairs of chromosomes and each pair has a characteristic length and staining pattern. The pairs have been given numbers as labels so that biologists can report their observations about particular chromosomes to each other.

Scientists have studied the occurrence of chromosome breaks in noncancerous cells for many years. In normal cells these breaks are rare, but when normal cells such as white blood cells are grown in culture dishes under certain conditions of deprivation, regular patterns of chromosome breakage can be detected in many cells.

Grant R. Sutherland, of Australia, discovered this phenomenon in 1977 through one of those seemingly unimportant alterations in laboratory procedure that can lead to surprising results. A simple change in the brand of culture medium used produced quite unexpected results and led to an important discovery. Sutherland found that cells grown in culture medium that lacked folic acid showed increased chromosome aberrations. Sutherland was studying chromosomal abnormalities associated with mental retardation. Several specific locations on chromosomes had been shown to be hereditary sites of chromosome breaks or nonstaining gaps, and these were called fragile sites. Sutherland was puzzled when a known fragile site in one patient could not be seen in the white blood cells after the cells were removed from a blood sample and cultured routinely for three days, then stained. More testing showed that different types of culture medium gave different results for the presence or absence of fragile sites, and further investigation showed that cells that were cultured without the presence of folic acid had more chromosome aberrations. To confirm the folic acid effect, Sutherland did methodical studies on specific fragile sites under controlled folic acid conditions. Many, but not all, of the chromosome breaks and nonstaining gaps disappeared when enough folic acid was used in the culture medium.[9]

Carlos Krumdieck of the University of Alabama, who probably understands the complicated biochemistry of folic acid better than anyone else, realized early on that the appearance of fragile sites in cells that were deprived of folic acid, as described by Sutherland, could be explained by decondensation (loosening of the coiled configuration) of the chromosomes from loss of methyl groups on the DNA. Methyl groups on DNA are important because they are involved in the binding of regulatory proteins to the DNA double helix and, possibly, binding of proteins that help stabilize the coiled configuration. (A lack of methyl groups is an early characteristic of tumors—see later in this chapter.)

In 1983, Krumdieck and Patricia Howard-Peebles offered their hypothesis on how folic acid deficiency could produce hypomethylated DNA when the deficiency results in impaired synthesis of the DNA precursors, especially thymine.[10] When folic acid is deficient, the thymine-containing DNA precursor is very scarce in the cells and uracil is incorporated into DNA in place of thymine. Thymine has a methyl group but uracil does not. Krumdieck and Howard-Peebles suggested that the loss of methyl groups if uracil is incorporated into DNA, in combination with a heritable defect in methylation of cytosines in DNA (see later in this chapter), could sufficiently alter the chromosome structure to produce the visible defects called fragile sites.

Jorge J. Yunis, pathologist at the University of Minnesota, was also studying fragile sites in cultured white cells. By careful study he found many more sites on the chromosomes of human cells that had a regular tendency toward fragmentation when the cells were cultured in medium that was deficient in folic acid and thymidine—a medium that provides a DNA-damaging environment. Yunis and his colleagues examined hundreds of stained cells for chromosome breaks after staining the chromosomes for microscopic examination. Chromosome breaks were common but, instead of occurring at random places, most of them were accounted for by fifty-one specific sites on the chromosomes.[11]

Yunis found a striking statistically significant association between the sites of these artificially induced breakpoints and the sites of known chromosome rearrangements in human leukemias, lymphomas, and malignant solid tumors, which also occur consistently at the same locations in tumors from different patients rather than in random locations. He speculated that there may be specific sites in the chromosomes that are prone to fragmentation and rearrangements when the cells are deficient in DNA precursor substances due to a lack of folic acid.

Yunis did an interesting experiment by giving one volunteer extra folic acid supplement before taking a blood sample for testing in the DNA-damaging culture medium. The volunteer took 5 milligrams a day (a nontoxic dose but 25 times higher than the RDA) for three days prior to donating a blood sample. The white cells of this sample were resistant to the DNA-damaging effects of the culture medium, again showing that folic acid had somehow reduced the tendency toward chromosome breaks.

As one would expect from the folic acid effects in megaloblastic anemia and in culturing human white blood cells, laboratory animals also show chromosome damage if their rations are deficient in folic acid. Scientists at the University of California tested blood samples from mice that were kept on a folate-free diet. After six or seven weeks on the diet, the folate-deficient mice had twice as much chromosome damage as control mice. The test for chromosome damage was a microscopic examination of red blood cells. Fragments of chromosomes called micronuclei in the cells are evidence of damaged chromosomes. This study added some new information on the question of possible harm to the chromosomes from caffeine. In the mice, caffeine produced an increase in the amount of chromosome damage in folate-deficient mice, but did not cause apparent damage in mice that received folic acid in their rations.[12] Caffeine in very high doses increases DNA damage because caffeine inhibits the DNA-repair enzyme. When enough folic acid is present, however, there is less need for DNA repair. Jorge J. Yunis, when studying cultured white blood cells, found the same type of results with respect to caffeine. Caffeine in the culture medium aggravated the chromosome damage caused by folic acid deficiency, but not when cells were tested from a volunteer who had received folic acid supplementation.

Another recent study on laboratory animals also showed damage to the DNA from folic acid-deficient rations, and also from methyl group deficiency. (A diet deficient in methyl groups can be arranged by giving the animals an artificial diet that lacks the essential amino acid, methionine, and the phospholipid component, choline. Without these sources of methyl groups, the complicated metabolic systems that use folic acid enzymes become unbalanced, with the result that DNA synthesis suffers particularly from a lack of thymine, even though the animal is given folic acid.) Jill James and Larry Yin at the University of California found striking biochemical evidence that deficiencies of folic acid or of methyl groups cause defective *de novo* synthesis of thymine and stimulate alternative metabolic pathways. They found that when rats were given any of the deficient diets for three weeks, the spleen cells contained DNA with considerably more strand breaks than cells from rats on a complete diet.[13]

These types of deficient diets have also been proven to cause cancer in laboratory animals—see later in this chapter.

Chromosome damage resulting from a marginal deficiency of folic acid was found in a human patient recently.[14] This patient did not have megaloblastic anemia, but he did suffer from a serious intestinal disorder that made it necessary for him to take vitamin supplements to compensate for poor absorption. His circulating red blood cells showed evidence of chromosome damage (micronuclei) that was observed to increase and decrease in close accordance with the stopping and starting of his folic acid supplement treatments. In normal people, these damaged red blood cells would be removed from the circulation by the spleen. But this patient had had his spleen removed following an injury; so his damaged red blood cells remained in the circulation.

His white blood cells also showed the effects of folic acid deficiency. When he was not taking folate therapy, his white blood cells showed chromosome breaks and chromatid gaps that were several times more frequent than in the normal population. Folate therapy lowered the frequency of these chromosome aberrations. Measuring the exact level of folic acid in his blood serum during these studies produced the somewhat startling information that the patient was producing new red blood cells with damaged chromosomes at a time when his serum folic acid level was not terribly low—it was in the low normal range and he had no outward signs of folate deficiency. It has been thought previously that DNA damage from folate deficiency would only occur after the folate level in the liver and other tissues drops to very low levels, but this may not be true in everyone after all.

This study showed that damaged chromosomes can be produced during cell replication long before the serious signs of folate deficiency, like megaloblastic anemia, are detected. A few other recent studies have also shown that some tissues in the body can suffer from folate deficiency symptoms long before a generalized deficiency becomes apparent. These studies make us wonder, how common is chromosome damage from low folate in the diet in the general population, and how closely related is the chromosome damage to the all-too-common problem of cancer initiation?

All of the scientists who have recently studied the chromosome damage that results from folic acid deficiency—in animals and in humans—were aware of the possibility of a connection between their studies and a partial explanation for human cancer. Cancer research since the 1970s has shown more and more convincingly that the cancer process probably begins either from mutations of certain genes (proto-oncogenes) or from chromosome alterations that damage the normal growth control mechanisms in the cells. Dr. Jorge J. Yunis, who studied chromosome breaks in cultured white blood cells, was among the first medical researchers to point out in 1984 the similarity of the chromosome damage caused by folic acid deficiency in human cultured cells and the chromosome damage that is seen in cancer cells. The possibility that folic acid deficiency might be the basic initiating factor in the majority of human cancers for which no specific cause can be found is a possibility that deserves serious consideration by the medical research community. In animal studies using folic acid-deficient rations, a direct connection has been seen between the folic acid deficiency and chromosome damage, and between folate-related methyl deficiency and cancer. In human studies, a direct connection between folic acid deficiency and cancer has not been established, but there is much circumstantial evidence that makes it seem likely that a direct connection will one day be found.

(The mutations that are involved in cancer are not the same as mutations that cause hereditary diseases. Hereditary diseases are caused by mutations that are present from the very beginning of development of a new individual, and the gene defect is present in all cells of the body throughout life. The mutations that are involved in cancer arise in a single cell sometime during the lifetime of an individual, and this can produce a clone of altered cells that exists at first in one small location. The goal of cancer research is to prevent or minimize these mutations that occur during adult life. Folic acid might help with this, but it would not be able to reverse or "cure" inherited mutations.)

In cancer cells some of the chromosomes usually show abnormalities in their structures. These chromosome aberrations have been studied intensively since the 1970s.[15] In 1960, Peter C. Nowell at the University of Pennsylvania showed that most patients suffering from chronic myeloid leukemia have in their malignant leukemia cells an unusual chromosome that contains parts of the normal chromosomes 9 and 22. One of the altered chromosomes, called the "Philadelphia chromosome," was the first chromosomal aberration to be correlated with a particular type of cancer. Another well-known altered chromosome in human cancer is the translocation between chromosomes 8 and 14 of Burkitt's lymphoma, where a promoter-enhancer region from one chromosome has been moved to a new location, with resulting changes in the nature of the cell.

There are now several dozen examples known where a particular chromosomal aberration can be seen consistently in the cells from a particular type of human cancer. The abnormalities can be translocations (rearrangements), deletions, inversions, or an extra copy of a chromosome. Scientists have suspected since about 1970 that these obvious changes in the chromosomes might be closely related to the causes of cancer. Along with other areas of cancer research that implicate the genes and the chromosomes—such as hereditary predispositions toward cancer and the mutating effects of carcinogens—the chromosome abnormalities suggest that cancer develops from these types of genetic damage.[16] This suspicion has been substantiated during recent years as newer techniques for studying DNA have shown that most of the proto-oncogenes and tumor suppressor genes are located very near the locations where chromosome breakpoints commonly occur in particular types of cancer.[17,18]

Scientists are excited about these new revelations coming from the chromosome and oncogene studies. As pointed out by Jorge J. Yunis and also by Janet D. Rowley in 1984, there is intriguing similarity in the chromosomal locations of some of the oncogenes and of fragile sites, and also similarity in locations of other oncogenes and the chromosomal translocations found in cancer cells.[19]

The studies on chromosomes and oncogenes are beginning to produce tantalizing glimmers of new understanding of some diseases. One type of leukemia called acute promyelocytic leukemia (APL) was shown to exhibit a translocation between chromosomes 15 and 17 in the leukemia cells. This translocation was discovered by Janet Rowley in 1977. In 1984, a human proto-oncogene related to the viral oncogene, erb-A2, was mapped to chromosome 17. This oncogene is the one related to the gene for the human retinoic acid receptor that was discovered in 1987. For several years, it has been known that patients suffering from APL could be helped if they were treated with high doses of retinoic acid. (This is the only type of leukemia that responds to retinoic acid treatment.) Now, scientists in London have identified the breakpoint in chromosome 17 in APL patients as being part of the retinoic acid receptor gene itself.[20] Although the complete explanation of how retinoic acid helps these patients is still not obvious, this work fills in parts of the puzzle. It shows something specific about how a chromosome aberration that disrupts a gene that is needed for normal growth control or differentiation is directly involved in the cancer process. Scientists expect that more research in this direction will lead to additional advances in treatment of cancer. For this to happen, they must discover the biochemical functions of the other genes that are disrupted in the altered chromosomes of cancer cells.

Jorge J. Yunis' suggestion that the fragile sites that are seen in white blood cells after culturing them in the absence of folic acid might be sites which are prone to breakage, with subsequent translocations or deletions like those seen in cancer cells, has been carefully considered by researchers in cytogenetics. A collection of research reports and editorial opinions about this hypothesis was published in the journal *Cancer Genetics and Cytogenetics* in 1988.

The locations of fragile sites in the chromosomes seem not to be exactly the same sites as the cancer breakpoint sites, but the two classes of chromosome abnormalities share the same general neighborhoods in the chromosomes. Both classes occur in sections of the chromosomes that contain active genes and are rich in guanosine and cytosine. Also, culturing cells under conditions that demonstrate the presence of fragile sites produces chromosome abnormalities that appear identical to cancer chromosome abnormalities under the microscope.

Although the research is intriguing, scientists are not sure how close is the relationship between the fragile sites and the cancer chromosome abnormalities. The research suggests there is a great deal of similarity in the way these two abnormalities can happen, but the question of whether fragile sites become the chromosome aberrations in cancer cells has not been settled.

There is much current research into the details of the chromosomal translocations and the frequent involvement of oncogenes. Some translocations involve the transfer of a promoter-enhancer region from one chromosome to a different chromosome with the result that a proto-oncogene becomes activated or is expressed more abundantly.[17] The proto-oncogenes are thought to be genes that play important roles in normal growth regulation and differentiation and, when their expression is increased by a mutation or translocation, abnormal growth of a cell is the result. In most cases so far, the identity of the gene that is being studied is known only in terms of its chemical sequence—the identity of an oncogene in terms of its biological function in the cell is usually unknown or only partly understood. For instance, some oncogenes are known to produce protein products that have some function in the cell nucleus, and other oncogenes produce proteins that function near the outer cell membrane. Finding out the biological functions of the oncogenes is a major goal of researchers. This knowledge will help explain how cells respond to external signals, divide or remain quiescent, or differentiate into specialized cells.

Whether or not the chromosome mutations and translocations that produce alterations in oncogenes were the very first defect in a cell that travels down the path of the cancer process is not proven, but this type of hypothesis for carcinogenesis is very common. Chromosome abnormalities can explain how cancer can be initiated by viruses in some animal cancers, by chemical carcinogens that interact with DNA, or by spontaneous chromosome breaks arising from a lack of folic acid.

Folic acid deficiency is thought to cause DNA damage by producing deficiencies of the DNA precursor substances—purines and thymine—that must be synthesized in the cell before normal cell replication can take place. (For a human adult it has been estimated that there are twenty million cell divisions taking place in the body every second. Most of these cell divisions are in epithelial tissues and blood-forming tissues.) When the DNA precursor substances are not in good enough supply, DNA synthesis may become a little out of synchrony with the cell cycle. If the deficiency is severe, cells are arrested at the part of the cycle when they are duplicating their DNA, and this is when they are most susceptible to carcinogens. This might result in the chromosome breaks and increased mutations that have been found in cells that are deficient in thymine. Another possibility is that uracil can be incorporated into new DNA where thymine was meant to be. If the uracil is removed by a DNA-repairing enzyme, the chromosome might develop a break at this point. The recent studies on how this happens have been discussed in several articles.[13,21,22]

So, possible mechanisms through which folic acid deficiency might cause DNA damage and cancer have been thought out and are at least as plausible as are possible mechanisms through which chemical carcinogens might cause cancer. Chemical carcinogens such as benzpyrene are known to cause cancer in animals. But, even after decades of intense study of experimental cancer in animals and investigation of the interactions between chemical carcinogens and DNA, the explanation of how cancer is initiated by some of these interactions is still lacking.[23] It is now known that chemical carcinogens can interfere with methylation of cytosine in the DNA (see later section in this chapter). The carcinogens could have this effect through a variety of mechanisms, and the result would be altered gene activity in a cell.

Medical researchers have learned a great deal about the altered chemistry of the cancer cell, but the details of how the process begins are not yet proven.

Folic acid studies in animals

Animals that are given artificial diets that lack the nutrients involved with folic acid develop cancer. This was shown originally in nutrition studies in the 1940s, and it was rediscovered more recently in studies on cancer at the National Cancer Institute and also at the University of Toronto and at the University of Pittsburgh. These studies deserve our attention because of the possibility that a similar deficiency might lead

to human cancer. Compared to the many studies on vitamin A in relation to cancer in animals, there have been relatively few studies on
the connection between folic acid nutrition and the occurrence of cancer in experimental animals.

The first report of the cancer-causing effect of a low-folate diet was
published in 1946. Scientists at the Agricultural Experiment Station in
Auburn, Alabama studied the effect of choline and methionine deficiency in rats, and found cancer in 58% of the animals after eight
months. Tumors developed in liver, lungs, and several other tissues.
None of the control animals that received supplements along with the
basic deficient rations developed any tumors.[24]

Giving a diet that is deficient in choline and methionine is tanta-
mount to giving a diet that is deficient in folic acid because extra demands are placed on the body stores of folic acid. Choline and
methionine are nutrients that have methyl groups that can be used for
synthesis of other necessary chemical components of the tissues that
require a methyl group. A diet deficient in choline and methionine is
called a methyl-deficient diet.

It was mentioned earlier in this chapter that folic acid and methionine have interrelated metabolic cycles. Folic acid is required for the
biosynthesis of three of the four bases found in DNA, and folic acid
and vitamin B12 are also used in the biosynthesis of methionine from
other amino acids. These two processes can compete for folic acid. A
deficiency of any of the major players results in imbalance in the interrelated metabolic processes, and the result usually observed is an
imbalance in the DNA precursor substances, which leads to the possibility of DNA damage when cells are dividing.[22] With a methyl-
deficient diet, the tissues must synthesize methyl groups from amino
acids in order to maintain the level of methionine, and this process
puts extra demand on the body's store of folic acid, which is needed
for the enzymatic conversions to take place. As the folic acid enzymes
work harder, folic acid may be lost faster through breakdown and ex-
cretion of folate, or folic acid may be distributed through the tissues in
a different pattern. Biochemists have recently measured a sudden decrease in the amount of folic acid in the liver of rats that were put on
a methyl-deficient diet.[25] Although the reason for this sudden decrease is not yet known, it is likely related to the metabolic difficulties
imposed on the animals by the methyl deficiency.

Although the folic acid enzymes work harder, there may not be
enough folic acid present for all of the body's needs on a methyl-

deficient diet. In 1946, when Salmon and Copeland put rats on a diet that was deficient in choline and methionine, the outcome was clear. The animals had to use their folic acid to synthesize all of the needed methionine instead of using folic acid for synthesizing DNA precursors (thymidylic acid and purine nucleotides), and for the rats, this meant cancer.

When Drs. William D. Salmon and D.H. Copeland did their studies on methyl-deficient diets in 1946, the likely mechanism of the diet as producing a DNA-damaging environment in addition to fatty liver was not realized. Salmon and Copeland did notice changes in the chromosomes, however. Their microscopic examination of the tumor tissue in the rats showed unusual giant nuclei in cells as well as other obvious abnormalities of the chromosomes. They also remarked about the similarity between the pathological changes in their methyl-deficient rats and the changes that were being reported by other scientists who were studying the effects of carcinogenic hydrocarbons in rats. And yet, Salmon and Copeland were not administering carcinogens, but were simply providing a deficient diet.

Prior to Salmon and Copeland's work, it was known that choline deficiency caused cirrhosis of the liver in experimental animals. It was also known that cirrhosis of the liver and liver cancer are two diseases that are often associated in humans, for instance, in alcoholics and also in other populations who suffered from malnutrition. Salmon did his studies on prolonged choline deficiency in animals in a deliberate effort to find out whether this would cause neoplasms, and he found that it did. Salmon had also heard of some intriguing earlier work where scientists injected lecithin (a choline-containing phospholipid) directly into tumors in animals and saw a diminished tendency of the tumors to metastasize. (Related experiments have been done more recently—see later in this chapter.)

After their original studies in 1946, Salmon and his associates continued to study the effects of choline deficiency. They found many neoplasms in rats, including mammary carcinomas and sarcomas. They did a study in 1950 that foreshadowed some recent work on experimental carcinogenesis. They showed that temporarily depriving the rats of an adequate supply of protein (and thereby depriving them of methionine, the essential amino acid) accelerated the development of liver tumors, but not if the rats were given adequate choline supplement throughout the experiment. (The methyl groups of choline and methionine are easily interchangeable in metabolism; as long as one or the other of these is in good supply, the animal will not suffer from methyl deficiency if the vitamins are also present.) This experiment showed that even a temporary disruption in the supply of DNA precursors or S-adenosylmethionine—we don't know which is more important—might produce DNA damage that could accelerate formation of tumors.

(In 1950, the fact that DNA damage is a consequence of depriving the animals of essential nutrients was not yet appreciated. The scientists could see that their artificial diets produced cancer in the animals, but they did not know why. Today, scientists can detect several different types of changes in animals that are deprived of choline and methionine, in addition to the DNA damage. Examples of this are: changes in the enzymes that detoxify foreign chemicals, impaired function in some parts of the immune system, and oxidative damage in cell membranes. Choline deficiency also stimulates cell proliferation in the liver, and cells that are proliferating and, thus, replicating their DNA are more susceptible to mutation. Some scientists have speculated that these changes might be related to the carcinogenic process somehow, but I think these changes most likely play a minor role compared to the damage to the chromosomes and alteration of gene activity that can be the result of methyl group or folic acid deficiency.)

Salmon and his associates did more work on the nutritional needs of animals. They studied the effects of choline, folic acid, and vitamin B12 by varying the levels of these nutrients in artificial diets, and showed how small amounts of all three of these nutrients could keep chickens and rats in healthy condition. But when any one of these three was deficient in the feed, the animals developed several obvious deficiency symptoms that could be ameliorated somewhat by giving larger amounts of the other two. They concluded that small amounts of all three of these nutrients are required, and that the three nutrients are closely interrelated in their effects on metabolism.[26] Today, scientists understand the biochemical details of the interrelationships between these nutrients, and they are indeed complicated.

In contrast to the carcinogenic effect of the methyl-deficient diets, other studies on animals and humans have shown that folic acid and vitamin B12 sometimes caused pre-existing tumors to grow more vigorously. When folic acid was given to a few leukemia patients in the 1940s, the vitamin made the disease worse. When the vitamins were given to anemia patients, there sometimes developed an apparently new case of leukemia. Studies on leukemia in mice have shown that folic acid in the diet made the disease more severe—mice survived longer if they were kept on a folate-deficient diet.[27] The study on human leukemia in the 1940s led to the development of folic acid antagonists—drugs that have been used successfully to treat some types of human cancer by interfering with the function of folic acid. So, folic acid plays a dual role where cancer is concerned. Adequate folic acid helps prevent the chromosome damage and mutations that are likely involved in initiation of cancer and, after the development of some cancers (at least, leukemia), excess folic acid can produce more rapid tumor growth.

During the 1970s, scientists who were studying cancer induced in rats by chemical carcinogens began to test the effects of dietary variations at the same time. Epidemiological studies were showing that human cancer is associated with low dietary intake of beta-carotene and fiber and high dietary intake of fat. When the effects of these dietary factors were tested in rats in experiments that also included chemical carcinogens, one consistent result was found. This was the cancer-enhancing effect of a high-fat diet that was also deficient in choline, methionine, and folic acid.[28] Rats that were given this diet (containing 30% of total calories as fat, like a typical American diet) and were also treated with a chemical carcinogen, produced more tumors than did rats who received supplements of the methyl compounds. Even marginal deficiencies of choline, methionine, and folic acid resulted in more tumors in several tissues in rats when they were exposed to a chemical carcinogen.[29] At this point in the story, scientists thought that the deficiencies, which caused several types of damage to cells, functioned through promotion, meaning the dietary deficiencies were thought to accelerate the cancer process after it was initiated by some carcinogen. The scientists knew that giving extra choline to rats along with a chemical carcinogen sometimes resulted in no tumors, but they did not realize that the methyl deficiency could initiate the cancer process.

The study of the carcinogenicity of a methyl-deficient diet has continued into the 1980s. During the early 1980s, three laboratories rediscovered the fact that deficiency of choline and methionine produces cancer in rats, even when no chemical carcinogen is used and even if the deficiency is temporary. This is the same conclusion that came from W.D. Salmon's studies, but during the 1970s this conclusion had been put aside because of the discovery of aflatoxin. Aflatoxin is a carcinogenic compound produced by some molds that can contaminate grains and other foodstuffs. It was suggested in the 1970s that the rations used by Salmon in the 1940s might have been contaminated with this carcinogen, causing cancer in his animals. (The new suggestion did not explain how choline supplementation prevented cancer in his animals.) In any event, Salmon's conclusions suffered from undeserved uncertainty until new studies were done in the 1980s. With the more recent studies that again have shown the carcinogenicity of methyl-deficient diets, this time using rations that were analyzed and were found to be free of contamination, it has become accepted, finally, that the methyl-deficient diet alone produces cancer in rats.[29]

Lionel A. Poirier and his colleagues at the National Cancer Institute were one of the groups involved in this rediscovery in the early 1980s. They were "somewhat surprised" to find in 1983 that a diet deficient in methionine and choline caused liver cancer in rats without the use of a chemical carcinogen. Poirier had been interested in studying the relative importance of the methyl compounds, methionine and choline, and the vitamins, folic acid and vitamin B12, in counteracting the effects of chemical carcinogens. To do this, he devised a diet for animals that was completely synthetic. Instead of giving the animals natural foods, he fed them a mixture of all of the essential amino acids, along with purified carbohydrates, fat, vitamins and minerals. Using this synthetic diet, he could control the amounts of both methionine and choline that were in the diet with more accuracy than would be possible using natural foods. The synthetic diet was analyzed and found to be free of aflatoxin.

The animals remained in good health on this diet (which contained 22% of calories from fat) unless one or both of the methyl compounds, methionine and choline, was omitted. When methionine and choline were withheld, 43% of the animals developed liver cancer during the 18 months of the experiment, even when no chemical carcinogen was used. If a chemical carcinogen was used in addition to a methyl-deficient diet, even more liver tumors were produced. Some of the malignant tumors spread to the animals' lungs, and this event was more common in the animals that received the more methyl-deficient diets. In those animals that had choline and methionine in their diet but developed liver cancer anyway from a high dose of chemical carcinogen, there were no lung metastases, in contrast.[30]

Scientists at the University of Toronto found the same kind of results with methyl-deficient diets although they did not use a completely synthetic diet. Amiya K. Ghoshal and Emmanual Farber fed rats a methyl-deficient diet that was based on a mixture of peanut meal and soybean meal with other nutrients added. These proteins are both low in methionine. When they found malignant tumors in two-thirds of the rats after several months, they concluded that this must have been caused by the methyl deficiency. They had analyzed the rations for aflatoxin and found none, and had tested the rations for mutagenic activity in bacteria and found this to be very low. Like Poirier and his colleagues, they realized that the deficient diet was solely responsible for the induction of liver cancer in the animals. None of the animals that received a choline supplement as a source of methyl groups developed the liver tumors. Ghoshal and Farber realized that these findings with methyl-deficient diets might be relevant to human health problems in some populations where there is a deficiency of good-quality proteins containing methionine. They recommended re-examination of the role of dietary deficiency in the causation of cancer.[31,32]

Scientists at the University of Pittsburgh also have found that liver cancer results from a diet low in choline. Benito Lombardi and co-workers had also been studying the interaction between methyl-deficient diets and chemical carcinogens in experimental animals. After they had studied for several years the seemingly powerful promoting effect of a deficient diet when this was superimposed on a dose of chemical carcinogen, they thought to try the deficient diet alone. Their diets were semi-purified and were analyzed for aflatoxins and for several pesticides. Their results also showed that liver cancer resulted from a diet low in choline, even when no chemical carcinogen was given.[33]

Poirier and his group at the National Cancer Institute have done additional work with the methyl-deficient diets. They showed in 1984 that even a brief time on the deficient diet caused the appearance of carcinogenic changes. They gave rats a methyl-deficient and folic acid-deficient diet for only a few weeks during the beginning of a year-long study and then switched to a normal diet. This produced precancerous changes in the liver and also produced liver cancer. If a small dose of chemical carcinogen was also given at the beginning of the study, only those animals that had the methyl- and folic acid-deficient diet for a while developed cancer, and this happened in 87% of the animals. Those animals getting the small dose of carcinogen and a normal diet had no cancer or precancerous lesions at the end of the year.[34]

Poirier and his colleagues also measured the amount of S-adenosylmethionine in tissues of rats that were kept on a methionine and choline-deficient diet for a few weeks. This compound is a regulator of folic acid metabolism and it is the compound that supplies methyl groups for DNA methylation and other areas in metabolism where methyl groups are needed. Poirier found that the methyl-deficient diet had a powerful effect on the S-adenosylmethionine level in the liver, slashing the amount present. This would be expected to have many deleterious effects on maintenance of healthy tissues and might play a role in carcinogenesis.

Poirier's group went one step further with their study of the effects of the methyl-deficient diet. They looked into the question of whether feeding a diet that is deficient in methyl groups would produce a difference in the amount of methylated DNA in animals. By the time they did this study, many experiments had shown that DNA methylation was inversely related to several cancer-related phenomena that could be examined in cell cultures, but it was not known whether dietary changes would produce altered DNA in a living animal. To find this out, they fed the rats the amino acid-defined, methyl-deficient diet for several weeks. They then isolated the DNA from nuclei of rat liver. Chemical analysis of hydrolyzed DNA showed a statistically significant decrease in the amount of methyl groups on the nuclear DNA (decreased methylcytosine). And chemical analysis of the quantity of S-adenosylmethionine again showed that this intermediate was greatly altered due to the methyl-deficient diet.[35] Together, these results meant that dietary restriction of the methyl compounds can have a definite, deleterious effect on one of the mechanisms that is probably involved in regulating and maintaining normal tissues. The results did not prove that the altered DNA is responsible for the carcinogenic effect of the methyl-deficient diet, but this is one possibility.

In a later section of this chapter, we will see that the methylation pattern in DNA is thought to be more or less permanent once it is established in a tissue. In other words, it is not thought to be easily reversible. This would explain how the brief use of the methyl-deficient diet used by Poirier in the 1980s and the brief use of a low-protein diet used by Salmon in 1950 could produce some permanently altered DNA. Either mutations or methylation pattern can be permanent changes in the DNA.

In the United States, most people have plenty of protein in their diet; so deficiencies of preformed methyl groups (methionine) are probably rare, occurring only in those who have poor general nutrition. But it is possible that we do not consume enough folic acid to prevent DNA damage. Some nutritionists say folic acid deficiency is common (see chapter 12). The preformed methyl groups are easily obtained from methionine and choline. Methionine is high in good-quality protein and choline is found in liver, egg yolk, wheat germ and plant foods, or it can be synthesized by the tissues if there is extra methionine available. Even though we have enough methionine and choline in the diet, we need folic acid from vegetables, legumes, whole grains, or milk for production of the DNA precursors. The pre formed methyl group in methionine is used for methylating DNA, but it is not used for production of DNA precursors. If we have enough methionine in the diet, we do not have to use folic acid and vitamin B12 for synthesizing as much methionine, but we still need folic acid from vegetables for synthesis of the DNA precursors. The animals on methyl-deficient diets had to use their folic acid stores for synthesizing both methionine and DNA precursors, a task that was too much for the metabolic system, and the result was DNA damage.

None of the three groups that rediscovered the carcinogenic property of methyl-deficient diets reported results for folic acid-deficient diets. Poirier's group did try to test rats that were kept on a folic acid- and vitamin B12-deficient diet superimposed on choline and methionine deficiency, but the diet was too severe. The rats all died early in the study. One would like to know whether a diet that is adequate in methionine and vitamin B12 and marginal in folic acid, like a common American diet, also has a carcinogenic effect.

An ambiguous role for folic acid

The role of folic acid in pre-existing tumors is complicated and there are puzzles and possibilities that have not been thoroughly investigated. Drugs that interfere with folic acid metabolism have been used successfully to stop the growth of some human cancers and, on the other hand, folic acid and the methyl suppliers, choline and methionine, have also shown anticancer effects when tested in some animal tumors. The explanation of how folic acid could have these opposite effects is unknown; the answer may lie in the biochemical nature of different types of cancer cells. Different cell types might have different requirements for the use of DNA methylation (see later section of this chapter) in setting the cells on the right path to normal functions. A great deal of medical research has gone into the effort to take greater advantage of the antifolate drugs for cancer therapy, but very little research has been done to look into the possibility that folic acid might have a therapeutic role in some types of cancer.

It was mentioned earlier in this chapter that the folic acid antagonists were invented after trials with folic acid in leukemia in the 1940s showed that folic acid made the disease worse. Sidney Farber and his associates in Boston were the group trying folic acid. Actually, in their first series of tests, giving high doses of folic acid to advanced cancer patients with several types of cancer, their conclusions were that the vitamin was not toxic and should be studied further because it produced temporary improvements in many patients.[36]

The story goes that these researchers subsequently found that young leukemia patients were dying faster than usual while on the folic acid treatment; so Farber then tried the opposite treatment, giving folic acid antagonists. The antagonists were new drugs that were chemically similar to folic acid and were synthesized for him by the chemists at Lederle Laboratories. These drugs, being similar to folic acid, were taken up by the cells, but the drugs blocked the action of a critical enzyme in folic acid metabolism, thus causing the cells to stop growing. Farber and associates reported in 1948 that the folate antagonists produced remissions in acute childhood leukemia.[37] This was the beginning of the successful use of chemotherapy to help leukemia patients, and Farber was widely recognized for his momentous discovery.

The folic acid antagonists include the well-known drug, methotrexate. This drug has been used successfully against some types of human cancer, in particular childhood leukemia, choriocarcinoma, and epidermoid carcinoma of the head and neck.[22] Methotrexate has also been used in many studies on animals and, in some types of experiments, methotrexate gave an unexpected result, producing more tumors instead of fewer. Human patients who have been treated with methotrexate were surveyed to see if methotrexate might sometimes produce new tumors in humans, but the survey results are not consistent; so there is no proof that methotrexate causes new tumors while it helps to control the original tumor.

There has been a relative lack of good-quality studies on animals to investigate how closely the level of folic acid in the diet is related to carcinogenesis.[22] As already mentioned, some early studies on leukemia in mice showed that folic acid made this disease worse. And folic acid or vitamin B12, when given to patients with anemia, may have stimulated the growth of leukemia cells.

But other early studies using folic acid or choline had results that showed anticancer benefits from these nutrients. Long ago in 1913, when the methyl-supplying compound, choline, was first being studied, scientists at the University of California found what appeared to be a beneficial effect. They injected lecithin (which contains choline) into tumors in rats and found that the tendency to metastasize was diminished, although there was not much slowing of the growth of the original tumor.[38] (Seventy years later, Lionel Poirier's work with chemical carcinogens and methyl-deficient diets also showed diminished metastasis from choline, this time when it was obtained in the diet.)

Another early study on experimental cancer in rats produced some intriguing results in animals that were given choline in their drinking water. The choline treatment resulted in much smaller incidence of tumors after rats were injected with cells from a transplantable sarcoma, and produced disappearance of some of the tumors that did develop. This was in comparison with a large group of control animals that did not receive the choline treatment. From one-third to two-thirds of the tumors that formed disappeared in the choline-drinking rats in several experiments.[39]

A study in 1952 from the Agricultural Experiment Station in Alabama tested the cancer incidence in rats on diets that varied in protein content. All of the rats were fed a chemical carcinogen in their rations. When one group of rats was fed extra folic acid and vitamin B12, they developed tumors earlier, but this was shown to be due to their greater consumption of food and, consequently, more carcinogen. A more significant result of this feeding study was the cancer-preventing effect of a high-protein diet. The protein that was used was casein, a milk protein, which is a good source of methionine. Groups of rats that received a high-protein diet (which contained the same amount of added carcinogen as the low-protein diets) but kept to a moderate food intake, had drastically lower incidence of tumors from the chemical carcinogen.[40] As if the high-protein diet had a folate-sparing and cancer-preventing effect.

In the mid 1940s, when the chemistry of the newly discovered vitamin, folic acid, was just being worked out, doctors at Mount Sinai Hospital in New York City tested the new vitamin in mice that had spontaneous mammary carcinomas. The vitamin produced complete regression of the tumors in one-third of the animals. The experiments were repeated because of some uncertainties surrounding the different activities of folic acid in its different chemical forms. The repeat experiment showed the same result, as well as a negative result for a different form of the vitamin. Folic acid having three glutamate residues attached produced complete regression in 40% of the mice, but folic acid with one glutamate residue had no effect at the same dose and caused more rapid tumor growth at a higher dose.[41]

This intriguing effect of one form of folic acid drew the attention of cancer researchers for a time—this work was the reason for Sidney Farber's interest in giving folic acid to cancer patients—but the interest waned when it was found that folic acid made human leukemia worse. Very quickly in the next couple of years, as many doctors tried the new antifolate drugs, positive benefits were found from therapy with these drugs and there was never a good explanation offered for the beneficial effect of folic acid in the mouse breast cancer study.

In the mouse study, the folic acid compounds were injected intravenously. The type of folic acid that produced the tumor regression was the triglutamate, which is not the type of folic acid that is included in multivitamins. Multivitamins contain the monoglutamate form. The extra glutamic acid residues are normally attached to folic acid after it has been taken up by the cells. It has been suggested recently that the variable effects of folic acid may reflect the natural variation in the chemical forms of folic acid, some of which may be antagonists for the vitamin or may block the normal vitamin-transporting proteins.[42]

In recent experiments with cancer cells growing in culture dishes, it was found that depriving the cells of folic acid caused DNA damage in the cells as would be expected and, at the same time, tremendously increased the ability of the cells to metastasize after they were injected into mice, but without increasing the growth rate of the cells. Richard F. Branda and colleagues at the University of Vermont reported these results in 1988.[43] The results relate to the dilemma that is often faced by cancer patients and the doctors trying to help them. Some of the anticancer drugs, such as the folate antagonists, have the capabilty of halting the growth of cancer cells by interfering with the cells' replication of DNA, but the drugs are not 100 per cent effective; so a small fraction of the cancer cells survive and these may contain new chromosome aberrations and mutations that eventually cause the cells to continue growing with even fewer of the growth control mechanisms that operate in normal cells. The tendency of advanced cancer cells to acquire more chromosome aberrations with time is thought to be directly related to the tendency of these cells to become more malignant with time. It is not certain what causes this tendency. The use of DNA-damaging drugs is one possibility; other possibilities are the "natural history" of the cancer cells, meaning their tendency toward increased alteration, or a selection process that allows some altered cells to grow more vigorously or invasively in particular tissues.

Branda and his colleagues at the University of Vermont were interested in studying the possible role of folic acid deficiency in the cancer process. They noted that blood tests for folic acid in a series of cancer patients in 1967 had shown that most of the patients had a low blood level of folic acid. The well-known effect of folic acid in preventing DNA damage and the large amount DNA damage that is seen in tumors that metastasize encouraged these scientists to study the effects of folic acid deficiency in mouse cancer cells grown in the laboratory. Their results showed a greater tendency of the cells to metastasize if the cells were cultured in a folic acid-deficient medium for three days before being injected into mice. The DNA from the cells was also tested and showed the same characteristics—chromosome breaks and delayed DNA replication—as the DNA of blood cells that develop in a folate-deficient medium. Branda's studies tend to confirm the idea that folate deficiency may contribute to the progression of some types of cancer cells to more lethal forms, and that this may occur partly because of more damage to the DNA in the chromosomes. This type of result showing enhanced metastatic capability is also seen in experiments that use various types of mutagenic agents to treat the cells.

So, it seems that more research into the connection between folic acid and the cancer process might well yield important new information that would help us deal with this problem, not only in the field of cancer prevention, but perhaps also in prevention of metastasis. As Branda points out, there has not been much recent research into defining the role of folic acid in cells that have become cancerous. It has not been carefully ruled out that using some form of folic acid might not be useful for counteracting the cancer process at some stage after it begins. We also need more epidemiological research into the role of folic acid in cancer prevention. In this book you will find only two studies that questioned whether cancer incidence is correlated with folic acid in human diets (see chapter 11). These studies were published in 1991. Most epidemiological studies that have been completed have not tried to calculate the folic acid content of people's diets. This might yet be possible for more of the completed studies; however, not many dietary surveys have included questions about the frequency of eating legumes. The legumes (such as lima beans, lentils, kidney beans, peas and soybeans) are an important source of folic acid. Multivitamin tablets, if they contain folic acid, might be another important source for some people. The studies that show lower cancer incidence correlated with more green leafy vegetables in the diet are the most important confirmation we have for the possibility that folic acid helps prevent cancer in man.

DNA methylation

DNA methylation is another property of the chromosomes in which differences are found between tumor tissue and normal tissue. The subject of methylation is important for cancer research and for many other fields of biology because methylation of DNA is now thought to be one way the cells control the activity of the genes—methylation can determine which genes are actively transcribed and which genes are not. The research on DNA methylation is at the leading edge of cancer research where there is much excitement being generated as the researchers find out more of the details about what goes wrong with the genes during development of cancer. In the last few years, scientists have made a start at studying the connection between DNA methylation in specific genes and the presence of certain diseases.

Folic acid may help in the maintenance of normal DNA methylation through its involvement in one of the two routes in metabolism for producing S-adenosylmethionine. It was mentioned earlier in this chapter that S-adenosylmethionine is used in several biosynthetic chemical reactions in metabolism. S-adenosylmethionine is the source of the methyl groups that are added to DNA after DNA replicates. It is also the source of the methyl groups of epinephrine and creatine, the source of the methyl groups that convert phosphatidylethanolamine to lecithin, and the methyl groups that are needed in nerve tissue to prevent the permanent damage that results from prolonged vitamin B12 deficiency (see later in this chapter). In addition to supplying methyl groups, S-adenosylmethionine has a regulatory function in the cell. If its level becomes too low, there is an additional damaging effect on DNA. There are changes in activity of the folic acid enzymes which result in disruptions in the supply of DNA precursors and possible damage to new DNA.[22]

Folic acid and vitamin B12 are needed to replenish the supply of S-adenosylmethionine after S-adenosylmethionine donates a methyl group in one of its reactions. S-adenosylmethionine can also be replenished without using vitamin B12 and folic acid through an alternate route that requires a constant source of methionine from good-quality protein in the diet. The alternate route has a potential drawback in that it bypasses the only method in the cell for removing a methyl group from folic acid. The result can be a disruption in recycling folic acid. The ideal situation is to be well nourished and able to use either route to S-adenosylmethionine—the route that requires protein or the route that requires folic acid.

To summarize, it is not known whether folic acid nutrition influences DNA methylation. However, the enzymic process that methylates DNA requires S-adenosylmethionine, and the folic acid metabolic cycle is linked to that of S-adenosylmethionine. The two metabolic cycles are interrelated and do not run smoothly and efficiently if there is a defect in one of the cycles. Because of the possibility that folic acid nutrition might have an influence on DNA methylation, I will describe here some of the research in this newer area of biological and cancer research.

When Lionel Poirier investigated the tissue levels of S-adenosylmethionine and the extent of methylation of DNA in animals that had been fed a methyl-deficient diet in 1983 and 1984, several types of studies had already shown that methylation of DNA might be related somehow to development of cancer. Specifically, the chemical, ethionine, known to interfere with S-adenosylmethionine function, could be used to produce cancerlike changes in cultured cells. Another chemical, azacytidine, a nucleoside analog that cannot be methylated, can be incorporated into DNA and also causes cancerlike changes in cultured cells as well as cancer in animals. Azacytidine also causes chromosome aberrations and hypomethylation of some oncogenes. Several known chemical carcinogens, when given to animals or to cell cultures, interfere with methylation of DNA. And, DNA methylation had been tested in human tumor cells and had been found to be different from that in normal tissue.[30,44,45]

Readers who are familiar with chemistry but who are not familiar with the laboratory techniques used by molecular biologists may

wonder just what is meant by methylation of DNA and how hypomethylation of DNA is detected.

The methyl groups in question are on cytosine, one of the four bases
in DNA. The only cytosines that become methylated are those that are
followed by a guanine residue in the 5' to 3' direction. DNA is a polymer of the four deoxyribonucleotides that contain adenine, guanine,
thymine, and cytosine. The two strands of DNA in the double helix
are held together by hydrogen bonding between the pairs, adenine and
thymine, and guanine and cytosine, one of each pair residing in either
strand. Approximately 4% of the cytosines in mammalian DNA have
been converted to 5-methylcytosine. This conversion takes place after
a new strand of DNA is synthesized. An enzyme, DNA methylase,
transfers the methyl group from S-adenosylmethionine to a cytosine
residue in a new strand of DNA, at a site that is opposite a methylated
cytosine on the original DNA strand, thus preserving the pattern of
methylation that existed before DNA replication took place.[46]

The methyl group at position number 5 of cytosine does not interfere with normal base pairing or with DNA replication. The presence
of 5-methylcytosine in DNA was known in the late 1940s but not much
attention was focused on this until 1975, when two scientists indepen-
dently suggested that a specific pattern of methylation in the DNA of
a cell could be passed on to a daughter cell during cell division. This
intriguing suggestion offered a possible explanation for the heritability
of information on the activity of different genes.

The ability to study the occurrence of 5-methylcytosine residues in
DNA was greatly aided by the discovery during the 1950s of a class of
bacterial enzymes called restriction endonucleases. These enzymes
chop up DNA strands at specific base sequences and the enzymes can
be used like a chemical reagent for analyzing the methylated property
of DNA. The restriction endonucleases have specificities of different
sorts for 5-methylcytosine in certain sequences and, when DNA is
treated with one of these enzymes, the pattern of DNA fragments that
is produced depends on the presence or absence of methylated cytosines in particular base sequences. The DNA fragments produced
can be visualized after being separated according to their molecular
weights by gel electrophoresis, and different patterns of fragmentation
appear for a sample of DNA depending on the pattern of methylation
of cytosines and the particular endonuclease used.[47]

The sensitivity of this type of analysis is being improved constantly.
Using cloned individual genes or parts of genes as hybridization

probes, biologists can study the methylation pattern in specific genes from different types of tissues.

The methyl groups on cytosines regulate gene activity by changing the interactions of proteins with DNA. In some cases, binding of activating proteins to DNA is prevented and a gene does not become activated. In other cases, the possibility exists that genes may be suppressed rather than activated by DNA-binding proteins, which, in this case, would function as blocking agents to stop gene transcription. The DNA-binding proteins, also called transcription factors, trans acting factors, or nuclear receptors, are produced in the cytoplasm of the cell through the expression of other genes and migrate into the cell nucleus to bind to DNA at specific sequences. DNA-binding proteins may also be involved in stabilizing the coiled configuration of the chromosomes.

The suggestion in 1975 that methylation might be a general mechanism for controlling gene activity was remarkable in view of the fact that very little was known about the DNA-methylating enzyme in higher organisms. In bacteria, enzymes were known that could methylate DNA, and the bacterial system for methylation had a purpose— protecting the organism's own DNA from the DNA-splitting enzymes (restriction endonucleases) that were present and that were used to destroy foreign DNA that might enter the bacterium. As already mentioned, the existence of methylated cytosines in the DNA of higher organisms (both plants and animals) was known, but the reason for their presence here was a mystery. Scientists had speculated about the role of DNA in the development of a mature plant or animal from the embryo and had suggested ways that changes in base sequence in the DNA or binding of cellular proteins might control gene activity, but none of the suggestions had led to confirming experiments.

The DNA methylation hypothesis for gene regulation was put forward by Robin Holliday, a geneticist in London, and by Arthur D. Riggs, a molecular biologist in California.[48,49] The idea was presented to explain how the stability of a differentiated cell line might persist unchanged through many cell divisions—how cells that were committed, for instance, to becoming bone cells by switching off some genes and activating others might replicate and pass on to a daughter cell the same pattern of gene activation. (Each of the cells in an organism contains an identical set of genes—approximately 50,000 genes in each human cell—but a cell only uses those genes that are needed for its specific functions. Bone cells use some genes that are not used in skin cells or liver cells, and vice versa. Genes that are not needed in a particular type of cell are present but they are silent.) Methylation of DNA as a controller of gene activity might also explain the orderly progression through stages of development in a new organism, and might explain the strict inactivation of one of the two X chromosomes in the cells of female mammals.

According to Riggs and Holliday, control of gene activity by methylation could allow for heritable states of differentiation, at the same time allowing for reversibility if a mechanism existed for removing the methyl groups prior to establishing a different pattern of methylation in a cell. This control over differentiation would take place without requiring any changes in base sequence in the DNA, or mutations. It does require the existence of an enzyme that methylates a new strand of DNA as it is synthesized, at the same sites where methyl groups existed in the parent strand of DNA.

Arthur Riggs' research interests had included both gene-regulating mechanisms in bacteria, which were elucidated during the 1960s, and the puzzle of how one X chromosome in females becomes inactivated. He realized that DNA methylation, as developed in the bacteria, had some characteristics that made the process potentially useful for other purposes. Nature sometimes finds more than one use for a good idea, and methylation of DNA could conceivably be used several ways by an organism.

Riggs said in 1975 that his ideas about the methylation hypothesis were not really new, that others had thought about a possible role for DNA methylation in regulating cell activity. It is true that others had thought about the possible function of DNA methylation and had begun to study the enzyme involved and had measured the amounts of 5-methylcytosine in many species, but other than vague suggestions that DNA methylation might be related to differentiation, the tentative suggestions they made as to function were mostly wrong. Some had suggested that methylation conferred species specificity on an organism, or greatly affected the conformation of DNA, or controlled differentiation through an accumulation of point mutations of cytosine to thymine.

None of these earlier efforts to explain the function of DNA methylation hit on the real advantages of the process, which were that the pattern of methylation could account for stable differentiation by influencing the effect of DNA-binding proteins, could be heritable without requiring mutations, could be reversible, and would not have much effect on DNA conformation.

Confirmation for the hypothesis that methylation of the cytosines in DNA plays a role in controlling gene activity came from three directions in the next few years. Evidence for the existence of an enzyme that maintains the previous state of DNA methylation after DNA replicates was found in several laboratories and characteristics of the enzyme were studied.[46] The enzyme functions just as the theory predicted. Also, using analysis of methylated cytosines in specific genes, it could be shown that a gene was active or inactive in different tissues according to whether the methylated cytosine content was low (where the gene was active) or high (where the gene was inactive). In other experiments, the degree of methylation of a gene was manipulated experimentally and this resulted in altered expression after the gene was placed into cells in tissue culture.[47,50]

In 1979, Robin Holliday extended the methylation hypothesis into a new theory of carcinogenesis.[51] The sites of the methylated cytosines in DNA were thought to be most likely located in control sequences adjacent to genes. These sequences would be methylated enzymatically during cell division if the original sequence was methylated, but if normal methylation were disrupted, the activity of the genes would be altered. Some examples of how the methylation pattern could be disrupted and possibly lead to cancer were explained by Holliday in connection with DNA damage, which results from UV light or from carcinogens. The cells have well-known mechanisms for the repair of damaged DNA. One mechanism is excision repair, where a section containing the damage is cut out of one strand of the double helix and the other strand serves as template for the patch. If a section containing methylated bases is removed with the damage and DNA replication of the double helix occurs before the patch is remethylated enzymatically, the pattern of methylation would be lost in one of the daughter cells at that part of the chromosome. So, DNA damage combined with the normal cellular repair mechanisms can theoretically result in a loss of the methylation pattern and changes in gene expression. This could have minor or major consequences depending on which genes were altered.[52]

Holliday pointed out that this theory offers an explanation for two of the puzzles in cancer research. In human cells grown in tissue culture, spontaneous mutations can be detected about as often as in rodent cells grown in culture, but the human cells in culture never acquire cancerlike characteristics spontaneously, although it is common for rodent cells to do so. As if something other than mutations is involved in transformation of normal cells to malignant cells. An explanation might lie in the known differences between man and mouse in the efficiency of their excision repair mechanisms. The human cultured cells have more of the enzymes for efficiently repairing damaged DNA than the mouse cultured cells, and this is likely to result in greater preservation of the established methylation pattern and less tendency toward malignant transformation.

Also, certain experiments on transplantation of cancer cells in animals show that the transplanted cells produce different kinds of growths depending on the environment in which they are placed. As if the cancer cells still have the ability to revise their gene activities under the influence of their surroundings. In some experiments the new growths are no longer malignant. This is difficult to explain if the cells were malignant because of several irreversible mutations.

Many laboratory studies on cells have shown that the genetic expression of the chromosomes in mature, specialized cells can be reprogrammed by transplanting the specialized nucleus into a different environment.[53] This means that some alterations in genetic expression are not caused by classical mutations; although mutations, of course, can be a cause of alterations in gene expression.

During the early 1980s, many studies were done to test the correlation between DNA methylation and gene expression in animal cells. In general, it was found in most experiments that the particular gene that was under study was more active after suppressing DNA methylation by administration of one of the chemicals that interferes with methylation. Studies on animal tumors that were caused by viral oncogenes showed the oncogenes to be undermethylated in active tumors and highly methylated in silent tissues. These studies support the idea that methylation at certain sites in the chromosomes plays an important role in gene control. However, scientists do not believe that DNA methylation is the only mechanism employed by the cells to control gene activity.[44,54]

Human tumors have also been analyzed for their degree of methylation and the results show a deficiency of methyl groups on the DNA. These results contribute to the idea that tumor cells are lacking some growth control mechanisms. Hypomethylation has been detected in specific genes, in oncogenes, and in the overall 5-methylcytosine content of tumor tissue when compared to normal tissue.[55]

The first work to be published on the 5-methylcytosine content of human tumors was done at Johns Hopkins Cancer Center by Andrew Feinberg and Bert Vogelstein. These two scientists were well on their way to achieving notable success using the techniques of molecular biology to study the gene defects in human cancer. They knew that theories about cancer suggested that a variety of DNA alterations, including altered methylation, might be involved in the cancer process. They tested the DNA methylation level in recently removed, malignant tumor tissue from colon cancer patients and, for comparison, they tested normal epithelial tissue that was adjacent to the tumors. Their analysis was limited to the methylation level in three specific genes—genes that would not be expected to have any function in the lining of the colon. (Their method made use of the restriction endonucleases to chop up DNA, gel electrophoresis to separate the fragments, and radiolabeled hybridization probes to detect the three genes.) Four colon cancer patients were tested. Three of the patients showed substantial loss of methyl groups in tumor tissue and even greater loss in a metastasis.[56]

This small study showed only that some genes in the tumors might have escaped from the normal gene control system; it could not give any information as to whether the hypomethylation was involved in initiating the cancer process, or whether it was a secondary effect.

These same researchers also detected hypomethylation in an oncogene from colon and lung cancers in eight patients.[57] The oncogene that showed loss of methyl groups in the tumors was one of the ras family of genes, which are known to be involved in normal growth control of cells. These results showing hypomethylation of a gene in tumors compared to normal tissue confer practical significance on the tissue culture work on gene methylation. In cultured cells, it had been demonstrated by many workers in the early 1980s that methylation of a gene controlled whether the gene was active or inactive.

Later in 1983, a much larger study was published that showed loss of methyl groups in the DNA of human tumors. In this study, the entire DNA content of the sample was tested rather than specific genes. Melanie Ehrlich, Miguel Gama-Sosa, and a group of colleagues at Tulane Medical School had earlier devised methods for enzymatically hydrolyzing DNA down to the deoxyribonucleoside level and analyzing the bases by high performance liquid chromatography. This method enabled them to calculate the amount of 5-methylcytosine in the DNA. They analyzed 103 human tumor samples of many types, including benign tumors and metastasized tumors. They compared the results with the 5-methylcytosine content of fifteen different types of normal human tissue. The 5-methylcytosine content of normal tissues varies from one kind of tissue to another; but in this study all of the results for normal tissues were pooled, as were the results for benign, malignant, and metastatic tumors, in order to see the higher incidence of hypomethylation in the more advanced tumors. The benign tumors as a group only showed hypomethylation as often as did normal tissues, but malignant tumors were more likely to be hypomethylated, and metastasized tumors were even more likely.[58]

These scientists speculated that the greater loss of methyl groups in the more advanced tumors might be related to the usual progression of tumors, which generally shows a greater variety of cellular characteristics in the more advanced cases. They suggested that hypomethylation might be related to the other chromosomal defects that are well known in cancer cells.

In 1985, Feinberg and Vogelstein extended their study of hypomethylation in colon cancer, this time analyzing benign tumors (polyps) as well as malignant tumors. Colon cancers were used in their studies for several reasons, including the nature of the tumor tissue and the fact that it is known that colon cancers develop from benign tumors, or polyps, that could also be studied. They tested miscellaneous genes that would not be expected to be functioning in colon epithelium—in normal tissue, in benign tumors, and in cancers. They found hypomethylated genes in benign tumors and in cancer in all of the patients tested. In fact, the benign tumors had nearly as much loss of methyl groups as did the malignant tumors. This means the loss of methyl groups happened prior to the development of malignant tumors and might be involved in the initiation of the cancer process.[59]

In order to straighten out some results that differed in these last two studies (do benign tumors have hypomethylated DNA or don't they?), Feinberg (now at the University of Michigan) and Ehrlich teamed up in another study of colon tumor DNA using the best features of both of their previous laboratory methodologies. In the new study, DNA samples were analyzed for 5-methylcytosine content using high performance liquid chromatography but, instead of pooling groups of samples according to diagnosis, each tumor sample was compared with normal colon tissue from the same patient, taking care to avoid samples that contained mixed normal and tumor cells. The results showed that, as far as the 5-methylcytosine content was concerned, there was no difference between benign tumors and malignant tumors. Both types of tumors had a statistically significant loss of methyl groups on the cytosine fraction of DNA, when the samples were compared with normal colon tissue. Every benign tumor and malignant tumor tested had the hypomethylation.[60] These results show again that alteration of DNA methylation happens early in the carcinogenic process; the benign tumors had as much loss of methyl groups as did the malignant tumors.

A study on human prostate tumors also showed hypomethylation of DNA in benign prostatic hyperplasia and in metastatic tumors, in comparison with normal tissue. In this study it was not possible to do same-patient comparisons between normal and tumor samples; so the results can only be taken as a suggestion that altered DNA methylation might be involved in changes in the prostate gland.[61]

Bert Vogelstein and his coworkers at Johns Hopkins have made additional discoveries about the gene alterations in colon cancer, following up on their first studies of hypomethylation in certain genes in the tumors in the early 1980s. This group has used the latest laboratory techniques for the study of DNA with their own innovations added, along with great persistence and determination, to study and explain quite clearly the accumulation of alterations in certain genes that develops during the progression of colon cancer. Cancer researchers have been applauding this work because it provides new, partial explanations for several long-studied ideas about factors involved in cancer, on a molecular basis. Scientists concluded some time ago that malignant tumors probably develop through a stepwise, progressive series of damaging changes in the chromosomes over a period of years. They hope that knowing more about the gene defects and the normal functions of these genes will eventually lead to new treatments for cancer. Vogelstein's work has added new knowledge in this endeavor.

Vogelstein's group, as well as another group from the University of Utah, has recently studied genes on chromosome 5 that are mutated in colon cancer. This location was shown by others to be important in the rare hereditary type of colon cancer. Mutation at these genes may be early gene defects in development of all colon cancers. But it remains to be seen whether mutations on chromosome 5 are found in all colon tumors, like hypomethylation of DNA, which was found in all colon tumors tested. The biochemical functions of the chromosome 5 genes are not yet known; preliminary testing shows some similarity to large proteins that make up the cytoskeleton of the cell and similarity to proteins used in the signal-transducing ballet involving G proteins near the cell surface.[62]

Vogelstein's gene studies have touched on several other areas of cancer research. His earlier work on oncogenes in colon cancer showed that H-ras is hypomethylated and K-ras is often mutated in colon cancer, but neither of these alterations happens at the initiation of the cancer process. Vogelstein showed that the loss or mutation of a tumor suppressor gene called p53, which is located on chromosome 17, could account for the previously known common involvement of chromosome 17 aberrations in colon cancer, but that this gene alteration is one of the later events in development of malignancy rather than an early event.[63] Vogelstein's coworkers have also identified and characterized another gene that is lost or mutated in colon cancer cells. They call this gene, which is on chromosome 18, DCC for deleted in colon cancer. This is another genetic event that happens late in the development of tumors rather than early. After cloning a part of the chromosome containing this gene and doing a large amount of analysis on the gene, they determined the base sequence of the gene and the amino acid sequence of the protein that is coded. By comparing the sequence with known proteins, they showed that DCC codes for a large protein that is similar to cell surface glycoproteins that provide adhesion between cells and between cells and the extracellular matrix.[64] Cancer researchers have long known that one of the characteristics of advanced cancer cells is lack of normal stickiness. This is not the only reason that cancer cells are able to migrate from their origin, but it is one of the prerequisites for this migration.

All of this recent work on the involvement of altered genes in the basic characteristics of cancer cells is extremely important. Scientists think that most of the common types of cancer in adults probably develop through the same kind of progressive and cumulative gene alterations and chromosome defects that have been described in colon cancer. For instance, approximately half of the samples in several other types of cancer (breast, lung, and bladder) contain mutations in the p53 gene.[65] Studies of chromosome defects in breast cancer are beginning to reveal several common gene losses and changes in gene expression in the tumor tissue, using the new techniques for studying DNA.[66,67] There is much still to learn about these gene defects. The tumor suppressor gene called p53 was studied first in 1979, but its biological function in normal cells is still not known except that it produces a nuclear protein. Recent work shows that the protein coded for by this gene is a transcription factor, which means that the protein binds to DNA at some specific sequence and thereby influences the activity of some unknown gene or group of genes.

The initial events in the colon epithelial tissue that first produce benign tumors are not known—hypomethylation of DNA is the earliest gene alteration that has been found so far in small benign tumors. But this could be a critical defect. Chromosome regions that are deficient in methyl groups on cytosine are known to exhibit decondensation— that is, they are not as compactly folded and coiled.[8] Several scientists have speculated that this might lead to the chromosome aberrations involved in the cancer process or it might result in increased and inappropriate activity of some genes.

Hyperplasia in colon epithelium—that is, accumulation of extra cells—precedes formation of benign tumors and, according to Bert Vogelstein, the hyperplasia tissue does not have the hypomethylation of DNA that is observed in benign tumors. If dietary factors are involved in these early changes in the colon epithelium, one can easily imagine that a deficiency of vitamin A or of calcium might produce proliferation of epithelial tissue similar to that seen in animal studies in the 1920s. The increased cell division would require extra folic acid for efficient DNA synthesis and DNA methylation. If folic acid were deficient, either from poor nutrition or perhaps only in the local tissue or only for brief periods, DNA hypomethylation might be the result, and this might be the beginning of the chromosome abnormalities.

The mutations and gene losses that are being described in the common types of cancer have, obviously, very sobering implications for the efforts to find ways to treat cancer. It would be unwise to say that scientists will never be able to replace the genes that are lost in cancer cells—the amazing feats that can be accomplished with modern techniques of biotechnology might include this kind of treatment someday—but no one expects this to happen soon. There is greater likelihood that the gene studies will lead to new kinds of drug therapy. But speculating about these possibilities should not divert our attention from the need to avoid cancer in the first place. The dietary studies that have already been done do not offer any hope that dietary factors can reverse the cancer process after it has a good start. It is only at the earliest stages of epithelial proliferation and benign tumors that vitamins and other dietary factors might make a difference. This is why good nutrition should be our first priority in the war on cancer. If the vegetable hypothesis is correct and cancer can be prevented by good diet, prevention becomes the easiest task in the world, treating cancer remains one of the most difficult tasks.

The study of DNA methylation has recently shown another new connection with an oncogene. As already mentioned, the cytosines that are methylated in DNA are only those that are followed by guanines and this combination is abbreviated CpG. Earlier it was mentioned that the degree of methylation of one oncogene, ras, was found to be altered in human tumors; whether the function of the gene was also altered was not studied. Another much-studied proto-oncogene is myc. This gene produces a protein that has some as yet unknown function in the cell nucleus; myc inhibits differentiation. Scientists at New York University have found that the myc protein, a transcription factor that normally binds to a specific sequence in the DNA in test tube experiments, is inhibited from binding DNA when the specific sequence, which includes a CpG dinucleotide, is methylated.[68] Methylation of this particular cytosine in the DNA might thus very well have an effect on cell differentiation in animal tissues.

Scientists in France have found new information about methylation of CpG at a fragile site that is associated with a particular disease. The fragile site is related to an inherited form of mental retardation. The fragile site in question is the same one that was the subject of Grant Sutherland's original studies in 1977 when he discovered that folic acid in the culture medium prevented the appearance of fragile sites in chromosomes of cultured white blood cells. The scientists have now shown that this fragile site is also a location of altered methylation in the DNA. Patients who suffer from this condition have a methylated CpG, but carriers of the defect and normals have unmethylated CpG at the same location.[69] This discovery is not the full explanation for the disease, but it does point to a specific chromosomal marker for the unknown mutation that must be involved. The complicated genetics of this disease remain a puzzle, but with the recent progress, scientists are hopeful of gaining more understanding.[70]

Earlier in this chapter it was mentioned that scientists recently found new information about acute promyelocytic leukemia (APL). The chromosomal breakpoint in this disease occurs in a gene for a retinoic acid receptor. This happens to be another example of a connection between CpG sites and chromosome damage. The section of the gene where the breakpoint occurs contains two areas that are rich in CpG dinucleotides.[20] Whether or not methylation was involved was not determined.

The studies on DNA methylation and its relationship to specific diseases are only beginning. There are many aspects of DNA methylation that are still a great puzzle. We are left with many questions about the connections between folic acid nutrition, chromosome aberrations, methylation of CpG dinucleotides and gene activation, the association of CpG-rich sequences in the DNA and chromosome breakpoints, and the possible role of nutrition in maintaining normal DNA methylation.

Some of the basic steps in DNA methylation are not yet understood by biologists. No one knows how the genes are first methylated or demethylated during early development of the embryo. The enzyme, DNA methylase, that functions to maintain the pattern of methylation in mature animal tissues has been studied, but no one knows how the pattern of methylation of the genes is reprogrammed if necessary during development. No one knows how or why tumor cells lose some of their DNA methyl groups—there are several possible explanations. Much more study of the biochemistry of the DNA methylase reaction is needed.

We do not know how much effect deficient folic acid nutrition has on DNA methylation or on chromosome aberrations in man. Nor do we know how much effect chemical carcinogens have on DNA methylation and mutations in the average person. It is possible that either nutritional deficiencies or metabolic errors related to folic acid could be causes of chromosome defects, but the epidemiological evidence for a major role of diet in carcinogenesis favors a focus on nutrition.

What we do know about folic acid and DNA methylation in connection with cancer prevention can be summarized:

1. Folic acid, vitamin B12, and preformed dietary methyl groups are all necessary for synthesis of S-adenosylmethionine for efficient transmethylations, and for synthesis of DNA precursors.

2. In animals, a methyl-deficient diet causes cancer and DNA hypomethylation.

3. Folic acid deficiency (even brief deficiency) causes DNA damage in animals and in human blood cells.

4. Human cancer cells have hypomethylated DNA and chromosome aberrations.

What we do not know as yet: Is folic acid deficiency the cause of the altered DNA methylation or the chromosome aberrations in human cancer? Does folic acid deficiency cause cancer in animals? In man? Finding out the relative importance of folic acid nutrition in human cancer, in comparison with other risk factors, will be an interesting task for cancer researchers.

The good sources of folic acid

Folic acid is called the vegetable vitamin because it is found in appreciable amounts in a wide variety of vegetables and in legumes. It is also high in wheat germ and in liver, and it is present in smaller amounts in milk, eggs, and many common foods. Folic acid is not high in all vegetables, however, and this can present a problem if you wish to select foods that have the larger amounts of folic acid. The legumes are always rich in folic acid, and the dark green leafy vegetables are often rich in folic acid.

In recent years, the nutritional advice that appears in newspapers and magazines always says we should eat plenty of the dark green leafy vegetables and more legumes. This theme has been an important part of the recommendations from the National Research Council in their 1982 and 1989 reports on diet and health (see next chapter). The recommendation is that we should have at least five servings a day of fruits and vegetables, emphasizing the yellow and dark green leafy vegetables, and citrus fruits.

This is wonderful advice for our general health, and it will help in the prevention of cancer more than any other advice could, other than quitting smoking, if we can improve our diets in this fashion. In chapters 3 and 4 we saw that almost every epidemiological study that questioned people about the frequency of eating dark green leafy vegetables produced the result that these vegetables correlated with lower incidence of cancer. The epidemiologists think beta-carotene is probably the most important anticancer factor in these vegetables, but they astutely point out that beta-carotene is not likely to be the only anticancer factor in vegetables. Their reason for saying this is that some of the calculations indicate there must be additional anticancer ingredients in vegetables. The correlation between dietary carotene and lower incidence of cancer is not as strong as the correlation between servings per day of all vegetables and lower incidence of cancer. The epidemiologists have speculated about the identities of the other anticancer factors that must be present in the vegetables. There have been many laboratory and dietary studies on the effects of vitamin C, vegetable fiber, carotenoids, and a variety of other chemicals that are found in vegetables. But the epidemiologists have not generally been aware that folic acid is an especially good candidate for explaining the cancer-preventing effect of vegetables.

The folic acid content of foods can be determined in the laboratory by food chemists, and the U.S. Department of Agriculture includes the results of folic acid analyses in their extensive publication, Handbook No. 8 "Composition of Foods." The USDA Handbook No. 8 might be found in the public library. It consists of twenty-two volumes that are updated from time to time; so not many consumers would want to have it in their home libraries. However, an excellent paperbook book was published recently that contains a large selection of the USDA nutrient tables in condensed version. This is *Jean Carper's Total Nutrition Guide,* Bantam Books, New York 1987, and it contains the folacin contents of the foods listed.

We can spot the foods that are rich in beta-carotene by their orange color or by the dark green color of the chlorophyll that is also present in the leafy vegetables, but for folic acid there is no such simple method for distinguishing those foods that are the best choices. We are thus dependent on the food composition tables from the U.S. Department of Agriculture if we want to make a comparison of different foods for their folacin contents. In the years to come, when raw fruits and vegetables in the supermarket are labeled with the amounts of nutrients present in accordance with the Nutrition Labeling and Education Act of 1990, perhaps we will see the folic acid levels listed on these labels. The new law has the potential to help consumers determine which vegetables contain more folic acid, but it is not at all certain that the law will accomplish this.

The Nutrition Labeling and Education Act was passed by Congress in response to consumers' requests for help in acquiring information about the nutritional values of various foods. Among the innovations to be made in accordance with the new law are nutrition labels for some produce and for some raw fish. Congress decided to help educate consumers by requiring that nutrition labels be displayed near the most popular fruits and vegetables and fish when these products are sold at retail for preparation at home. The program specified by Congress for labeling raw fruits, vegetables, and fish is a voluntary one at first, and will remain voluntary if supermarkets follow the FDA guidelines for the new labels.

An unfortunate aspect of the new law is that it requires nutrient labeling not for all raw vegetables, but only for the twenty most frequently consumed vegetables in the United States and, according to research by the FDA, this does not include very many of the dark green leafy vegetables.[71] Thus, broccoli, green cabbage, and leaf lettuce will be labeled, but the nutritious green vegetables listed below will not be labeled. FDA, constrained by the deadlines imposed by Congress for setting up the new program and lacking the resources to review thoroughly all of the nutrition research, will not require any information about folic acid content on the new labels (56 FR 60880).

In time, the situation may improve. FDA will review regularly the sales figures for fruits and vegetables in the United States, and the list of vegetables that must have labels may change. FDA can also make changes in the vitamins and minerals that must be listed on the labels. Perhaps Congress will expand the program to include more of the most nutritious vegetables that consumers should know about. Or, the supermarkets can do this on their own. Supermarkets can provide information about the folic acid content of any vegetable if the nutrition label also lists the FDA-specified nutrients and if the nutrient data have been reviewed and accepted by the FDA. This type of labeling for the green leafy vegetables would certainly show their value compared to many of the more popular vegetables.

Among the dark green leafy vegetables, spinach has the most folic acid. The other familiar green leafy vegetables that are good sources of folic acid are collards, turnip greens, and mustard greens. In contrast, kale, beet tops, Swiss chard, and dandelion greens are low in folic acid although they are rich in beta-carotene.

A variety of other popular vegetables are good sources of folic acid. These are artichokes, asparagus, green beans, beets, broccoli, Brussels sprouts, bok choi, cabbage, cauliflower, corn, okra, parsnips, and winter squash. The folic acid contents vary considerably among these vegetables. Asparagus and Brussels sprouts are rich in folic acid; cabbage and green beans are somewhat lower.

Only a few of the fruits are good sources of folic acid. Fruits that contain folic acid are avocado, banana, blackberries, boysenberries, cantaloupe, loganberries, oranges, plantain, raspberries, and strawberries. These fruits vary in their folic acid content. They range in value from 13 micrograms of folic acid in one-half cup of strawberries to 56 micrograms in half of an avocado.

The legumes are all very good sources of folic acid. Various types of legumes have been popular foods in different parts of the world for centuries. They go by different names in different regions. In Europe, legumes as a group are called pulses and in India they are called grams. The mung beans that originated in India and the soybeans that originated in eastern Asia are legumes, as are chickpeas (garbanzos) that are common in India and the Near East. Lentils from the Near East and black-eyed peas (cowpeas) from the southern United States are very good sources of folic acid. So are lima beans and peas (but not the peapods).

In the United States, the most familiar legumes besides peanuts are the common beans, *Phaseolus vulgaris,* that are native to Central and South America and were introduced into Europe by the early explorers of the New World. Different varieties of *P. vulgaris* are known as black beans, great northern beans, kidney beans, pink beans, navy beans, pinto beans, and white beans.

Approximately one-half cup of one of these legumes—that is, about 100 grams, measured after boiling and draining—will provide from 50 to 200 micrograms of folic acid, depending on the type of legume. The current RDA for folic acid in the United States is 200 micrograms. (See chapter 9 for discussion of RDA and its significance.)

Soybeans are used in several forms in our food supply, and they are a very good source of folic acid—whole soybeans that is, that have been roasted or boiled. Tofu, made from soybeans, is very low in folic acid; but the fermented soy products, natto and tempeh, are rich in folic acid.

Soybeans are important in the Chinese diet, where the beans are processed different ways to make derivative foods, such as soy sauces, bean curd or tofu, and bean sprouts. According to USDA Handbook No. 8-16, soybeans are rich in folic acid, but bean curd is almost devoid of folic acid. The tofu loses folic acid during the processing. Some areas in China have high rates of cancer, and epidemiologists in China are investigating the role of dietary variables in cancer risk. If the scientists were to include soybean in its various forms in the diet surveys, they might discover whether whole soybean products have an advantage in reducing the risk of cancer.

We have many other sources of folic acid in our diets besides vegetables and legumes. Other sources of folic acid are egg yolk, liver, wheat germ, grains, milk, and multivitamins. Milk and grains are low in folic acid compared to the vegetables and legumes, but if you consume enough of these items, they do contribute to your folic acid nutrition. I have calculated my own daily intake of folic acid using several one-day food records and the food composition tables, and I find that my usual quart of milk a day and four slices of whole wheat bread contributes about one-third of my total dietary folic acid.

In the United States, the average dietary intake of folic acid is estimated to be 280 to 300 micrograms per day.[72] This was calculated from the folic acid content of the food supply in the United States, according to U.S. Department of Agriculture data of 1988.

Considering its wide distribution in foods, it might seem odd to suggest that we should be concerned about getting enough folic acid in our diets. The problem of low-folate diets arises because of the low popularity of many of the best food sources of folic acid and our frequent failure to follow the recommendation to have at least five servings a day of fruits and vegetables. There are many people who seldom eat beans, milk, wheat germ, yeast or liver, and many who avoid eating eggs. There are others who assume they are eating a good diet if they have one serving of vegetable a day and one piece of fruit. This is generally not enough to provide the vitamins needed. If the vegetable is sauteed zucchini with tomatoes and the fruit is an apple, you have added only 25 micrograms of folic acid to your diet. If the vegetable is cooked spinach and the fruit is an orange, you have had 170 micrograms—much better.

The small amounts of folic acid that are found in most foods do add up during the day, but it is important to consume a variety of good foods to improve your chances of getting the folic acid and other nutrients you need. When I calculated my own folic acid intake from some of my usual daily diets, I found it to be close to the amount predicted by the U.S. Department of Agriculture 1988 data. (This was before I had begun eating more beans.) But my diet is quite varied and rich in nutrients due to my longtime interest in nutrition and my determination to consume less than two thousand calories a day. I am concerned about people who have not followed the dietary guidelines and have not made the effort to plan variety into their meals. There are several good ways to make sure you get enough vitamins. You can educate yourself about nutrition, or you can take a good multivitamin tablet occasionally, or you can eat a good variety of foods. If you can do all of this, you will surely be ahead of the game. I suspect that if nutritionists and government agencies provided more details in their publications about the interesting biological functions of the nutrients in our foods, we might make more of an effort to follow the dietary guidelines.

The RDA for folic acid has been the subject of some disagreement among the experts because of uncertainties in some aspects of folic acid utilization. The RDA for folic acid was set at 400 micrograms per day for normal adults in 1980. This was calculated from studies on volunteers where different doses of pure vitamin were given daily for several weeks while the blood levels of folic acid were being monitored. A dose of 100 micrograms per day maintained the blood level in the normal range. After allowing for cooking losses and incomplete absorption, the RDA was set at 400 micrograms. This explains why multivitamins that include folic acid contain 400 micrograms (see also chapter 9).

In 1989, the Food and Nutrition Board changed the RDA for folic acid after reconsidering several older studies and some recent studies on folate requirements. They still think that 100 micrograms per day, in the form of a pure supplement, is adequate for adults. But after allowing for absorption losses from foods, the RDA was set at 200 micrograms per day for men and 180 micrograms per day for women (or 3 micrograms per day per kilogram of body weight).

This RDA is supported by a dietary study where forty men lived in a metabolic ward for six months and consumed a controlled diet that averaged about 3 micrograms of folic acid per day per kilogram of body weight (or about 200 micrograms of folate per day).

According to this RDA, 200 micrograms per day on the average is a completely adequate intake of folic acid from foods for a person who weighs 67 kilograms, or 148 pounds. But what about the person who weighs 220 pounds (100 kilograms)? Should this person be consuming 300 micrograms per day on average? Yes, absolutely, this would be the prudent thing to do. One of the more mysterious risk factors that has been found in some epidemiological studies of breast cancer and colon cancer is a higher risk of developing cancer in those individuals who have larger body size. It seems reasonable that larger people, who have more cells in their bodies and, therefore, more cell divisions every day in the normal course of the continuous regeneration of many tissues, would require more vitamins and minerals as well as more calories and protein than smaller size people. More cell divisions may be necessary for the larger individual, but this automatically imposes greater risks because cancer only begins in cells that are dividing. If the folic acid intake is too low, some of the cell divisions may produce new cells with damaged chromosomes and this could lead to harmful mutations. In the United States, the average folate intake is about 300 micrograms a day, enough to supply the RDA, but there will be some who consume more than this and some who consume less. I wonder if those who consume less than the RDA are the same people who develop cancer.

Folic acid is not toxic. This was shown during the 1980s at the University of Alabama where women were given high doses of folic acid for four months in a study of nutritional remedies for cervical dysplasia. The women took 10 milligrams a day of folic acid, which is fifty times higher than the RDA, and had no ill effects from the vitamin.[73] Such high doses would be unwise and unjustified for normal, healthy people. There are some people who should definitely avoid taking high doses of folic acid, because of the possibility of serious consequences. Folic acid interferes with the absorption of a drug used for epilepsy; so epilepsy patients should be warned about this.[72] Strict vegetarians—those who avoid eating milk products and eggs—would run a serious risk if they took high doses (more than one milligram per day) of folic acid without taking the vitamin B12 that they need to compensate for avoiding animal foods. A long-term lack of vitamin B12 can produce degeneration in the nervous system and permanent paralysis, as well as megaloblastic anemia. If folic acid were to be consumed without any vitamin B12 in the diet, the megaloblastic anemia would not develop, but the nerve degeneration would continue to develop silently and irreversibly.

A few of the dietary surveys have questioned people about whether they took a multivitamin tablet, and there has not been found much correlation between multivitamins and cancer rates. Until recently, multivitamins did not contain beta-carotene and even now they usually contain only ridiculously small amounts of beta-carotene (see chapter 9). But with 400 micrograms of folic acid in a multivitamin tablet, one would think this would provide some measure of protection against the chromosome damage that is detected in human cancers. A few minutes of browsing through the multivitamins in two local drugstores showed me a possible explanation. I was shocked to find that many brands of multivitamins do not contain any folic acid. At one drugstore, I found nine brands (not counting the children's brands or those meant for pregnant women) and only three of these contained folic acid. At another drugstore, there were twenty-seven different formulations of multivitamins or B complex with vitamin C, and eight of these had no folic acid. This is a rip-off of consumers who may have thought they were buying some bargain-priced health insurance. So, be warned: multivitamins are not all alike.

Comparing the folic acid intakes in the United States and Puerto Rico with the rates of cancer incidence in these two countries shows some interesting contrasts. In Puerto Rico, the overall cancer rates are low compared to the United States and the folic acid intake is high. Beans are a popular item in Puerto Rican diets. It is not unusual for people in Puerto Rico to have a serving of beans every day. A good variety of vegetables and fruits is also available. Fat in the Puerto Rican diet is about 35% of total calories—about the same as in the United States—and vitamin A intake is just barely adequate. Puerto Rico experienced rapid improvements in economic development beginning around 1950 and since then, meat and dairy products have become an important part of the average diet. Beef is popular and also pork, chicken, and codfish.[74] Rafael Santini and Jose J. Corcino found that a typical diet in Puerto Rico contains from 1300 to 2300 micrograms of folic acid per day—several times higher than the estimate for the United States. This was from actual chemical analysis of cooked foods. Dieticians at the University of Puerto Rico prepared the meals for typical Puerto Rican diets, and the food was analyzed for folic acid.[75] The work was only meant to give some background information on the amounts of several specific nutrients in the Puerto Rican diet before the scientists proceeded to more specialized nutrition studies, but this report certainly should stimulate more inquiries into the folic acid contents of various people's diets. To date, the information on the high level of folic acid in the Puerto Rican diet has been neither confirmed nor refuted—the study has been largely ignored.

The specific types of cancer that occur much less often—with half the frequency, or less—in Puerto Rico than in the United States include cancer of the lung, colon, breast, ovary, pancreas, bladder, kidney, and prostate. Lymphoma and leukemia are about half as common in Puerto Rico as they are in the United States.[76] In Puerto Rico, a cancer registry was established in 1950 to track the frequency of different types of cancer in the island. A comparison was made between Puerto Rican data and a national cancer survey in the United States (covering seven cities and two states where cancer registries also operate) for a three-year period around 1970. In Puerto Rico, colon cancer was only 26% as frequent as in the United States. Breast cancer was only 40% as frequent as in the United States. And prostate cancer was 50% as frequent as in the United States.

In other parts of Central and South America, cancer rates are also much lower than in North America and Europe. The International Agency for Research on Cancer, based in France, sponsors epidemiological research on cancer and calculates estimated incidence rates for different parts of the world. According to recent IARC estimates, Central America (Mexico, Costa Rica, Panama, and other countries) has a combined rate of incidence for sixteen types of cancer that is only one-fifth as high as the combined rate in North America. (The native corn and beans of Central America are both good sources of folic acid. Might the low incidence of cancer be related to a high average intake of folic acid in the diet?) In Brazil, the most popular dish is a tasty stew called feijoada made with black beans, beef and pork, and usually eaten with a side dish of collards. According to the IARC estimates, this part of South America has cancer rates that are only half as high as the overall rates in North America.[77]

There are many possible explanations for differences such as these between countries in their rates of cancer incidence. The amount of folic acid in the diet should be considered as one of the possible explanations. For instance, it might be worthwhile to find out whether the diet in Finland is high in folic acid, perhaps due to rye bread and berries. The Finns have a high-fat diet and low rates of cancer, and scientists have wondered whether the Finns' high fiber intake from unrefined, coarse rye breads might be responsible for the low cancer rates. But fiber may not be the explanation—rye grain is a good source of folic acid.

In previous chapters I have mentioned the scientists' question about whether beta-carotene is the cancer-preventing factor in vegetables, or whether other factors in the vegetables might be the true cancer-preventing ingredients. Our study of folic acid involvement in the integrity of the chromosomes and the involvement of folate-related nutrition with cancer in animal studies provides good reason to suspect that folic acid is very likely involved in preventing mutations, chromosome damage, and cancer in man. Folic acid may be equally important with beta-carotene for cancer prevention. Studies that might address this possibility through dietary surveys are only now beginning to be planned and carried out. At present, we simply do not know which of these vegetable factors plays the stronger role in prevention of human cancer. Folic acid may help to prevent the chromosome abnormalities that may be involved in the initiation of cancer, and beta-carotene probably plays a secondary role by promoting differentiation and by suppressing proliferation in epithelial tissues. The result is a synergistic cancer-preventing effect from these two important vitamins.

Chapter 11

Five Servings a Day

Someone at a party asked me, "What are your favorite vegetables?" I answered, "Broccoli, kale, carrots, and lettuce." My friends knew I was writing about the value of vegetables and I was telling them about some of the recent studies on diet and cancer. Given a little more time to think, I would have to include a few others on my list of favorites. I would include cabbage, Brussels sprouts, green peppers, Swiss chard, beet tops, mustard greens, sweet potatoes, peas, corn, tomatoes, butternut squash, collards, and spinach.

I have been paying a great deal of attention to the amount of vitamin A in my diet for the past twenty years, but studying the epidemiological evidence for a role for vegetables in preventing cancer has made me even more aware of my daily vegetable consumption. I have started counting the number of servings I eat each day. The National Research Council strongly recommends at least five servings a day of fruits and vegetables, emphasizing the yellow and green vegetables and citrus fruits. One serving consists of approximately half a cup of most fruits or vegetables.[1] In my case, it required only a little extra effort to have five servings a day. Taking the time to peel and eat an orange in midmorning and sometimes taking the time to prepare an extra vegetable with dinner did the trick, because I was already in the habit of eating quite a lot of vegetables, both raw and cooked.

Cooking and eating well have always been among my favorite pastimes. I have long derived particular pleasure from my weekly trip to the supermarket. Choosing the produce I will need for the week is a treat, a fun outing, and such a bargain. The selection of luscious vegetables in our supermarkets all year round would have amazed my grandparents, who did not live in a time when planes and refrigerated trucks helped supply the produce section. I am like a child in a candy store when I pick out the vegetables I want and I have to keep reminding myself that I can only eat three meals a day and more vegetables will be here next week.

I mentioned Swiss chard as one of my favorites. Swiss chard is not available often in my supermarket, but I grow my own. Three plants keep me well supplied from July through November. Collard greens is another good vegetable for home gardens, as the plants produce continuously and can still be harvested after a frost. These greens and the others—spinach, kale, beet tops, mustard greens—are so nutritious, they should be eaten several times a week. They should be boiled only briefly in a small amount of water to avoid losing or destroying very much of the folic acid.

In addition to my favorite vegetables, I also buy onions, mushrooms, zucchini, eggplant, celery, parsnips, rutabaga and several others for preparation of my favorite dishes and for variety, but I don't regard these "second tier" vegetables as being especially valuable for nutrition. Rather, I use them for flavor or fiber or garnishes. Lest anyone feel provoked to quibble, I am well aware that tomatoes, squash and many other vegetables that contain seeds are really fruits, botanically speaking, but I choose to use the everyday designation of vegetables as the U.S. Department of Agriculture does in its publications.

The U.S. Department of Agriculture publishes a large amount of information on the composition of foods in handbooks that might be available in your library. Much of their data is also compiled in tables in some of the popular paperback books on nutrition that are widely available in bookstores. See the list of suggested readings at the end of this chapter.

U.S. Department of Agriculture Handbooks No. 8-1 through 8-22 are updated every few years as new data become available, and the handbooks are one of the most authoritative sources in the world for this type of information. The handbooks contain information on nine vitamins and nine minerals as well as amounts of protein, carbohydrate, fats, calories, water, ash, fatty acids, cholesterol, and amino acids in all classes of foods. The handbooks list these components of vegetables in all their normally consumed forms—raw, boiled and drained, canned, and frozen.

Are frozen and canned vegetables equally as good for you as fresh vegetables? Yes, they are, generally speaking. This can be seen in the USDA handbooks, which contain nutrient data for many vegetables in the raw state and also for the same vegetables after cooking, canning, or freezing.

What about organically grown vegetables? Some people believe that organically grown foods are free of pesticides or that they are more nutritious in some way, but neither of these beliefs is really correct—Nature's way of growing plants ignores such misinformed ideas. Organically grown vegetables are grown on composted fields without the use of chemical fertilizers or pesticides, but plants—including those plants that we use as food—produce their own natural pesticides which become part of our regular diet.

The purpose of organic gardening is to prevent deterioration of good soil or to improve the quality of inferior soil by returning composted plant material and manure to the fields. There is always tremendous interest from farmers and agricultural scientists in finding better farming methods, and composting benefits the soil so much that it seems that all farmers who try composting like the results. The exuberant growth of well-nourished plants is a joy to every farmer and gardener who provides adequate nutrients for the plants.

Composted soils contain a greater number of beneficial living things because the soil contains more humus (partly degraded plant material). The living plants and animals in the soil—the algae, yeasts, protozoans, mycorrhizae, and earthworms—help supply the farmer's crops with minerals and water by breaking down the organic humus into the mineral forms that can be used by plants. Aeration is improved by earthworms, and the mycorrhizae (a type of fungus) grow in contact with the roots of plants and transmit water and minerals into the roots. Farmers find that composted soils have better mechanical properties, allowing easier plowing in the spring and better water retention in dry spells. But crops grown on composted fields are no more nutritious than chemically fertilized crops. This is because all of the components of the plant tissues are synthesized within the cells of the plant according to its natural genetic blueprint. The crops will be as nutritious and disease resistant as their genes allow as long as they obtain the necessary minerals and water in the proper amounts. The nutritive qualities of a vegetable can vary with different growing conditions and mineral fertilizers, but whether the minerals came from compost and manure or from chemical fertilizers does not matter to the plants. This is why organically grown foods do not have any direct advantage for the consumer.

When plants have high levels of disease resistance, it is often because Nature has endowed them with the ability to poison their attackers, the grubs and insects. These plants have evolved complex mechanisms for synthesizing toxic chemicals which have helped ensure the plants' survival through eons of seasonal onslaughts by Nature's hungry hordes. Doesn't it follow that the workings of evolution—survival of the fittest—have provided us the most toxic plants—the best survivors—to use as our daily bread?

How do we and the animals survive if we must eat the natural pesticides in plants? Well, there are many plants that we have to avoid. For the rest, we unknowingly rely on our own detoxifying enzymes, which are synthesized in many of our tissues, especially the lining of the intestinal tract and the liver. Our cells contain many enzymes that convert noxious foreign chemicals and drugs into water-soluble derivatives that can be easily flushed out of the body. These enzymes are well known to biochemists in the pharmaceutical industry, who must find out the details of how the body gets rid of a dose of a new drug. The reason we have these enzymes is to enable us to get rid of toxic chemicals that are produced during our own metabolism *and* to get rid of the toxic chemicals produced by the plants we eat. An example is the enzyme called polycyclic aromatic hydroxylase, which is produced when we eat cruciferous vegetables and which works to detoxify many noxious chemicals found in foods. The detoxifying enzymes have been part of our metabolic machinery for much longer than chemists have been around, busy devising drugs to help treat various diseases.

The vegetables grown in Hunza were analyzed for their nutrient content in the 1960s because of the legendary good health of the Hunzukuts. Chemists at the West Regional Laboratories in Lahore, Pakistan analyzed cereals, legumes, and vegetables from Hunza and found the Hunza foodstuffs to be similar in nutrient content to Pakistani and British foods. No special qualities were found in the foods from Hunza.

The Hunza foods analyzed were the grains barley, buckwheat, millet and wheat; the legumes lentils, linseed, poppy and sesame; and the vegetables lettuce, turnips, coriander, and the important group of

Mustards called *Brassica oleracea*. In the United States we grow several varieties of *B. oleracea* including kale, cauliflower, broccoli, cabbage, collards, kohlrabi, and Brussels sprouts. These and other *Brassica* species such as turnips, mustard greens, mustard spinach, pak-choi, and rutabagas are all members of the group called cruciferous vegetables. Most of the cruciferous vegetables are good sources of folic acid and the dark green members of the group are good sources of beta-carotene as well. Cruciferous vegetables also contain small amounts of non-nutritive chemicals that can be shown to inhibit cancer in laboratory studies. These include the indoles, flavones, and isothiocyanates, all of which have been studied from time to time since the 1960s. These chemicals have been shown to either stimulate production of enzymes that convert toxic chemicals to less toxic forms or interfere with the reaction of carcinogens with DNA.

In previous chapters we reviewed some of the epidemiological evidence that what we eat has an effect on the development of cancer of many types. Many of the epidemiological studies showed an apparent protective effect associated with milk in the diet, but did not offer any conjecture on the mechanism. Whole milk contains vitamin A in both of its forms—retinol and beta-carotene. The amount of beta-carotene in milk depends on the feed of the cows, and the ratio of retinol to carotene depends also on the breed of cow. A quart of milk in a day provides approximately 40% of the Recommended Dietary Allowance of vitamin A. Milk also contains folic acid, which is a difficult vitamin to measure; the folic acid content of a quart of milk is thought to be about 50 micrograms, or approximately 25% of the RDA. Milk is also the best source of calcium and vitamin D. Some researchers are investigating whether calcium or vitamin D might play a role in preventing colon cancer and breast cancer. Epidemiological studies have shown this connection. The magnitude of the calcium effect and the possible mechanisms for a calcium effect in preventing cancer are being studied by a few scientists at the present time.

In previous chapters we saw evidence that beta-carotene and, in addition, other vegetable factors that have not yet been completely identified have a protective effect against carcinomas, including adenocarcinomas. We saw evidence for a protective effect of vitamin C against carcinomas of the upper digestive tract and of the cervix. We saw some evidence that fried and grilled meats are probably carcinogenic. Most of our foods have been analyzed for their nutrient content, but the chemistry of foods is incredibly complicated. We cannot be sure which of the nutrients and which of the non-nutrient chemicals such as indoles or fiber are the most important anticancer ingredients in fruits and vegetables. This is why we should not expect to obtain all of the necessary vitamins from supplements. All of the evidence we have so far points to the value of a variety of vegetables in the diet for prevention of most types of cancer.

In the study on lung cancer in New Jersey, eating vegetables more than 2.4 times a day was associated with only half as much lung cancer as eating only one serving a day of a vegetable.

In the Los Angeles study on lung cancer in women, eating carrots three times a week cut the risk of lung cancer by one-third compared to seldom eating carrots.

In the Hong Kong study on lung cancer in women, eating fresh fruit at least once a day was associated with one-half as much risk for lung cancer as seldom eating fresh fruit. Eating more carrots and leafy green vegetables also was associated with lower risk.

In Japan, daily consumption of green or yellow vegetables reduced the risk of dying from lung cancer, stomach cancer, or prostate cancer.

People over sixty-five in Massachusetts who had the highest scores for fruits and vegetables in their usual diet had only one-third the mortality rate from cancer compared to people who ate little fruits and vegetables.

Bladder cancer was twice as common in low vitamin A eaters as it was in high vitamin A eaters at Roswell Park. Eating more carrots or drinking more milk also correlated with lower risk.

In Washington, DC there was a significantly reduced risk for cancer of the esophagus in men who ate plenty of fresh meat or fish, fruits and vegetables, and dairy products compared to men who ate these foods less often. Risk reduction was achieved by eating three to six servings per day of fruits and vegetables.

In Milan, Italy the risk of cancer of the esophagus was related to carotene intake. Those with carotene intake approximately equal to the RDA level had less than half as much risk for cancer as those with low intake of carotene.

Ovarian cancer was only half as likely to occur in women who had high amounts of beta-carotene in their diets as it was in those who had low levels of carotene intake, in studies in Utah and at Roswell Park Memorial Institute.

Abnormal conditions of the cervix were found with two- or three-fold higher frequency in women who had low levels of beta-carotene in their diets than in women with higher levels of beta-carotene in the diet, in a study in the Bronx.

Consuming a high level of vitamin A (more than the RDA) from fruits and vegetables reduced the risk of breast cancer for women over fifty-five years of age in the Roswell Park study.

In the Athens, Greece study on breast cancer there was a ten-fold difference in risk between the highest and lowest quintiles for frequency of eating a variety of vegetables.

In Italy, eating eight servings per week of green vegetables reduced the risk of breast cancer by more than half compared to eating less than seven servings per week, but the correlation between beta-carotene and reduced risk was not as strong as the correlation between green vegetables and reduced risk.

In Buffalo, NY eating vegetables twice a day was associated with only half as much risk of colon cancer as eating a vegetable only once a day. Raw vegetables were especially good.

In Israel, reduced risk of colon cancer was associated with more frequent consumption of several fruits and vegetables.

In northern Italy, lower risk of colon cancer was associated with eating more green vegetables, tomatoes, melon, and coffee; and in Marseilles lower risk was associated with eating more vegetables, cooking oil, and milk.

In Sweden, pancreatic cancer was associated with frequently eating grilled foods and seldom eating carrots and citrus fruits.

New epidemiological studies continue to turn up in the medical journals. In Melbourne, Australia an eight year-long, population-based study on diet, drinking, and incidence of colorectal cancer was carried out beginning in 1979. Australia has a high rate of colorectal cancer, but there is not much variation in the dietary customs in the country; so it is difficult to determine whether certain dietary factors are related to illness. But if a large enough group of people can be studied with sufficient detail, then it becomes possible to look for statistically significant differences even though the population is mostly homogeneous in their style of eating.

The researchers at the University of Melbourne interviewed more than seven hundred people with colorectal cancer and an equal number of age- and sex-matched people from the community about their diets.

They collected frequency and serving size estimates for three hundred food items used in Australia. The overall average of vitamin A in the diet was just about equal to the RDA level.

Subjects were divided into quintiles according to their consumption levels of the various foods. Foods that were found to be related to lower risk of colorectal cancer were: total fiber if it was combined with high vegetable consumption, vitamin C, total vegetables, and cruciferous vegetables. This was another study that showed a protective effect from vitamin supplements—supplement users having only one-third the risk of colorectal cancer as non-users. Foods that were not related to risk included fats, carbohydrates, vitamin A from animal foods (retinol), meats, eggs and cereal.

The Melbourne study did show some positive association between high fat in the diet and higher risk for colorectal cancer, but the results were not clear cut and only showed up after adjustments were made for meat and vegetable consumption. In contrast, the protective effects of a high-fiber, high-vegetable diet were very clear from the data.

> Gabriel A. Kune et al., "The Nutritional Causes of Colorectal Cancer: An Introduction to the Melbourne Study," *Nutr. Cancer 9*, 1 and 21 (1987).

The idea that high fiber in the diet might actually be related to lower risk of colon cancer, like the idea that a high-fat diet might be related to higher risk, had its origins in comparisons of countries with differences in cancer incidence and dietary habits.

The fat hypothesis came from analysis of international data collected by the United Nations during the 1960s which showed striking correlation between the mortality from colon cancer or breast cancer in a country with the per capita consumption of fat for that country. Countries where a lot of fat was used were also the countries where there was more colon cancer and breast cancer. However, the fat hypothesis for cancer causation has not held up for all types of cancer in the types of studies we have seen in this book where the diets of large groups of individuals are inspected and compared with cancer incidence.

Many studies have been done to find out whether fat intake by individuals correlates with the occurrence of colorectal cancer or breast cancer, and the results have not been consistent. In breast cancer, some studies have found a weak positive correlation but just as many studies have found no correlation or an inverse correlation.[2,3,4] The most recent reviews on this question conclude that fat in the diet has not been proven to be related to risk of breast cancer—see also chapter 14.

For colon cancer and cancer of the ovary or endometrium on the other hand, most studies have shown higher risks for those individuals who have more fat in their diets, but at the same time, the studies show lower risks from consuming more vegetables. It appears that fat in the diet is not the major culprit that it appeared to be from the international statistics—there must be other factors present in those countries that have a high-fat diet which are equally responsible for the higher mortality from these types of cancer.

The fiber hypothesis, however, which also started from international observations has held up somewhat better than the fat hypothesis through many epidemiological studies on the diets of individuals. Many studies on fiber have found some protective effect from dietary fiber, although the effect of fiber is not always very pronounced. (Neither fat nor fiber in the diet is as consistently correlated with cancer incidence as is total vegetables.)

The importance of fiber became apparent from reports on cancer incidence in Africa. Several papers appeared during the 1950s and 1960s describing the types of cancer seen in hospitals in different parts of Africa. Colon cancer accounted for only 2% or 3% of all the cancer cases seen at the hospitals, making colon cancer very rare in the rural communities. A British doctor, Denis P. Burkitt, questioned the hospitals further to verify this fact during the next few years. His conclusion that the ten-fold lower rate of colon cancer in Africa, compared to the highly developed Western countries, is due to a large amount of fiber in the diet has been widely read and discussed since 1971. Although he did not study the diets of individuals, he believed that the high incidence of colon cancer and other bowel diseases in the developed countries is due to a diet containing too much refined food such as flour from which the bran has been removed and not enough fiber.

Burkitt's conclusions echo the fifty years earlier exhortations of Sir Robert McCarrison, whose contacts with the people of Hunza had so impressed him with the importance of unrefined foods for maintaining freedom from bowel ailments.

How could dietary fiber, or roughage as we used to call it, help prevent colon cancer? The modern-day, proposed explanations involve such things as bulkier stools when there is a lot of fiber in the diet which would dilute any carcinogens that might have been produced by bacterial action on bile acids, for instance, making it less likely that a molecule of carcinogen could come in contact with the mucosal lining of the colon. It is also well known that more fiber in the diet helps speed the transit of feces through the intestines, which might have a similar effect by reducing the amount of carcinogens produced by bacteria. Or, the custom of eating a lot of foods containing roughage might result in a different spectrum of bacteria that normally reside in the large intestine. All of these ideas are merely speculations which have been given some consideration and study during the past twenty years. In any event, a high consumption of fiber, vegetables, and bran are doubtless of great benefit for long-term better health. As Burkitt remarked in 1971,[5] whether or not we know the exact mechanism whereby an environmental factor, in this case dietary fiber, helps to limit a disease is less important than the knowledge that it does! With this knowledge we have the power to improve our diets and our health prospects.

The realization that dietary fat has relatively little influence on development of cancer in humans is a recent event in the long struggle to find out whether and how dietary factors have any influence on this disease. The fat hypothesis is well known and has been discussed and tested for twenty-five years or more, but for most human cancers the possible role of dietary fat is still uncertain. Also, a great deal of laboratory research has been done with mice and rats fed different types of dietary fat, but this avenue of research has also yielded results that are difficult to relate to human situations.

What we have here is an example of the difficulties in searching out the answers to human health problems. The fact that cancer incidence at different sites in the body is very low in some countries and perhaps ten times higher in other countries is one of the strongest arguments behind the statement that environmental factors have a powerful effect on the development of cancer. Exactly what it is about the different environments in these countries that has this effect is the mystery we need to solve. The newest research consistently points to our need for large amounts of vegetables for preservation of our health throughout our hoped-for threescore and ten.

The newer research in the epidemiology of cancer that has turned up in the medical journals lately includes some additional studies on diet in relation to ovarian cancer and cervical cancer. In Milan, Italy a case-control hospital study on ovarian cancer was done during 1983-86. Dietary interviews were completed in addition to medical and gynecological histories. The scientists found several statistically significant associations between diet and ovarian cancer, the strongest correlations being with green vegetables and with meat. Higher consumption of green vegetables—eight or more servings per week—was associated with reduced risk, compared to less than seven servings per week. More frequent meat eating—seven or more servings per week— was associated with increased risk, compared to less than four servings per week. Eating wholegrain bread or pasta was related to reduced risk, and eating more butter was related to increased risk.

Carlo LaVecchia et al., "Dietary Factors and the Risk of Epithelial Ovarian Cancer," *J. Natl. Cancer Inst. 79*, 663 (1987).

The same group of researchers at Albert Einstein College of Medicine in the Bronx who reported more frequent abnormalities of the cervix in women whose diets were low in beta-carotene have done a more recent study, this time analyzing blood samples for beta-carotene and for retinol. When they compared the average beta-carotene levels for the various diagnostic groups, they found a very striking and highly significant ($p < .0001$) trend in the beta-carotene levels. Normals had the highest blood level, mild through severe dysplasias had lower levels, and cervical cancer patients had the lowest level, which was only one-third as high as the beta-carotene level in normals. The implication of all this is that low beta-carotene level in the blood is a risk factor for developing cancer of the cervix. Retinol was also analyzed in the blood samples. The circulating level of retinol in most well-nourished people is thought to be controlled by homeostatic regulatory mechanisms and, in fact, the circulating retinol levels were the same in all of the diagnostic groups in this study.

Prabhudas R. Palan et al., "Decreased Plasma beta-Carotene Levels in Women with Uterine Cervical Dysplasias and Cancer," *J. Natl. Cancer Inst. 80*, 454 (1988).

Other groups of researchers in Birmingham, Alabama[6] and in London, England[7] have also found lower levels of beta-carotene in the blood of patients with cervical cancer or preinvasive disease. These results do not prove that beta-carotene is the only protective factor from foods, because other protective factors such as folic acid and vitamin C can be found in some of the foods that are good sources of beta-carotene. Blood samples would have to be analyzed for all of these vitamins in studies of this type to find out which vitamin is more important. The researchers in Birmingham, Alabama did analyze blood samples for folic acid and they found that it was below normal, but their patients all had advanced disease. A large study in Latin America[8] has found that more vitamin C and beta-carotene in the diet are related to lower risk for cervical cancer, but folic acid in the diet is not related to risk.

The epidemiologists in Milan, Italy who have been studying the relation between diet and nineteen types of cancer during the 1980s have published a summary of their findings regarding the value of vegetables. Their summary shows three important points which are in nice agreement with the observations by scientists in various other parts of the world over the last few years. They find that there is a long list of specific carcinomas for which the risk is definitely lower in those individuals who consume larger amounts of green vegetables. While fruit is also associated with lower risk of some cancers, especially in the upper digestive and respiratory tracts, the protective effect of fruit is not as strong and widespread as that of vegetables. And, they find that there is another group of specific types of cancer that is not associated with low intake of fruit and vegetables. The diseases not related to fruit and vegetable intake were cancers of the non-epithelial, lymphoid tissues, lymphoma and myeloma.

The cases and controls who had been interviewed for all of the previous studies in Milan were combined and divided into three groups according to their usual frequency of eating green vegetables—less often than once a day, averaging one serving a day, and averaging more than one serving a day.

For all of the carcinomas (cancers of epithelial tissues) in the study, risks were found to be significantly lower in people who usually had more than one serving a day of green vegetables compared to those who ate less than one serving a day. The risk reduction was especially large for cancers of the upper digestive tract, the prostate gland, and the bladder. For instance, those in the top third for green vegetable consumption, who averaged more than one serving a day, had only one-fifth the risk of liver cancer as those in the bottom third, who ate green vegetables less than once a day. For several other types of carcinomas such as pancreas, colorectal, ovary, kidney, and thyroid the risk reduction was about one-half. For breast cancer the risk reduction was statistically significant, but was only about one-third. The scientists were impressed with the consistently strong risk reduction that was associated with eating more green vegetables, even though they could not decide which of the many possible explanations for the effect will ultimately be the most important explanation.

Eva Negri et al., "Vegetable and Fruit Consumption and Cancer Risk," *Int. J. Cancer 48*, 350 (1991).

Two recent studies on colorectal cancer, published in 1991, have produced the first epidemiologic evidence that folic acid from foods can lead to lower risk for cancer in man. The studies were done on people living in two very different environments: the western part of the state of New York, and the island of Majorca in the Mediterranean.

In New York state, epidemiologists from the State University of New York at Buffalo had conducted lengthy interviews with cases and controls a few years earlier, during 1975 to 1986. Some of their original findings were described in chapter 4. These scientists later became interested in the possibility that folic acid might play a role in cancer prevention. They had become aware of the several avenues of research that show that a deficiency of folic acid can produce abnormal DNA synthesis and possibly also, impaired DNA methylation. Another reason for their interest in folic acid was a recent clinical study on patients with colitis that demonstrated that folic acid supplements protect these patients against precancerous changes in the colon.

To find out whether folic acid intake was related to risk for colon cancer or rectal cancer, the epidemiologists reviewed their earlier studies and made additional calculations. They calculated the amounts of several specific nutrients in the diets of their sixteen hundred subjects by making use of food composition tables, and estimated the calorie intakes of the subjects. For colon cancer they did not find any significant risk reduction associated with more folic acid in the diet, but for rectal cancer there was a statistically significant trend in lower risk associated with more folic acid in the diet after adjusting for calorie intake. Those subjects in the highest quartile for folic acid consumption, who consumed more than 385 micrograms per day, had only one-third the risk for rectal cancer as did those who consumed less than 250 micrograms per day. The risk reduction was not really specific for folic acid, as carotenoids, vegetable fiber, and vitamin C—which are found in many of the same foods that contain folic acid—were also related to lower risk for rectal cancer.

The epidemiologists suggested that more such studies on the possible correlation between folic acid intake and incidence of colorectal cancer should be carried out. Many people in the United States have a low intake of folic acid due to the low popularity of vegetables in the American diet, and this might produce DNA damage in some tissues, especially in the lining of the gastrointestinal tract where new cells are constantly being produced at a high rate.

Jo L. Freudenheim et al., "Folate Intake and Carcinogenesis of the Colon and Rectum," *Int. J. Epidem. 20*, 368 (1991).

A study on diet and colon cancer in the island of Majorca has produced specific evidence that folic acid from foods is associated with lower risk of cancer in man.

Majorca is an island in the Mediterranean and is part of Spain. The population is about 600,000. A case-control study was done during the 1980s using a dietary questionnaire that asked about the frequency of eating ninety-nine food items. The participants in the study were well nourished and consumed a high-fat diet, most of the fat being from olive oil. Fruit, vegetables, meat, white bread, fish, and dairy products are important parts of the diet. Legumes are part of the diet but are not eaten every day. The average intake of folic acid is 194 micrograms a day.

When the different food groups were analyzed for statistical association with risk of colon cancer, meats were found to be associated with increased risk and cruciferous vegetables were associated with decreased risk. Having a cruciferous vegetable daily gave one-half the risk of either colon cancer or rectal cancer compared to never eating these vegetables. Fat (mostly olive oil) was not related to risk, but a local pastry made with lard and eggs was related to increased risk.

Following up on their analysis of the various food groups, the scientists decided to calculate the amounts of specific nutrients in the participants' diets. Using food composition tables, they calculated the amounts of calories, protein, different types of fats, different types of fiber, and vitamins and minerals. Like many other studies on colorectal cancer, they found higher risks associated with higher calorie intakes. They also found that fiber in the diet was related to lower risk, and fiber from legumes (pulses) was associated with the greatest risk reduction of any of the twenty-nine specific nutrients that were calculated in the individual diets. After controlling for total calories in the diet as well as for age, sex, and weight, those who were in the top quartile for consumption of legumes had only four-tenths of the risk for colorectal cancer as those in the bottom quartile. This was in spite of the legumes not being a major part of the diet. The average amount of fiber in all of the diets was about fifteen grams a day, and legume fiber accounted for only 5% of this. (The other sources of fiber were vegetables, grains, and fruit.)

Folic acid was the only one of the seventeen vitamins and minerals calculated in the diets that showed a statistically significant trend of lower risk from higher intake. Folic acid in the diets came from both legumes and cruciferous vegetables. To my knowledge, it is only in 1991 that scientists have begun to test the hypothesis that folic acid might help prevent cancer in man. This epidemiological study in Majorca showing significant protective effects of folic acid and legumes should encourage more scientists to study the correlation between dietary folic acid and risks for other types of cancer. The scientists who worked on this study may have included folic acid in their list of nutrients to be calculated because of the clinical study that showed folic acid supplements can protect colitis patients against precancerous changes in the colon—more about this in chapter 14.

> E. Benito et al., "Nutritional Factors in Colorectal Cancer Risk: A Case-Control Study in Majorca," *Int. J. Cancer 49,* 161 (1991).

The scientists who have labored over these studies that I have described here so briefly and uncleverly are actually well aware of the potential value of their work for preventing one of the most serious chronic health problems of our time. They have even gotten together to do a little shouting from the rooftops—albeit in their own style.

In 1989 the Committee on Diet and Health of the National Research Council in Washington, DC published the opus, *Diet and Health: Implications for Reducing Chronic Disease Risk,* wherein a committee of nineteen leading scientists carefully reviewed the interrelationships between diet, health, and chronic diseases and made nine specific recommendations that Americans should follow.[1]

The committee was pulled together in 1984 by the Food and Nutrition Board, a division of the National Research Council, and given the job of analyzing all the newer pertinent studies on diet and health in order to evaluate the strengh of the evidence for associations between diet and health and to help Americans distinguish between fact and fallacy in dietary recommendations. Dietary guidelines from many authoritative sources have been published repeatedly during the past twenty years. Various groups from different countries have mostly given very similar recommendations, especially in regard to cutting down on animal fats and avoiding obesity.

The new committee was made up of nutritionists, epidemiologists, and experts in a variety of biomedical fields from universities and the NIH. Several of the nineteen have long been involved in some of the studies in this country that I have reviewed in this book and others have been involved in research on metabolism of fats, vitamins and other nutrients, or on the mechanisms involved in disease processes. Their mission was to set up standards for the evaluation of scientific studies on diet and health, and to use these standards to assess the evidence on diet in its relation to health, and then to suggest dietary guidelines that might help reduce the risk of chronic diseases.

Chronic diseases are those that usually develop over a period of time and turn into long-term conditions that require regular medical help. The committee focused its work on *all* of the major public health problems in the United States where diet is suspected to play some role. These problems are atherosclerosis, cancer, high blood pressure, osteoporosis, obesity and eating disorders, diabetes mellitus, liver-gall bladder disease, and dental caries.

The committee members tackled a very large job when they set out to review the scientific literature on the relation between diet and health. There are thousands of published studies in this field on both humans and experimental animals. The committee held several workshops where they listened to suggestions and opinions from other scientists as to what topics should be covered, listened to newer ideas and controversial data, and heard a variety of points of view. They studied the original data in the published studies and also considered earlier government reports on diet and health.

The standards they decided on for evaluating scientific studies are perfectly reasonable. They realized that international comparisons can provide clues to disease mechanisms but do not inform as to how important a dietary factor might be for individuals. What they looked for in evaluating scientific studies was consistency in the findings from various studies, the strength of the association between a dietary factor and incidence of disease, dose-response relationships, and biologic plausibility.

After three and a half years of work, the committee concluded there was strong enough evidence to make a number of recommendations to the American public. As the committee says in their final recommendations, " . . . although much remains to be learned . . . it would be derelict to ignore the large body of evidence while waiting for absolute

proof of benefit from dietary change. . . ." Before making their recommendations, they considered the degree of uncertainty in various
possible conclusions and the amount of risk engendered if people were
to alter their diets, compared to the potential benefits that might be
gained—for instance, would consuming more fiber interfere with intestinal absorption of minerals? According to the best available knowledge, following the committee's recommendations should not impose
any new risks to health. Their report, *Diet and Health: Implications
for Reducing Chronic Disease Risk,* explains their final recommendations in detail, with extensive discussions of how their recommendations should help the public health in many ways and should not
produce any negative effects. There is no better place to find a thorough analysis of the evidence for the effects of diet on the chronic
diseases.

What does the committee recommend? They make nine specific
recommendations. The recommendations are deliberately designed to
be quantitative; that is, definite numbers of servings or percentages or
grams of salt or protein are listed rather than indefinite suggestions to
merely cut down on salt or fats or to eat a variety of foods. This should
enable people to get a better idea of how well they are following the
recommendations.

The first and most important recommendation is to reduce total fat
intake to 30% or less of calories, and to reduce saturated fatty acid
intake to less than 10% of calories and keep cholesterol intake below
300 milligrams per day. This can be accomplished by choosing low-fat
meats and dairy products, by substituting fish and skinless poultry for
fattier meats, by eating less high-fat baked goods and fried foods, and
by eating more vegetables, fruits, cereals and legumes.

This first recommendation confirms the rules we have heard for
twenty years now. The concern about too much total fat and too much
saturated fat in American diets comes from their proven association
with cardiovascular diseases, heart attacks, and obesity. The committee explains their recommendations about the various types of dietary
fats in a most thorough and readable discussion that should be of great
interest to much of the public.

The second most important recommendation is to eat five or more
servings per day of vegetables and fruits, especially green and yellow
vegetables and citrus fruits. At the same time, increase starches and
complex carbohydrates to six or more daily servings of bread, cereals,
and legumes.

A "serving" of a vegetable generally means one-half cup. A serving of cooked cereal, fruit, or legumes is also about one-half cup. (Examples of legumes are lentils, lima beans, baked beans, kidney beans. A serving of beans can be counted as a serving of carbohydrate *and* as a serving of vegetable.) One slice of bread or one roll or muffin counts as one serving.

The committee did not mention whether white potatoes should be counted in the five servings per day of vegetables and fruits. White potatoes are a good source of complex carbohydrate (starch), akin to bread, pasta, rice, and cereals. White potatoes should be counted as a serving of starch, not as a serving of vegetable. Sweet potatoes, however, are so rich in beta-carotene that they should be counted as one of your vegetables and also as a serving of starch.

The remaining seven recommendations in the 1989 report will be mentioned here only briefly.

The committee recommends that total protein intake should stay about where it has been and should not be increased further. The average American diet already includes more protein than is usually needed, although there may be some individuals, most likely the elderly, who don't eat enough protein. The advantages to long-term good health from having a near-ideal weight are many. The committee recommends maintaining normal weight by balancing food intake with physical activity. They do not recommend alcohol, as many chronic diseases can result from excess alcohol. Salt should be limited to no more than six grams a day (as sodium chloride) in order to help avoid the common problem of hypertension. (This is the same as 2360 milligrams a day of sodium.) Calcium intake should be maintained at the RDA level; and fluoride intake, either from properly fluoridated water or from supplements, should be continued in order to avoid tooth decay.

The committee acknowledged that a large percentage of Americans take multivitamins on a regular basis, but since there are virtually no proven benefits or drawbacks from this practice, they recommend that, if vitamins are taken, the amount taken daily should not exceed the RDA level.

The Committee on Diet and Health believes that their nine recommendations have the potential to greatly reduce the risk of many chronic diseases. They also stated their confidence that these dietary changes are well within our ability to accomplish within our current life style, even though the nine rules will mean quite a few changes in diet for many people. They know that the American people have already made many improvements in their dietary habits during the last twenty years, and today we are better informed and more widely interested than ever before in nutritional matters.

Suggested Readings in Nutrition

1. Food and Nutrition Board, National Research Council, *Recommended Dietary Allowances, 10th Edition,* National Academy Press, Washington DC 1989. Concise, readable, updated information on all known nutritional needs of young and old, growing children, pregnant women and most healthy people. Explains how RDAs are set and discusses those situations where uncertainties exist.
2. Jean Carper, *Jean Carper's Total Nutrition Guide,* Bantam Books, New York 1987. Contains the U.S. Department of Agriculture data on nutrient content of 2500 common foods and includes fruits and vegetables, mixed dishes, lunch meats, popular fast foods and boxed cereals. Explains how nutrients work in the body and discusses recent research.
3. Robert H. Garrison, Jr. and Elizabeth Somer, *The Nutrition Desk Reference,* Keats Publishing, New Canaan, Connecticut 1990. Describes basic nutrition and recent research, with references and discussion. Written for both general readers and health professionals.
4. Patricia Hausman, *Foods That Fight Cancer,* Warner Books, New York 1983. Diet advice from a nutritionist, based on the dietary guidelines for preventing cancer. Contains cooking tips and recipes.
5. Susan Finn and Linda Stern Kass, *The Real Life Nutrition Book,* Penguin Books, New York 1992. Written by a nutritionist to explain how busy people can follow the dietary guidelines. Includes lively advice on shopping, understanding labels, weight control, and managing stress.
6. Adelle Davis, *Let's Eat Right to Keep Fit,* Signet, New York 1970. The classic, popular book about nutrition and the links between diet and health. The food composition tables are from old editions of the USDA handbooks, but the stories remain profoundly important for our nutrition education.

Chapter 12

Do We Eat Enough Vegetables?

Government surveys show that, on the average, women in the United States have one serving of vegetable each day and one serving of fruit or fruit juice. This is far short of the fruit and vegetable intake that is recommended, and this low intake of fruits and vegetables by many Americans might very well be the explanation for the high rates of cancer incidence in this country. Fortunately, there is a lot we can do to change this situation and, with some planning and a little effort aimed at improving our diets, we should be able to turn the statistics around and improve our prospects for avoiding this disease.

The small quantity of vegetables in the diets of many Americans probably has several explanations. The hectic pace of modern life contributes to some of our health problems. We are often forced to take shortcuts in household chores, including meal preparation. When pressed for time, we are likely to postpone making home-prepared meals, where vegetables might be included automatically, and instead make use of convenience foods, snacks, or fast-food restaurants. None of these alternatives to home cooking puts much emphasis on vegetables.

In the rather short period of a few recent decades, the life style and eating habits of many families have changed. We use many more convenience foods today than our grandparents did as food suppliers have put literally thousands of new, often highly processed, food items into the supermarkets. We have easy access to sugary, refined grain, fatty desserts and high-calorie, low-nutrient convenience foods that satisfy the appetite briefly but do not provide as much vitamins and minerals and fiber as do meals that are prepared from unprocessed foods.

Even enriched wheat flour (white flour) is deficient in vitamins and minerals as a result of processing. We consume much of this product without realizing that we are missing part of the nutrients we should be getting from wheat. The designation "enriched wheat flour" is federally sanctioned and goes back to 1941 when this product was first defined. In 1941, knowledge of nutrition was much less sophisticated than it is today—some vitamins had not been discovered and the effects of deficiencies were not as well known. According to modern nutrition, this product would be better named today as "deficient wheat flour." The milling of wheat to produce white flour removes the bran and wheat germ and variable amounts of vitamins and minerals at the same time. The "enrichment" process adds back three B vitamins and iron (sometimes calcium is also added), but the enriched wheat flour remains deficient in vitamin B6, folic acid, pantothenic acid (another B vitamin), vitamin E, magnesium, and chromium because these nutrients are not added back. This is the reason nutritionists recommend whole grain products rather than refined grain products. As we shall see, the recent government surveys on diet show that American diets are usually deficient in vitamin B6, folic acid, and magnesium. This deficiency could be partly overcome by choosing whole wheat products whenever possible.

Enriched wheat flour is the main ingredient not only in most bread and rolls, but also in most of our pasta, noodles, doughnuts, cookies, cakes, and the like. There have been no improvements in the "enrichment" process since 1941. Why not, after fifty years of nutrition research? Roger J. Williams, the distinguished biochemist from the University of Texas who spent his entire long career in nutrition research, said in 1971 that it was a disgrace that the flour and baking industry had made no effort since 1941 to improve the nutritional quality of its product. Williams contrasted this strange behavior with the continuous advances in other industries such as communications, transportation, textiles, and coatings.[1] Although the 1941 plan for enrichment of white flour was reasonable at the time, it has long been outdated. Williams hoped that a better-informed public would realize that better-quality foods are necessary for our cells to have a healthier internal environment. Today, an informed public should be aware that deficiencies of magnesium, chromium, and vitamin E have been linked to heart disease and hypertension in newer research, that deficiency of chromium is also linked to diabetes, that vitamin B6 is needed in protein metabolism and in folic acid metabolism, and that folic acid might be important for the prevention of mutations. A grain as nutritious as wheat has been the prize of civilizations since the beginning of history. Because of the knowledge that is now emerging about folic acid, vitamin B6, and minerals like chromium and magnesium, it is high time for us to switch back to the healthier forms of the wheat that mankind has so long treasured. Knowing a little about nutrition makes it easy to choose whole wheat products rather than deficient white flour products as a prudent step toward better nutrition.

According to *Nutrition Desk Reference,* only half of the calories consumed in the United States come from whole grains, fruits and vegetables, lean meats and legumes, and milk products. The other half of our calories are from sugars, white flour and other processed grains, and fats—all of which are low in vitamins and minerals. Even if you are sufficiently active to be able to eat a lot of the high-calorie foods without gaining weight, your body requires vitamins to carry out the metabolism of these high-calorie foods. Consuming a lot of high-calorie, processed foods without taking the vitamins that are needed for metabolism contributes to malnutrition by putting a drain on the body's stores of vitamins.

There are other reasons for our low intake of vegetables besides time constraints. Everyone has heard by now the recent recommendations to consume more vegetables, but there exists a certain amount of public skepticism about the scientists' abilities to determine exactly what changes in our habits and our environment are truly needed to make an appreciable difference in the cancer statistics. We have heard over the years a variety of stories about the causes of cancer. Many of these stories have been exaggerated in the news media in order to exploit an emotional subject. Some stories have continued for years as investigators have tried in vain to find proof that some environmental factor such as pollution causes cancer in man. It is not easy for the public to decide which news reports are trivial and which should be taken seriously; the body of evidence that supports the reports is not usually described. For each new story about something that "causes" cancer, it must be remembered that the true explanation for this disease will have to be compatible with some well-known facts. The facts are that the cancer problem has existed for thousands of years and, in our society, one out of four people develops cancer at some time. The available records tell us that, except for tobacco-related cases, the age-adjusted mortality rate for cancer has changed very little since the early years of this century.

Now, since the early 1980s, government agencies and private organizations are offering some genuine, good advice. They are advising us to improve our diets for better health, and one of their recommendations is to eat more vegetables of certain types to help prevent cancer. The public must decide whether or not to accept this advice. Some of us have already accepted this message and have adopted the habit of including more fruit and vegetables in our diet, but many others will remain skeptical about the new recommendations until they have the opportunity to read some of the background information and until they hear additional explicit advice from authoritative sources. Health professionals could help by including advice about diet in all of their routine contacts with patients.

Another reason for slighting the vegetables in our diets is a lack of education about nutrition. Many people would welcome reliable information on nutrition and the importance of good diet for staying healthy, but acquiring this education in nutrition is not easy. Much of the diet advice we see every day is in the form of advertising, or comes from special-interest groups or incomplete news reports. This kind of advice should always be considered carefully for one-sidedness and to see whether the advice is compatible with good nutrition practices. We sometimes see unfounded ideas being offered to the public under the guise of advice for better nutrition, but not all of the advice is based on good nutrition or on good studies.

Government agencies aim to help educate the public about nutrition. A helpful publication is entitled *Nutrition and Your Health: Dietary Guidelines for Americans.* This important little pamphlet contains all of the basic dietary advice most people need. It was prepared for the Department of Agriculture and the Department of Health and Human Services by a committee of nutrition experts. The pamphlet gives clear advice about diet without going into the details of nutrition research. The pamphlet is available free for the asking. You can write to: Nutrition and Your Health, Dietary Guidelines for Americans, Consumer Information Center, Pueblo, Colorado 81002 to request a free copy. How much more convenient it would be if this pamphlet were available in the supermarket or other public places. The public has made it clear to our lawmakers that we desire more nutrition information—witness the new law, the Nutrition Labeling and Education Act of 1990—but there seem to be unnecessary obstacles to distribution of the nutrition information that is available.

The U.S. Department of Agriculture has a longtime, traditional concern with the dietary habits and nutritional status of the American population. The USDA began taking national surveys in 1935 to find out what Americans eat. In the 1930s, the main reason for the surveys was the economic question—the aim was to find out what economic resources were required to feed a family in different parts of the country, and what general quality of diet was achieved. So, the surveys only asked what foods were brought into the household and they did not inquire about what the individual family members actually ate. Eventually, the surveys were deemed useful by the USDA for their mission of nutrition education and ensuring the availability of a nutritious diet for Americans. In the 1960s, the surveys began to focus on the foods consumed by individuals because of the increasing demand for information on the relationship between diet and health.

The USDA surveys have continued on a regular basis. By means of personal interviews and telephone interviews, the surveys attempt to record everything that was eaten by a participant on the day before the interview. Representative samples of households are selected from all regions of the country, from all economic levels, and from both urban and rural areas. The households are contacted by trained interviewers who are nutritionists or home economists, who explain how the survey works and invite participation. The USDA surveys aim to complete four days of diet information for each participant, with the four days spaced at two-month intervals in the most recent surveys. Surveys are designed to study three types of people in particular—women between the ages of nineteen and fifty and their small children, low-income women in the same age group with small children, and men. The interviewers collect information on household income, size of household, what foods are eaten away from home, and other information that might be related to their general health.

These surveys by the USDA are called the Nationwide Food Consumption Survey and the Continuing Survey of Food Intakes by Individuals. The U.S. Department of Health and Human Services also has completed some nutrition surveys, with medical exams and blood tests included. These are called the National Health and Nutrition Examination Surveys (NHANES). NHANES I covered 1971-1974; NHANES II was done in 1976-1980; and NHANES III will run from 1988-1994.

There are many uses for the data gathered in these surveys.[2,3] The data can serve as a foundation for maintaining and improving the nutrition education of the public, as scientific background for programs to fortify certain foods, as a means for identifying groups who are at high risk for deficiencies, and for describing and understanding the wide variety of dietary patterns in the United States. The surveys are used for economic research and market research by government agencies and the food industry. Government agencies depend on the surveys to help them design school lunch programs and food stamp programs. The dietary surveys are also the basis for the FDA study called the Total Diet Study, where the FDA analyzes foods for pesticide residues, industrial chemicals, and minerals. The FDA purchases foods in different parts of the country in the same stores used by consumers and in accordance with the food patterns described by consumers in the USDA surveys. The foods are analyzed several times a year.

So, the diet surveys are valuable for several kinds of research efforts in the fields of public health and nutrition education. At the same time, there are limitations to the conclusions that can be drawn from the surveys.[4] The diet surveys often show low intakes of some nutrients by some groups but, because of individual variation in requirements, it is difficult to predict whether this has damaging effects on these people. The RDAs are the commonly used standard for nutrient intakes, but RDAs are deliberately set about 30% higher than the amount needed by the average person (see chapter 9). Nutritionists often use a lower standard—perhaps seven-tenths of the RDA level—when they calculate how many people in a survey consume an amount of a nutrient that probably meets their needs. There are other types of uncertainties surrounding the results of the surveys such as questions about whether the survey is truly representative of the population that is investigated and whether the nutrient intakes can be accurately calculated from the food intakes that are reported.

Although nutritionists face many difficulties when they try to interpret the surveys, they believe the surveys should continue. The surveys are not as accurate or complete as desired and they do not answer all the questions that nutritionists might have, but they can be used for many purposes. The surveys can be used to monitor trends in dietary habits that might be related to public health. For instance, the U.S. Department of Agriculture survey of 1965 showed that some nutrient intakes had declined from ten years earlier due to declines in consumption of milk, vegetables, and fruit. Educational efforts by the Department were then stepped up to try to reverse this trend.[3] Another reason to continue doing dietary surveys is a continuing need for information about certain groups. Nutritionists say there is still a lack of information on dietary habits of the poor, of migrants, and of people in institutions, as these groups have not been properly represented in the surveys to date.

Although it is difficult to assess the adequacy of nutrient intakes for individuals by studying the diet surveys, the average nutrient status for large groups of people can be estimated from the surveys. The surveys usually produce concern among nutritionists rather than complacency. This is because the typical American diet appears to be deficient in several vitamins and minerals. The surveys show that some groups, most often women, seldom consume recommended amounts of the nutrients they need. The nutrients that are usually thought to be too far below the RDA are folic acid, vitamin B6, magnesium, calcium, iron and zinc. In the Nationwide Food Consumption Survey of 1977-78, only 20% of the participants consumed vitamin B6 at the RDA level and only 25% consumed magnesium at the RDA level. Forty-three per cent consumed iron at the RDA level.[4] The majority of those surveyed were below the RDA levels for these nutrients.

A joint committee of the Department of Agriculture and the Department of Health and Human Services prepared a report for Congress in 1986 covering the nutritional status of Americans as far as could be determined from the surveys up to 1980. They recommended continued investigation of several nutrients because some groups appear to have low intakes or else because not enough data are yet available to draw conclusions about our nutrient status. The nutrients they thought should continue to be monitored are vitamin C, vitamin B6, folic acid, calcium, iron, fluoride, magnesium and zinc.[5] The committee concluded that vitamin A intake appears to be adequate but, of course, they meant the total vitamin A intake which, in the United States, is more than half retinol and less than half beta-carotene.

A recent USDA survey, part of the Continuing Survey of Food Intakes by Individuals for 1985-86, showed that the average American woman has slightly more than one vegetable serving per day and slightly more than one serving of fruit or fruit juice.[6] Not counting white potatoes, the average intake of vegetables was 118 grams, or a little over half a cup, and the intake of fruit or juice was 119 grams. Not surprisingly, 70% of the women consumed less than RDA levels for seven of the fifteen specific nutrients that were calculated in their diets. This was found in all income groups and all regions of the country. The seven nutrients that appeared to be low in the average reported diets were vitamin E, vitamin B6, folic acid, calcium, magnesium, iron and zinc. As already mentioned, being below the RDA level is not necessarily dangerous because of people's different requirements and because the RDAs are deliberately set about 30% high. What really matters is how far below the RDA the habitual intake is for an individual. The farther below the RDA level is the intake of one of these essential nutrients, the more likely it is that a deficiency will develop that could contribute to a chronic disease. In reading these USDA reports, one should keep in mind that some RDAs have been changed since the diet surveys were analyzed. The RDA for folic acid has been cut in half since 1980 and the RDA for vitamin B6 has been reduced by ten to twenty per cent. So, comparisons of average intakes of a nutrient with RDAs can become obsolete. Nevertheless, the data on absolute quantities of vegetables and nutrients in diets remain valuable.

If the average American woman has only two servings a day of fruits and vegetables combined, it is easy to understand why we could develop chronic diseases that are vitamin related. Even if the two servings were chosen carefully from a good knowledge of nutrition, it would be very difficult to obtain the recommended amounts of the vitamins from only two servings. Increasing the fruits and vegetables to five servings a day makes it easy to get enough vitamins, if we emphasize the deep yellow and green leafy vegetables. In this survey from 1985-86, the deep yellow and green leafy vegetable intakes averaged only 15 grams per day, out of the total vegetable intake of 118 grams. So it appears, sadly enough, that we have not paid enough attention to the most valuable vegetables such as spinach, broccoli, mustard greens, carrots and sweet potatoes that we should be eating every day.

The USDA survey calculated the amount of folic acid in the women's diets and the average intake was 189 micrograms per day. At first glance this might seem reassuring because the current RDA for folic acid is 180 micrograms for women. But averages also mean that approximately half the population studied will be above the average and half will be below the average value. In the case of the women's folic acid intake, 65% had intakes of folic acid that were less than 200 micrograms per day (excluding intakes from vitamin supplements). Twenty-five per cent of the women had intakes of less than 124 micrograms of folic acid per day (these are the 25% who are jeopardizing their chromosomes), and 10% reported intakes of less than 95 micrograms per day (very dangerous indeed). So the diet surveys do explain why nutritionists are concerned about Americans' diets. The surveys clearly demonstrate that nutritional deficiencies can be found even in a land of plenty.

The amount of vitamin A in the women's diets was 23% higher than the RDA, on the average, but again a sizable fraction of the diets were far below the average value. Twenty-five per cent of the women had only half the vitamin A in their diets that is recommended. And only about one-third of the total vitamin A consumed was in the form of beta-carotene. Two-thirds of the vitamin A was from foods where the vitamin A is mainly retinol such as liver, eggs, milk and cheese, butter and margarine, and fortified cereals.

The men who were surveyed by the USDA in 1985 fared better in their vitamin intakes than the women. The average intake of folic acid was 305 micrograms per day. Not counting white potatoes, the men averaged three servings a day of fruits and vegetables, or 328 grams, but the deep yellow and dark green vegetables only accounted for 15 grams of this. There was no information in the published report about the percentage who were far below the average in their intakes of vitamin A or folic acid.[7]

A large earlier survey on American diets also showed a rather dismal record of vegetable intake. The NHANES II survey of 1976-80 (mentioned earlier in this chapter) questioned almost twelve thousand people between the ages of nineteen and seventy-four about their food consumption during the day before the personal interview. The survey was done before dietary guidelines for cancer prevention were published by the National Research Council and the American Cancer Society in the early 1980s. In 1988, epidemiologists at the National Cancer Institute reviewed the survey just to find out how the respondents in the NHANES II survey had selected foods that are now thought to be useful for cancer prevention.[8] They found that, when all possible vegetables were considered, most of the respondents had had at least a serving; but when white potatoes and salad were excluded, only half of the respondents had had some other vegetable on the day of the interview. Only one out of five people had had any serving at all of a fruit or vegetable that is rich in beta-carotene, and only one out of five had had a cruciferous vegetable. These results were much the same in all age groups and income groups. Thus, the epidemiologists concluded there is a widespread need for public education to encourage better food choices for better nutrition and cancer prevention.

Many smaller surveys on limited populations have shown deficiencies of folic acid or vitamin A. Deficiencies have been found in the poor, in adolescents, in the poor elderly, and in cancer patients. In Canada, a nutrition survey in the early 1970s found that folic acid deficiency was the most common nutrient deficiency, with 60% of the elderly showing signs of low intake of folic acid. Several studies on older people in Great Britain have shown that low blood levels of folic acid are common in the elderly.

The Ten-State Nutrition Survey that was done in 1968 to 1970, partly to find out how much malnutrition and hunger existed in the United States, showed that deficiencies of folic acid and vitamin A were common among the poor. The results of this survey in Massachusetts showed that 25% of the women whose red blood cells were tested for folic acid had levels so low that they could be assumed to have deficiencies of folic acid in their tissues. The Massachusetts director of the study warned that dietary deficiency of folic acid might be a major problem. He noted that blood levels of vitamin A were also low in many people, probably from a lack of green leafy vegetables in the diet. Green leafy vegetabless can provide both vitamin A and folic acid.[9] (The folic acid level in blood serum changes according to the recent diet; so the folic acid level in the red blood cells is used instead as a measure of folic acid nutrition during the previous few months. The level of folic acid in the red cells cannot give any information on deficiencies that might have occurred in the more distant past.)

Nutritionists at Auburn University in Alabama recently studied the dietary intake of folic acid and the blood levels of folic acid in adolescent girls in order to find out how common deficiency might be during a period of growth when extra nutrients should be ingested. Food intakes during twenty-four hour periods were recorded and the dietary intakes of folic acid were calculated from food composition tables. The average values of serum and red blood cell folic acid for the entire group were close to normal and the dietary intake was close to the RDA of 180 micrograms per day but, again, averages do not tell the whole story. Red blood cell folate levels were below the safe, normal range in 38% of the twelve year-olds, in 46% of the fourteen year-olds, and in 65% of the sixteen year-olds, showing that deficiencies of folic acid existed in approximately half of these subjects. None of the girls who took a vitamin supplement containing folic acid had below-normal levels in the blood tests. There was not much difference between those from higher and lower income families.[10]

Many other studies have also demonstrated that adolescents, especially girls, often have signs of folic acid deficiency that can be detected by blood tests and can be corrected by folic acid supplements.[11] The significance of these deficiencies in the young can only be speculated. The teen-agers who were studied all appeared to be in good health, but those with folate-deficient red blood cells probably suffered from folate-deficient cells in other tissues as well and, possibly, some damaged chromosomes. Most of the teen-agers were consuming dietary folic acid at about RDA levels; so their signs of deficiency may have been due to their going through a period of rapid growth. It may be that adolescents, like pregnant women, need extra folic acid to maintain normal levels of this vitamin.

Nutritionists in Florida studied the folic acid status of 193 people over sixty years of age from an urban, low-income area in Dade County. Blood samples were analyzed for several components that could be related to anemia. One-fourth of the subjects had folic acid levels in their red blood cells that were so low as to indicate dangerously low intakes and stores of folic acid.[12]

The same group of scientists have done another study, this time comparing the folic acid status of older women from two income levels. One group of subjects were white women living in a middle class retirement community in Florida that stressed health maintenance. The other group of subjects were black women living in a densely populated, urban poverty neighborhood. None of the subjects took folic acid supplements. Among the middle class women, the prevalence of dangerously low levels of folic acid in the red blood cells was low—only 6% of the subjects had this problem. But among the poor women, the prevalence of low folic acid in the red blood cells was high—60% of these women had dangerously low levels. Brief analysis of the dietary habits of the two groups confirmed that there were considerable differences in their customary frequency of eating vegetables.[13]

A survey of healthy, older people in New Mexico in 1982 also showed that diets low in folic acid are common, even among well-off, health-conscious people. The participants in the survey were middle income people over sixty years of age, with above average educational level, who had volunteered for a study on nutrition. The study required them to record in detail their food intakes for three days and to provide information about vitamin supplement usage and about their life styles. The long-range purpose of the study was to follow their health status for five years. Approximately 40% of the study participants were found to be consuming folic acid in their diets below the RDA level of 200 micrograms per day. Presumably, these were health-conscious people in the first place to have volunteered for the study (more than half took vitamin supplements) and, yet, they had not become educated about the specific nutritional reasons for eating plenty of legumes, whole grains, and green leafy vegetables. Other nutrients besides folic acid that were low in their diets—less than half of the RDA was consumed—were vitamin B6, vitamin D, vitamin E, and zinc. Their vitamin A and vitamin C intakes were good.[14]

All of these surveys that show low intakes of the vegetable vitamin, folic acid, or low blood levels of folic acid serve as ample warning that many people do not eat enough vegetables. The nationwide surveys that have found that many people have only one serving a day of vegetables confirm our suspicion that we need to make an effort if we want to achieve the 1989 recommendations of the Committee on Diet and Health in regard to vegetable consumption.

This is the kind of effort for better health that we can only enjoy. Eating more of the good fruits and vegetables must surely be one of the most pleasant and satisfying dietary changes that we could be asked to make. For many years the public interest in foods and nutrition has been on the rise because of our acceptance of the connection between diet and health. During these years many of us have learned to count calories. Some of us have even learned to count grams of fat and milligrams of cholesterol. Now we must learn to count servings of vegetables in a day. This should be easy—everyone can count to five. It does require a new habit. Before sitting down to dinner, you must pause and reflect back through the day. Ask yourself: did you have any fruit for a snack, how many vegetables for lunch? If it doesn't all add up, you will have to reach into the freezer for a quick-cooking package of carrots or spinach or lima beans or fix a bowl of greens and other raw vegetables. Some days you will have to do both. You will be doing your digestive system a favor, your vitamin-craving cells a favor, and you can be a little less apprehensive the next time you go for an annual physical.

The Food and Nutrition Board of the National Research Council is preparing more reports on nutrition as guidance for restaurants, airlines, schools, and other institutions with suggestions on menu improvements that would benefit the public by implementing the nine specific recommendations in the 1989 report from the Committee on Diet and Health. My own feeling is that restaurants will change their menus faster if the public demands change. Many of us have many meals at fast-food franchises, delicatessens, and restaurants, and we are usually not offered enough vegetables. Too many restaurants serve a plateful of a pasta dish or a large hamburger and fries and think they have served you well. But, to my mind, it is not a well-balanced meal unless there are two vegetables in addition to any white potatoes, rice, or noodles.

We could encourage better menus by demanding more vegetables. Why don't we ask for a scoop of carrot salad or bean salad with a delicatessen lunch instead of a scoop of potato salad or French fries? Why don't we ask for steamed broccoli with a little oyster sauce or lemon sauce instead of green beans or zucchini? (Both of these are low in beta-carotene.) Why don't we ask for some old-fashioned peas and carrots for a good helping of beta-carotene and folic acid? Why don't we ask for a salad of raw kale or spinach instead of so often white lettuce? Why don't we ask for sweet potatoes with the chopped sirloin? A better choice of vegetables when eating out would make a great improvement in our vitamin intakes.

When meals are prepared at home, it is only necessary to remember the variety of ways of including more vegetables. If there is not much time to cook, vegetables can be used in a convenience form. Mixed dishes such as casseroles can usually accomodate an extra can of corn, peas, or lima beans for some added nutrition. Stir-fried dishes are better with added peas or thin-sliced carrots. Lentils are a good way to add folic acid to vegetable soups. Dried apricots go well with everyone's breakfast and are a convenient way to include beta-carotene in the morning meal. Dried fruits, bananas or oranges, a wedge of raw cabbage, raw carrot or other raw vegetables should be included in a carried lunch along with a cooked vegetable.

We should not forget the legumes with their high content of folic acid and other valuable nutrients. Almost everyone loves baked beans. It is hard to imagine a family gathering or potluck dinner that does not include a casserole of beans, and there are seldom any leftovers. Why should we wait for special occasions to enjoy some of the most nutritious old favorites like baked beans, sweet potatoes, or collards? We would be better able to avoid the chronic diseases if we ate beans more often—they are a good source of fiber, protein, complex carbohydrate and, most important, folic acid. Even when you are having a quick meal alone and don't have time to cook from scratch, you can open a can or jar of baked beans and count this as one of your five vegetable servings for the day. Baked beans and bean salads would probably be popular items if they were offered by fast-food restaurants. The legumes and the green leafy vegetables deserve our frequent indulgence whether they come from a can, the freezer case, or are prepared in a favorite recipe. The important thing is to get in the habit of including something from all of the major food groups in every meal. The scientists who have investigated the nutritional value of vegetables and the mysterious diseases like cancer have given us solid reasons to devote plenty of attention to what we eat.

Here is some old-time advice from Elmer V. McCollum, professor in the School of Hygiene and Public Health of Johns Hopkins University, who said, "There are dietary properties in the leafy parts of vegetables which differ entirely from the properties of potatoes and the root vegetables such as beets and turnips. Eating leafy vegetables in liberal quantities provides the body with invaluable substances, which it cannot secure in adequate amount from milled cereals, potatoes, and . . . meat. . . . They are of great advantage also because they leave a bulky residue, which aids the intestine to empty.

"Remember that the leafy vegetables are important for both their vitamins and their inorganic matter. The most important of them are spinach, lettuce, cabbage, chard, cauliflower, Brussels sprouts, collards, kale, beet tops, turnip tops, dandelion, water cress, and lambs-quarters. The onion bulb is really a mass of thickened leaves, and so may be included in this list."[15]

When McCollum said this in an interview for *American Magazine* in 1923, only four vitamins had been discovered. (Three of the four had been discovered by McCollum.) The discovery of folic acid was more than twenty years in the future. McCollum realized that the deficiency diseases (xerophthalmia, beri-beri, and scurvy) were not common in the United States, but he thought many people had tendencies toward deficiency diseases; and he thought eating more leafy vegetables, raw fruits and vegetables, and milk would guard against the deficiency diseases and greatly improve the general health of most people. This advice has never been faulted and remains one of the most important rules for good diet. In the words of the most cautious of today's scientists, it is defensible.

Chapter 13

Another Deficiency Disease

The deficiency diseases that result from lack of certain vitamins were the cause of great suffering in the past and great perplexity among the medical profession as they considered, sometimes for centuries, what might be the causes of these diseases. Cancer is another perplexing disease that has caused great suffering for a long time and whose true causes have yet to be completely defined. Many possible causes of cancer have been considered and studied during the twentieth century—viruses, X-rays, hormones, chemical carcinogens, and heredity come to mind. Each of these agents has been found to play a role in the development of some cases of cancer, but none of these agents has been implicated in as many types of cancer as has been the deficiency of vegetables in the diet. Because the dietary factors that we obtain from vegetables—beta-carotene and folic acid being of greatest importance—have functions in metabolism that theoretically can help prevent cancer and because the vegetables appear to have cancer-preventing effects against so many types of carcinomas in dietary surveys, I choose to call cancer another deficiency disease.

The idea that cancer incidence is somehow related to dietary habits is not new. In earlier years, well-known physicians including Sir Robert McCarrison and Denis Burkitt pointed out that cancer was rare in some areas of Asia and Africa where people had plenty of vegetables in their normal diet. These physicians knew diet had something to do with the absence of cancer in these peoples, but they also knew the story was probably very complicated and might involve any number of other factors not yet even imagined. They could not make any absolute claims that better diet alone would prevent the chronic diseases—cancer, heart disease, diabetes, and digestive disorders—that are common in the developed countries because they knew they did not understand the complete etiology of these diseases. They could only encourage people in Western, developed countries to look to their own dietary customs and question whether they were eating the kinds of foods that are needed for the best health.

McCarrison wrote in 1921 that the subnormal health experienced by many people in Europe was due to diets that were high in sugars and white bread and low in green vegetables, fresh fruits, fresh eggs and meats, and other natural foodstuffs that could supply needed vitamins. He believed better health would be attained if people could be instructed to adopt a better diet. Campaigns to improve diets were carried out in England. Better diet—which means plenty of milk, vegetables, salads, whole grains, fish, fruits, and meats—was advocated by local physicians in some communities in England during the 1920s and 1930s. The physicians wanted to see healthier patients; so they gave out dietary rules and watched as the general health of their patients became much improved. During the Second World War, the whole of England was strongly encouraged by the Ministry of Food to follow good nutritional habits as an essential part of the war effort. A comprehensive campaign to fortify the home front was carried out. Radio shows, newspaper ads, and pamphlets were used to educate the public in nutrition and to teach the best ways to cook the foods that remained available. Children's health statistics became much improved as a result and many people appreciated their increased nutritional knowledge and sense of better health.[1]

But when community efforts toward better health slack off and people are without enough nutritional background, the concern with diet gives way to the other demands of time and attention and diet takes a back seat.

During the past 150 years there have been many advocacy groups who espoused good diet for better health. A few of the better-diet advocates have taken on the trappings of food faddists and have made claims for which they had little evidence or have promised cures from better diet in situations where dietary changes alone could not possibly provide a cure. Nothing rankles the scientific and medical professions more than groups who make claims for curative methods without having any evidence. To the scientists it is obvious that you must have some evidence before making your claims. The scientists have not always understood that non-scientists may be unfamiliar with this rule, may be unable to search out the evidence, or, in some cases, may even be willing to believe just about anything.

Scientists now know that dietary changes can ameliorate a few of the chronic diseases such as coronary heart disease, diabetes, and some digestive disorders, and doctors give strict dietary rules to patients who have developed these illnesses. However, dietary changes will probably not provide much benefit for cancer patients once the cancer cells have become established—the advanced cancer cells have extensive alterations in the chromosomes that make the disease usually irreversible.

Prevention, however, is another matter. This is the area of cancer research that is beginning to look so hopeful from the results of the epidemiological studies that have been done so far. The studies imply that good dietary habits that include plenty of vegetables will help us to counter the development of cancer cells. Nowhere in this book have you read any suggestion that better diet can cure cancer. But we have seen consistent scientific evidence that diets that include large amounts of vegetables are associated with fewer cases of carcinomas.

Many of the earliest epidemiological studies that showed this result were originally health surveys designed to find out whether or not there was some relationship between illness and several life style factors. We saw studies in Norway, Singapore, and the Western Electric study in Chicago that were examples of this. When various aspects of diet were tested statistically for relevance to disease, the vegetable intake often showed the strongest correlation of any dietary factor when cancer was considered. More recent surveys of diet and specific types of carcinomas continue to show this correlation.

Correlations between vegetables and less cancer don't tell us anything definitive about what causes cancer, but the correlations do encourage scientists to study the ways the body makes use of vegetable factors such as beta-carotene and other carotenoids, vitamin C, and folic acid to find out how these factors might play a role in normal cell division and differentiation, in the immune defense system, and in other potential mechanisms for guarding against the neoplastic process. The biological chemists know quite a bit about the functions of these vitamins, but a great deal more remains to be discovered about the functions of vitamins in the cells and tissues.

A new hypothesis, called the vegetable hypothesis so far, is being formulated which should provide a new slant on research to understand how cells and tissues maintain their normal phenotypes and resist potential damage from carcinogens. More research is needed before scientists can discover the mechanisms of action of beta-carotene in the maintenance of normal cells and the role of folic acid deficiency in carcinogenesis. They will seek plausible mechanisms that lead to new understanding of cellular processes, consistent with past understanding of cellular functions.

We do not have to wait for all of these detailed mechanisms to be sorted out before improving our diet. Doll and Peto, in their 1981 review on the causes of cancer, noted: "Of course, what ultimately matters from a public health point of view is not so much the *mechanism* whereby dietary factors may affect cancer, but rather the *nature* of the dietary factors that are important determinants of cancer."[2]

In the early years of this century the lack of a particular familiarity with the vitamins resulted in a great deal of skepticism and confusion when biochemists suggested that there were disease-preventing factors in foods. It required decades of work before chemists could isolate and measure the small amounts of vitamins needed to prevent some diseases. The story of the unraveling of the terrible deficiency diseases of past centuries has been told and retold many times by popular and scientific writers. The story is not yet finished.

The search for understanding of the causes of cancer resembles in a startlingly similar way the efforts to understand some of the other mysterious diseases that plagued mankind not too long ago. Scurvy, beriberi, rickets, pellagra, and goiter were all terrible public health problems and exceedingly mysterious diseases until it was proven after long arguments among the wisest of the medical scientists and experimentation on the sufferers that each had a dietary deficiency as the primary cause.

During the late 1800s and early 1900s many diseases were found to be caused by specific infectious agents (viruses, bacteria, or parasites) and were eventually brought under some control by means of better sanitation, quarantine, avoidance of insect carriers, vaccination, or later on, antibiotics. The list of infectious diseases that were subdued by these efforts included yellow fever, typhoid, cholera, polio, plague, diphtheria and TB.

Infectious agents or environmental factors such as tainted foods became such popular explanations for disease in the early years of this century that infectious agents were also the prime suspects in the early efforts to understand the deficiency diseases. Infectious agents had become the normal way of thinking about a disease, and some of the characteristics of the way deficiency diseases seemed to "spread" resembled infectious diseases.

Scurvy is a deficiency disease that became a serious problem when European explorers in the fifteenth and sixteenth centuries began spending months at a time on sailing ships without any fresh provisions. Scurvy could develop after going two months without fresh foods and it was often a killer. Scurvy had decimated the armies of the Crusaders, and it continued to wreak havoc with the shipbound explorers. Some expeditions suffered 80% or more incidence of scurvy, and the disease was naturally spoken of as if it were a spreading infection. By the year 1600, it was known by some Europeans and by the Indians of Canada that fresh foods or citrus fruits could ward off the disease, but another two hundred years of experimentation, false economies, and occasional disasters went by before fresh fruits for sailors became *de rigueur.* Even in the nineteenth century, disasters from scurvy happened on some expeditions for reasons that are uncertain—the limes employed may have been of poor quality or the lime juice may have been heated before using, thus destroying the vitamin C.[3]

It wasn't until the late 1920s that vitamin C was finally isolated and shown to be the antiscorbutic ingredient in fresh foods. Albert Szent-Gyorgyi, a young Hungarian biochemist working temporarily in Cambridge, England, isolated a crystalline compound, later to be called ascorbic acid, from oranges, lemons, cabbages, and adrenal glands in the course of his studies on oxidative enzyme systems. After the crystals were later tested by an associate for vitamin activity and found to be identical to vitamin C, he managed to extract and purify a couple of kilograms of ascorbic acid from a ton of Hungarian red peppers (the paprika-type peppers) for distribution to researchers around the world for further study.[4] In the course of his vitamin C work, Szent-Gyorgyi also discovered that another component of the red peppers, flavones or bioflavonoids, cured the subcutaneous bleeding seen in scurvy cases even though the vitamin C itself did not help this symptom. Szent-Gyorgyi later received a Nobel prize for his vitamin C work and for his many contributions to the new science of biochemistry.

Rickets was another deficiency disease for which the proper cure was slow to be recognized. Rickets caused terrible sickness in babies and children who did not get enough vitamin D, which they desperately needed in order to be able to absorb the calcium from milk.

Vitamin D is produced from a cholesterol-related compound in the skin when sunlight reaches the skin. In summer, a baby would be assured of getting enough vitamin D if he was taken outdoors to get some sun. Mother's milk contains only very low levels of vitamin D; so winter babies—those born in the fall and winter—often died from lack of vitamin D, even in the early years of this century in spite of one hundred years of medical experience showing that cod liver oil could prevent and cure the disease. (One of my uncles died from rickets in infancy in 1920.)

Cod liver oil was an old home remedy for rheumatism in northern Europe and a Dutch physician, Dr. Bodel, thought to try it on the sickly victims of rickets in 1817. He found that it cured rickets like a miracle drug. The treatment became accepted medical practice during the 1800s even though the active ingredient in the oil was not known. Not all children who could have benefited from cod liver oil received it and rickets remained a common problem into the 1920s, while some medical authorities continued to debate whether rickets might be caused by an infectious disease or by a parathyroid deficiency. The search for external causative agents for specific diseases was the normal way of thinking when tackling a medical problem.

In 1922, Elmer V. McCollum, the chemist who had discovered the vitamins "fat-soluble A" and "water-soluble B" and who also would later show the necessity of magnesium in animal diets, while working at Johns Hopkins, proved that a specific vitamin in cod liver oil cured rickets.[3] He was experimenting with rats that had rickets on account of being on an experimental diet that contained none of the vitamin. This method of inducing rickets had been used by Edward Mellanby in London to produce rickets in dogs. McCollum was able to show that cod liver oil contained a specific antirachitic factor, which he named vitamin D. He bubbled hot air through the cod liver oil, thus destroying the vitamin A that was already known to be present, and showed that the antirachitic factor remained still active in a bioassay using the rats, and so was a separate component from the vitamin A. In the 1930s, dairies in the United States began adding vitamin D to milk upon the advice of the American Medical Association after many studies had shown the benefits of adequate vitamin D intake for children's health, and rickets finally became a rare disease.

Beriberi was another mysterious and debilitating disease in the last century that turned out to be a deficiency disease. Beriberi resulted in nerve damage, sudden heart failure, and paralysis; and spread through armies, prisons, and ships like an epidemic, causing battles to be lost and shipping businesses to languish. The cure was found fairly quickly, perhaps because of its commercial importance.

The disease became a widespread problem in the Far East during the last three decades of the nineteenth century after polished white rice became available from a new milling process. The new mills removed the pericarp covering and the germ from the rice grains, and removed the B vitamins at the same time. With no B vitamins in the diet, soldiers on restricted diets eating rice and not much else or sailors on long voyages eating fish, vegetables, and polished rice developed beriberi in ninety days.

Physicians were divided in opinion as to whether the disease might be caused by an infectious agent or by a dietary problem. The Director-General of the Japanese navy, Takaki, thought it might be a dietary problem. He noticed that the British sailors came down with the illness less often than the Japanese and the British were eating more protein. In the 1880s, Takaki substituted barley for part of the polished rice in the Japanese sailors' rations, and added some evaporated milk and meat to their fish and vegetables. This cured the Japanese sailors and Takaki thought the additional protein had effected the cure.

The concept of deficiency disease was still a few years in the future; so the potential causes of beriberi that were most often considered revolved around the possibility of a toxin in rice or a toxin in the soil on which the rice was grown or on some taint in salted meats.

A young Dutch surgeon, Christian Eijkman, was sent to the Dutch East Indies in 1886 to study the beriberi problem. He stayed ten years, setting up a colony of birds as experimental animals. He tried to induce the disease in the birds by means of inoculating them with infectious material but this didn't work. The birds finally developed avian beriberi after they were fed the "better quality" polished white rice for a while instead of their regular feed, by mistake. Eijkman followed up this accidental discovery, proving that birds (and later prisoners) developed beriberi on a white rice diet but not on a whole rice diet. He still clung to the toxin idea for a few more years, believing that white rice contained or produced a toxin that was neutralized by the pericarp covering of the rice grains. (In 1915, McCollum showed the rice did not contain a toxin. He fed some of his rats polished rice and some of them a smaller amount of polished rice with purified starch added to make up the difference in calories. Cutting back on the amount of polished rice in the diet did not alleviate the symptoms of beriberi, proving that a toxin was not to blame.)

The concept of deficiency disease developed slowly from the beriberi investigations and from similar studies in animals within a few more years. Although chemists still could not isolate any of the vitamins in the first two decades of this century—the vitamins were present in such small amounts—they began to believe that protective substances were present in many foods that could prevent specific diseases. F. Gowland Hopkins' theory about the "accessory factors of the diet" made this idea clear, but general acceptance of the true nature of some specific diseases was painfully slow.

Pellagra was another mysterious disease that was seen only in the poor and the undernourished. It caused severe skin lesions, nerve disabilities and, eventually, insanity. The disease was first described in 1735 by a Spanish physician whose observations convinced him that the disease was caused by poverty and by the spoiled corn that was eaten by the poor as a last resort before starvation. Corn-growing had been introduced to Europe by the Spanish who had found many new crops being grown in Mexico, and corn became popular for a while in southern Europe because it grew well in warm humid areas, but the Indians' methods of preparing corn had never been taken to Europe.

Corn has a low content of the amino acids, tryptophan and lysine, and the niacin in corn is tied up in high-molecular weight complexes that are not readily broken down in human digestion. Niacin is the B vitamin that prevents pellagra, but this was not understood until 1937. Corn was used successfully as a staple grain by the Indians in America because their customs of either roasting the corn before storage or treating cornmeal with an alkaline solution of potash extracted from wood ashes or with limewater resulted in release of the niacin from the complexes.

Poverty-stricken Europeans or Americans who tried to live on corn that wasn't properly prepared became deficient in niacin and some developed pellagra. Not much attention was paid to the disease until a meeting of the American Medical Association in 1907 where George Searcy described seeing the disease in an insane asylum in the South and identified it as pellagra, having seen a description of the disease in an old European medical text.

More reports of the disease in other parts of the United States soon followed. Pellagra was made a reportable disease by the Public Health Service because the disease was thought to be an infection carried by an insect. The nutritional basis of the disease was eventually figured out by Dr. Joseph Goldberger who was commissioned by the Public Health Service in 1914 to turn his considerable investigative talents to studying the etiology of pellagra.[5]

Goldberger visited an orphanage in Jackson, Mississippi and quickly noticed that only the undernourished children showed symptoms of pellagra and never the better-fed adults looking after them. He spent several years in the South, proving by means of many experiments that pellagra was a nutritional deficiency and not an infectious disease. He cured the children in the orphanage by augmenting their meager diet with meat and milk, and produced the disease in volunteer convicts by giving them a low-protein diet with no B vitamins for a period of six months.

Goldberger's experiments did not tell him the exact nature of the nutritional deficiency, and several years passed before the deficiency theory of pellagra was fully accepted by everyone in the medical field In 1937, eight years after Goldberger's death, niacin (vitamin B3) was identified as the missing nutrient through experimental work on pellagra in dogs at the University of Wisconsin. Niacin was already known to be part of a coenzyme and was being studied as a growth factor in the metabolism of certain bacteria. A discussion among biochemists working on growth factors for bacteria and a group working on pellagra in dogs resulted in the niacin being tested in the dogs. And it cured them dramatically.

The pellagra story had many interesting puzzles in it. The disease may have become more common in the United States after the 1905 invention of a machine for making cornmeal that removed the germ from the grain, eliminating a substantial fraction of the niacin value. As the new type of cornmeal was shipped across the country by rail, cases of pellagra seemed to spread along the rail routes. Of course, no one understood then that there was something wrong with the cornmeal, so people naturally suspected all manner of other causes. The association of the disease with extreme poverty led some people to think that poor sanitation was to blame, when the real cause was lack of enough good-quality protein in the diet. Milk or eggs could cure the disease even though milk and eggs contain little niacin, another puzzle. Laboratory experiments showed that either niacin or tryptophan could cure pellagra in corn-fed rats, an intriguing result that was finally explained in 1945 when research at the University of Wisconsin showed that tryptophan could be converted into niacin in the rats. Milk was able to cure pellagra in humans because it is a good source of tryptophan, not because it contains much niacin.

Although pellagra has disappeared because of improvements in nutrition and social welfare in the United States, the story bears repeating. The complications involved in solving the pellagra puzzle rival the complications involved in solving many other diseases, even cancer. Providing scientific proof of what seemed so obvious to Goldberger from his investigations at the orphanage, and convincing others of the real cause of pellagra were difficult endeavors. The unsolved puzzles in the pellagra story made many physicians reluctant to believe the nutritional basis of the disease, and Goldberger spent several heart-breaking years trying unsuccessfully to isolate the unknown nutrient that cured pellagra.

In all these stories of the deficiency diseases it seems that the traditional assumption that a disease is likely to be caused by an external agent, along with the lack of biochemical knowledge of the mechanism of a disease process, delayed the needed understanding of how to deal with the disease. The absence of plausible mechanisms to explain the details of how some minor, unknown components in foods could prevent specific illnesses was the reason behind a great deal of skepticism and polarized opinions when the deficiency diseases were first described as such. It was only after years of debate and experimentation that the importance of diet in overcoming these terrible diseases became finally acknowledged. Detailed mechanisms to explain the deficiency diseases have always been difficult to come by. The role of vitamins and minerals in preventing specific diseases required years of complicated research to understand and for most of the vitamins and minerals, there is still a great deal yet to learn.

Is cancer another deficiency disease? The epidemiological evidence that shows that people who consumed larger amounts of fruits, vegetables, and legumes suffered fewer cases of carcinomas of many types points to this conclusion. The functions of vitamin A and folic acid in maintaining normal epithelial tissues and normal chromosomes in dividing cells explain how the vegetables could have a cancer-preventing effect and support this conclusion. The dietary surveys that show low consumption of vegetables by most people in the United States are compatible with this conclusion. The incidence of carcinomas, which account for 80% of cases of cancer in adults, should be greatly reduced when we all adopt the kind of diet that includes a truly adequate amount of the vegetable factors that are associated with lower rates of cancer. When this happens, we will finally see progress against this deficiency disease.

It appears that deficiencies of the vitally important ingredients in vegetables can set the stage for development of cancer in at least two important ways. If vitamin A is lacking, epithelial tissues may proliferate at a higher than necessary rate in many parts of the body (but in the human colon, calcium serves as an antiproliferation agent), and if folic acid is also lacking, the proliferating cells are likely to slowly accumulate damage of several types in the chromosomes. One would expect that much of the damage would be repaired by DNA-repairing enzymes and that any permanent damage would be distributed in a more or less random manner throughout proliferating tissues. Only if one particular cell accumulates several alterations in important genes would it be transformed into a malignant cell that could no longer respond to the normal growth control mechanisms and which could invade other tissues. Such a process could happen without the involvement of any other risk factors such as external carcinogens or heredity; but if these conditions also exist, the process could be accelerated because of additional damage to the chromosomes.

The sad truth is that deficiency diseases can become irreversible in advanced stages, and this is what happens in cancer. Advanced cancer cells have a large number of abnormalities in their chromosomes. Instead of twenty-three pairs of intact chromosomes that replicate in orderly fashion only when commanded by the cells' chemical communications, there are extra chromosomes that were left behind in previous disorganized replications and changes in the coiled structure of the chromosomes. There are broken and rearranged chromosomes and missing or mutated genes that may have been needed for normal growth control. The damage is so extensive that medical researchers have little hope for ever being able to restore the chromosomes to their normal condition—their efforts are aimed instead at halting the growth or killing the outlaw cells. The inability of advanced cancer cells to respond to normal growth control mechanisms explains why taking large amounts of certain vitamins has not been effective against

advanced cancer. It is only in the early stages of chromosome alterations that maintaining enough vitamins in the diet could have an inhibiting effect on the damage process.

Vitamin deficiencies should not be taken lightly. In the United
States, it is often said that we need not worry about vitamins as long
as we consume a well-balanced diet. And this is so true! It was true
also in England in 1921 when Sir Robert McCarrison, in his book
Studies in Deficiency Diseases, deplored the same common platitude
because he saw many patients who often made a meal of white bread,
tea, margarine, and jam, and suffered all manner of ills because of
their ignorance and poor habits. As he put his conclusions, ''Access to
abundance of food does not necessarily protect from the effects of
food deficiency, since a number of factors . . . often prevent the
proper use and choice of health-giving foods.'' Instead of being lulled
by the statement that we need not worry about vitamins, we should
scrutinize this common remark to make sure we understand its full
meaning and importance. Perhaps it is time that we did worry about
the vitamin content of our diets, at least for the time it takes to educate
ourselves about the nutritional values of different classes of foods and
to make changes in our dietary habits if we decide this is necessary.

The truth is a many-sided story and does not always tell us what we
might have wanted to hear. There is good news and bad news in these
epidemiological studies. The good news is that we have it within our
power to prevent at least 35% of the cases of cancer in our Western
societies by improving our diets and eating adequate amounts of vegetables (and to prevent another 30% by not smoking). Some scientists
have estimated 60% of cases could be prevented by improved diet.
The bad news is that we have to assume the responsibility ourselves to
accomplish this. We can no longer point to the high level of industri-
alization in our country as the cause of this common illness. We can
no longer blame businesses for being the main culprit in causing cancer. We can no longer bemoan the medical profession's slowness in
finding a cure. We can no longer waste our energies worrying that
traces of pollution or pesticides are the explanation for the continuing
cancer problem.

The problem of pollution and the problem of cancer are closely connected in some of our minds, but these are entirely separate problems
that will have entirely different solutions. There seems to be a widespread suspicion among the public that some of the hazardous waste
disposal sites have been the cause of higher incidences of cancer. But

in fact, the efforts to prove that hazardous wastes, or air and water pollution, are associated with cancer have met with little success so far, except in the case of pollution from radioactivity or arsenic.[6]

In some of the most notorious cases of environmental pollution from chemicals, namely Love Canal, Times Beach, and Seveso, investigators could not find higher than normal rates of cancer in these areas even though the pollution caused terrible personal and economic problems.

In the section of Niagara Falls, New York called Love Canal, old, buried chemical wastes that were contaminated with dioxin, a highly toxic chemical in animal tests, percolated into the soil and contaminated homes. Love Canal was evacuated in 1980. The town of Times Beach, Missouri was purchased by the federal government and evacuated in 1983 because dioxin-contaminated waste sludge had been sprayed on roads for dust control in the early 1970s. In 1976, a chemical-manufacturing plant in Seveso, Italy had an accident that resulted in release of chemicals to the atmosphere. The plant produced the chemical intermediate, trichlorophenol, which was contaminated with dioxin, and approximately one to four pounds of dioxin rained down on the town. The residents suffered from a severe skin rash known to be caused by dioxin. Studies have been done on people who had lived in these three areas to find out whether their rates of cancer incidence are higher than in the general population, but no overall excess mortality from cancer has been found as yet. These studies continue.

Cancer in man has not been proven to be associated with exposure to dioxin even after many studies, and yet journalists continue to call dioxin a cancer-causing chemical. Do they say this because of high-dose testing in animals that results in cancer, or is it because previous news stories have called dioxin a cancer-causing chemical? Or, because the assumption persists that cancer must be caused by noxious external agents and we might as well blame it on dioxin as anything else? Environmental Protection Agency officials are reconsidering all the studies on dioxin and now say that dioxin may be only a very weak human carcinogen, if it is a carcinogen at all. Some of the environmental activists should study more of the scientific literature as well as their own propaganda. It will not be helpful in the efforts to prevent cancer to continue to promote unproven or false ideas about chemical residues—this produces myths about cancer and causes confusion. We need to reduce pollution, but we should not allow those who know nothing and fear everything to dictate our concerns, whatever their reasons may be.

This is not to say that these problematic aspects of our environment should be ignored. We know from the pioneering research of Rachel Carson and those who came after her that pollution damages the living plants and animals and the streams and lakes and now even the atmosphere. The environmental pollution problem needs the best engineering know-how we can recruit in order to improve our ability to maintain the atmosphere and the water supply in their natural condition. But even if we could solve all the environmental pollution problems, we would not have made much of a dent at all in the cancer statistics if we continue to ignore the importance of a high vegetable content in our individual diets.

Even though pollutants have not been shown to cause the more common types of human cancer, they can still have other toxic effects. Some small studies have found higher rates of leukemia and lymphoma associated with heavy exposure to various solvents and pesticides—these forms of cancer need more epidemiological studies. Governments have developed regulations that restrict, quite rightly, the dumping of many pollutants into air or water. The regulations are often established after toxic effects of some kind are found in laboratory testing or in the workplace.

The fraction of cancer cases that can be ascribed with certainty to external causes today (other than tobacco) is very small. In the past, occupational exposures in the mining, smelting, and chemical industries were directly responsible for many cases of cancer. Doll and Peto[2] have estimated that 4% of cancer cases in the United States are due to occupational causes, but these causes are declining as awareness of specific dangerous situations develops. The first dangerous situation to be observed to cause cancer was that of chimney sweeps, who used to develop cancer as a result of saturating their skin with soot. (Soot contains polycyclic aromatic compounds.) Chimney sweeps now avoid contact with soot and no longer develop cancer. Poly(vinylchloride) workers no longer develop angiosarcoma of the liver because they no longer climb into polymerization vessels to scrape chemical buildup out of the tanks. Rubber and synthetic dye workers no longer develop bladder cancer from using 2-naphthylamine. Ventilation improvements and changes in solvents are expected to reduce occupational exposures to benzene and formaldehyde.

A great deal of research continues on occupational exposures to potentially toxic materials. When chemical substances are even suspected of being associated with a toxic effect in workers, it is not unusual these days to see changes in the chemicals that are used or changes made in production methods to reduce the risky exposure. It is often easier to make changes in the workplace than it is to make changes in people's personal lives.

Most of us do inhale chemical fumes along with the fresh air at times. Such things as diesel exhaust, gas station fumes, passive cigarette smoke, and insecticides used around the home have been subjects of concern as potential contributors to the development of cancer. It is not possible for us to completely avoid exposure to these chemical vapors and to the natural toxic chemicals in our foods; so it behooves us to do what we can to maintain our natural defense mechanisms in tip-top shape.

The cancer statistics tell us that currently one out of four Americans can expect to encounter this disease during his lifetime. What can we do to counter these statistics? Is there any way to improve our chances of enjoying a healthy old age? Obviously, what we can do is continue protecting ourselves from unnecessary chemical exposures, even though these exposures do not account for a large part of the cancer statistics. And the epidemiological studies teach us that we can do a great deal to improve our own long-range health prospects by consuming the larger amounts of vegetables that appear to have protective effects against many of the most common types of cancer.

Fortunately, the interest on the part of the general public in their own nutritional needs continues to increase steadily. People are more concerned than ever before with their blood lipids, the amount and types of fat in their diet, their calcium and fiber intake, and choosing the very best fortified or wholegrain cereals. Many people try to educate themselves in the field of nutrition and the bookstores do a lively business trying to fill the public's demand for information. Our nutritional literacy increases.

Food processing companies help when they make an effort to provide vitamin-enriched and high-fiber cereals, and taste the wrath of the nutritionists when they promote sugary cereals for the young.

Employers are jumping onto the health-craze bandwagon by installing exercise equipment on their own property, by offering after-hours exercise classes and lunchtime lectures on nutrition and stress management. Dieticians and nurses are invited in to business establishments to teach brief classes on common health problems.[7] Employers, of course, hope that health education for their employees will keep down medical costs and boost productivity, and their efforts should really help the health statistics if they can generate the enthusiasm, the peer pressure, and the discussion that produce more interest in nutrition and encourage the more knowledgeable among the workforce to share their information with their coworkers.

Keeping health costs down and fitness levels up is a reasonable and serious goal for individuals, too. An important way to keep feeling fit for a lifetime is smart shopping at the supermarket. Paying attention to selection of adequate amounts of the most nutritious foods is probably the most important thing we can do (other than quitting smoking) to change the cancer statistics. Most of us get enough protein and vitamin B12 in our diet from meat and fish, and most of us get adequate carbohydrates from bread, rice, potatoes and pasta. But there are several questions you could ask yourself as you plan your grocery shopping. Do you buy enough vegetables and fruit to get your requirements for beta-carotene, vitamin C, vegetable fiber, minerals, folic acid, and the five servings per day now recommended to help prevent chronic diseases such as cancer? Do you buy enough wholegrain bread, cereals, or wheat germ to get your requirements for vitamin B1 (thiamine), vitamin B3 (niacin), vitamin B6 (pyridoxal), folic acid, cereal fiber, vitamin E, and magnesium? (Remember, more than half of the natural folic acid in wheat has been removed in the production of "enriched wheat flour.") Do you buy enough milk to get your requirements for calcium, vitamin D, vitamin B2 (riboflavin)? Do you buy polyunsaturated oil and monounsaturated oil (both are good sources of vitamin E) to cook with or to use in salads?

This is not to say that these foods contain only the nutrients mentioned. They all contain a bigger variety of nutrients than we may realize. Milk, for instance, contains small amounts of all the known vitamins, even traces of vitamin C, and is an important source of protein and simple carbohydrate. Chicken and turkey are good sources of vitamin B6, and nuts and legumes are good sources of magnesium, vitamin B6, and folic acid.

We have always known that good diet is important. Now, the epidemiological studies that show better diet to be associated with fewer cases of the common forms of cancer in adults confirm our beliefs about the importance of diet and extend our understanding about the causes of cancer. We have an obligation to ourselves and our families to eat more of the most nutritious foods because ultimately the responsibility for making use of the epidemiological and laboratory evidence for the nutritional deficiency aspect of cancer causation is the responsibility of each of us. Implementation of our newer knowledge of the importance of diet should not be postponed. We have waited long enough for the good news about good diet.

Chapter 14

Clinical Trials

Scientists love to speculate about what might be the explanations for their observations in the lab and in the field. Speculation is part of the normal process that scientists use in gathering new information and designing studies or experiments to clarify their understanding. Speculation is fun, but scientists know that it is important to be able to design an experiment that will test their proposed explanations. Curtis Mettlin, an epidemiologist at Roswell Park Memorial Institute, has pointed out that epidemiology, like astronomy, is not an experimental science because epidemiologists can only gather information and make measurements on their subject matter; they do not put people in controlled, defined environments to see what happens to their health. Their studies can provide intriguing clues about the causes of disease, but the conclusions from epidemiologic studies always include some questions about unsuspected, important factors that might have been overlooked and might have influenced the results.

The task of testing the hypotheses that arise from epidemiologic studies lies within the bailiwick of the clinical medical scientists. In order to overcome the unknown, confounding factors that can produce erroneous conclusions in epidemiologic studies, medical scientists use randomized, clinical trials to look for proof of a hypothesis. In such a trial, volunteers are recruited and are placed at random in one of two groups—either a group that will take a drug, vitamin, or diet that is being tested or a placebo group that takes a dummy capsule without the drug. By assigning recruits at random to either group as they enter the program, the scientists hope to even out the confounding factors such as heredity or life style habits that could somehow influence the course of a disease. Participants are not told which group they are in and the physicians who monitor their health status during the study do not know who is in which group.

Conducting randomized trials in the cancer prevention field is an especially daunting task because cancer is thought to develop slowly over many years in most cases. This means the volunteers in the trial must be willing to continue their dietary supplement or their new diet for many years. The costs of organizing and monitoring such trials can be steep. Many of the clinical trials that have been set up have used special strategies to shorten the time required for finding out whether a treatment will produce some benefit. These trials started with volunteers who already had some type of precancerous condition or who were at high risk because of smoking or because of having had a previous case of cancer.

Although they are difficult to plan and expensive to carry out, clinical trials are needed because of the uncertainty that remains after studying the cancer statistics and general dietary habits among different countries and after studying individuals and their diets. Public health policy makers would like to know with greater certainty whether or not a specific dietary change or some nontoxic drug or vitamin will be effective for preventing cancer and how much benefit can be expected. There is no guarantee that clinical trials will always give the answers sought, but they are a good way to begin to settle these questions.

Vitamin A and a class of synthetic drugs related to retinoic acid have both been tested in patients with a variety of precancerous conditions.[1,2] Generally, improvements have been found in at least half of those people treated, but there are also some side effects such as skin peeling. Skin cancer (other than melanoma) and precancerous lesions in the mouth are conditions that have responded to treatment with drugs that are related to retinoic acid. For actinic keratoses more than half of the patients treated had regressions of the precancerous skin lesion. For basal cell skin cancer improvement has been seen in some of the people who were treated. Several small clinical trials have tested the synthetic drugs on a precancerous lesion in the mouth known as leukoplakia. More than half of those treated experienced at least some regression of the leukoplakia. Additional trials on skin cancer using drugs related to retinoic acid or beta-carotene or vitamins C and E are under way at medical centers around the country. Vitamin A and the drugs related to retinoic acid have also been tested against other precancerous conditions such as cervical dysplasia and benign tumors in the bladder, also with improvements in about half of the patients.

Beta-carotene is being tested in about a dozen different clinical trials which are funded by the National Cancer Institute.[3] Most of these are large studies that are recruiting thousands of participants who have higher than average risk for some particular type of cancer. For instance, there are several trials being carried out on people who have been diagnosed with benign tumors in the colon. Several other treatments besides carotene are also being tested in these trials—vitamins C and E, wheat bran, calcium, and an antiarthritic drug are also being evaluated in the colon studies. Long-term heavy smokers are participating in several trials to test for benefits from beta-carotene and retinol. People with asbestos-related lung damage from working in the asbestos industry or in shipbuilding are participating in a clinical trial to find out whether treatment with carotene and retinol will reduce their high risk of developing lung cancer or mesothelioma. Another large study recruited thousands of physicians who did not have any high risk for cancer but who were willing to participate in a study to test for possible long-range effects on cancer incidence from taking high doses of beta-carotene. Results from most of these studies are not expected until the mid-1990s.

A large clinical trial on beta-carotene and skin cancer finished in 1990. The study found that a high daily dose of beta-carotene for five years had no effect at all in preventing the development of new skin cancers in patients who had already had at least one occurrence of either basal cell or squamous cell skin cancer.[4]

Another study found that 13-cis-retinoic acid was very effective in preventing new cancers in the upper respiratory tract in patients who had already suffered from one occurrence of such a cancer. These types of carcinomas are often associated with long-term smoking, and the patients are at high risk for developing a second cancer. The researchers plan to study the effectiveness of the drug at lower doses in order to have less toxicity, and they suggest the possibility of using the drug in all high-risk tobacco users.[5] It remains to be seen whether treatment with beta-carotene or with retinol might also be effective in these high-risk patients.

Beta-carotene was first employed in smaller trials by Hans F. Stich, who studied precancerous changes in the mouth in populations in the Philippines, in India, and in Alaska.[6] Oral cancer is common in many parts of the world, and especially in developing countries in Asia. The oral cancers are thought to be caused by the widespread habit of chewing a quid of betel leaf mixed with tobacco and other ingredients. The chewers also have the common precancerous lesion in the mouth, leukoplakia, and cells scraped from the inside of the mouth show evidence of damaged DNA. Stich and coworkers give high doses of either beta-carotene or retinol, or both together, for several weeks or months and find improvements in tests for precancerous lesions in most of those people treated, even though the chewing habit continues. Another carotenoid, canthaxanthin, which is said to be a quencher of singlet oxygen, has no effect in the test for improvement of DNA damage, while carotene and retinol have protective effects according to the test.[7]

The interest in testing canthaxanthin came from suggestions from chemists that beta-carotene might have anticancer effects because it is a quencher of singlet oxygen (high-energy oxygen). Canthaxanthin is a carotenoid that also quenches singlet oxygen; but unlike carotene, it is not converted to retinol in animal tissues. A compound that quenches singlet oxygen may be called an antioxidant.

In the popular press and in some scientific reviews there has been frequent discussion of antioxidants and free radicals in connection with cancer during the last few years. We read that free radicals race through the body wreaking havoc and causing damage that leads to cancer. We also read that eating too much fat and not enough antioxidants causes the formation of lipid peroxides in cell membranes which somehow leads to cancer. These ideas are quite fanciful as there is little evidence that membrane peroxidation or free radicals cause human cancer. Hereditary or experimental conditions that produce extra high doses of oxygen radicals can damage DNA and can cause cancer, but under normal conditions our enzymes deactivate the oxygen radicals that are produced during metabolism. Free radicals and lipid peroxides entered the arena through the side door and got into the discussion about causes of human cancer by mistake. They are relevant to the study of experimental cancer in animals, but they are not known to be relevant to human cancer.

The talk about free radicals, singlet oxygen, and peroxides comes up because these are the types of chemical species that can be deactivated by antioxidants. The antioxidant theory for beta-carotene and other carotenoids began as a speculative suggestion to try to explain how beta-carotene could have anticancer effects in man although retinol does not. Speculation is a legitimate part of the scientific process, but after a few years we should ask whether any evidence has been found to support the notion. We should not be repeating the suggestion with embellishments added as if it were fact.

The problem of imagining how extra carotene might have anticancer effects even though it does not produce higher circulating levels of retinol in well-nourished people was known to PDB&S. In their 1981 paper in *Nature*, PDB&S recommended consideration of several possible mechanisms whereby beta-carotene could have anticancer effects in man similar to the cancer-inhibiting effects in animals and cultured cells that had been demonstrated for retinol. One of the mechanisms that might be considered was quenching (deactivating) of singlet oxygen. Chemists at UCLA had demonstrated that carotene quenches singlet oxygen that was artificially produced by irradiation of a solution containing an olefin and a photosensitizing dye.[8] This work offered a possible explanation for the antioxidant effect of carotenoids in photosynthesizing plants. In plants carotene is known to function as an antioxidant; but so far, carotene has not been shown to have an antioxidant function in normal animal cells. (PDB&S also recommended testing human tissues to see whether carotene can be converted into retinol in tissues other than intestine and liver and thus serve as a localized source of retinol. As described in chapter 8, very little of this work has been done. But where the experiments have been done, it was found that carotene can indeed be converted into retinoic acid.)

Free radicals and peroxides are potentially damaging types of chemicals whether they occur in plants or animals or in synthetic materials such as rubber and plastics. Animals have evolved methods to take care of these bad actors when they are formed as by-products of normal oxidative metabolism. We have enzymes that convert oxygen radicals and hydrogen peroxide into harmless oxygen and water. The enzymes are superoxide dismutase, glutathione peroxidase, and catalase. These enzymes, along with vitamins C and E, are our natural antioxidants.

Epidemiologic studies have shown that vitamin C and vitamin E in the diet are correlated with less cancer. Vitamin C has been quite consistently associated with lower incidence of many types of cancer. A few studies have also asked whether higher intake of vitamin E is associated with lower incidence of cancer. Most of these studies have found a slightly lower level of vitamin E in cancer patients than in controls, indicating that vitamin E, which is the main antioxidant in cell membranes, might play a role in cancer prevention.[9] The antioxidant enzymes have not been associated with higher or lower incidence of cancer except in some hereditary conditions where an enzyme is lacking.

If singlet oxygen occurs in animal tissues, there are methods for deactivating it that are more effective than beta-carotene. Experiments using normal human plasma showed that the plasma proteins are far better quenchers of singlet oxygen than beta-carotene when singlet oxygen was added by means of a photosensitizing dye and laser irradiation.[10] Beta-carotene may have some antioxidant function in cell membranes, but whether it does and whether this has any relevance to human cancer is still speculation.

Another hypothesis that remains unproven is the suggestion that breast cancer is caused by a high-fat diet. One clinical trial that was planned but was not set up was a randomized trial on breast cancer to test whether a low-fat diet can prevent this disease. The trial has not been approved; but if it were carried out, it would be one of the largest and longest clinical trials. The participants would be women who have some of the risk factors for breast cancer such as heredity or a biopsy that showed atypical hyperplasia.

In chapter 11 I mentioned that it has not been demonstrated through case-control studies that fat in the diet contributes to the incidence of breast cancer. This is one of the many reasons that the trial was not approved. The question of fat and breast cancer has been a very controversial subject in the epidemiologic literature. Studies on dietary fat in animals support the idea that a high-fat diet produces more mammary tumors, but there are some anomalies in the results of the animal studies (carried out by giving certain chemical carcinogens to sensitive strains of rodents) that have produced uncertainty about their relevance to human disease, and there is a general lack of correlation with the results of human dietary surveys. The human dietary surveys have not produced consistent evidence for fat being related to higher risk, nor have they shown that higher intake of polyunsaturated fat is related to higher risk as it is in the animal studies.

Two prospective studies have also failed to show an association with dietary fat. Thousands of women who had filled out dietary questionnaires were contacted a few years later to find out how many cases of breast cancer had occurred. It was found that fat had not increased their risk; in fact, it seemed to have decreased their risk.

As explained by Walter Willett and his associates at Harvard School of Public Health, the hypothesis that a high-fat diet contributes to breast cancer has not held up in studies on the diets of individuals. As mentioned earlier, this hypothesis came from the observation that countries with high-fat diets had greater incidence of breast cancer. Willett and also several other researchers have reviewed the studies on diets of individuals and have concluded that there is no good evidence to support the hypothesis that dietary fat is related to breast cancer.[11,12,13] And there is no established biological mechanism whereby fat could have such an effect.

This conclusion has important implications for public health efforts to reduce the scourge of breast cancer. No one would recommend that women should indulge in high-fat diets recklessly because this could increase the chances of atherosclerosis, overweight, and some forms of cancer. But if the goal is to reduce the incidence of breast cancer, some other dietary changes must be recommended instead of low-fat diets. According to Willett's analysis, we cannot expect that reducing the amount of fat in the diet will alter the breast cancer statistics. Women who adopt a low-fat diet will be improving their health prospects in some ways, but they should not be lulled into believing that breast cancer will be less likely.

There is evidence from clinical trials that folic acid is effective for reversing precancerous conditions. Trials using folic acid have been done in connection with precancerous changes in the cervix, in the lungs, and in the colon.

In 1982, scientists at the University of Alabama reported that folic acid produced improvement in women who had cervical dysplasia. They compared the effect of vitamin C, given in a small dose as a placebo, with that of folic acid and found significant improvement from taking folic acid. Cervical dysplasia is a common condition that occasionally improves spontaneously, but doctors monitor the condition because it sometimes becomes more severe over time, leading to cervical cancer.

The interest in testing folic acid for treatment of cervical dysplasia goes back to a 1973 study where folic acid was proven to be effective in producing normal Pap smears in women who had abnormal appearing cells. The abnormal cells resembled blood cells of people who suffer from megaloblastic anemia due to deficiency of folic acid or vitamin B12, in spite of these women having normal levels of folic acid in the blood. Folic acid treatment caused the cells to revert to normal appearance. It was suggested that, in tissues that use a lot of folic acid because of hormone stimulation, localized deficiencies of folic acid might develop even though the level of folic acid in the circulation is normal.

The group of scientists at the University of Alabama have long been involved in the application of nutrition research to public health problems. Their understanding of folic acid biochemistry has lead them to discuss the hypothesis "that differences in folate status modulate the risk of malignancy in human tissues . . . "[14] This hypothesis arises from the effectiveness of folic acid for improving megaloblastic changes in the cervix and from the theoretical susceptibility of DNA to cancer-causing damage when folic acid is deficient. These scientists realize that folic acid might play an important role in restoring normal cell characteristics to abnormal, proliferating cells. Their understated suggestion probably applies to a wide range of human cancers.

The 1982 folic acid trial on cervical dysplasia was considered to be a preliminary trial because only a small group of women who were all using oral contraceptives were treated. A much larger study has been completed in which patients were compared for a variety of risk factors for cervical cancer. The scientists found, among other things, that infection with human papillomavirus increased the risk of cervical dysplasia and increased the risk much more in those women who had low blood levels of folic acid. The explanation for this may be that DNA in folate-deficient tissues is more easily altered by the oncogenic virus.

Women in this study who had cervical dysplasia were recruited to participate in a randomized, placebo-controlled trial designed to find out whether six months treatment with folic acid would have an effect on their precancerous condition. The results of Pap tests showed that folic acid had no effect on the six month test results. Approximately half of the patients, all of whom had cervical dysplasia at the beginning of the trial, had normal Pap smears after the six months, whether they had taken folic acid or the placebo. So, folic acid in the diet may have helped prevent the incidence of some cases of dysplasia but it did not affect the subsequent course of the disease.[15]

Another clinical trial conducted by the researchers at the University of Alabama involved giving supplements of folic acid and vitamin B12 to smokers. The smokers all had abnormal-appearing cells being sloughed off from the lining of the bronchial tubes, as determined by microscopic examination of sputum samples. This type of altered cell is frequently a forerunner of lung cancer. Carlos L. Krumdieck, at the University of Alabama, has hypothesized that the chemicals in cigarette smoke, some of which can inactivate folic acid coenzymes, might produce folic acid deficiency in the bronchial epithelium. To find out whether the abnormal cell condition responds to vitamin supplements, the researchers carried out a controlled, randomized trial where participants were given high doses of folic acid and vitamin B12 for four months. At the end of the trial there was more frequent improvement in the appearance of sloughed off cells in those who received the vitamins than in those who received a placebo.[16]

In chapter 11 I mentioned a recent clinical study that showed that folic acid supplements protected colitis patients against precancerous changes in the colon. This was not a controlled, randomized trial but, rather, was an inquiry into the medical records of ninety-nine patients who suffered from ulcerative colitis and had been monitored for more than seven years in a surveillance program at the University of Chicago. Ulcerative colitis is a serious, chronic disease that increases the risk for colon cancer, but about three years before cancer develops, dysplasia consisting of abnormal epithelial cells with enlarged nuclei can be detected in the colon. Doctors monitor these patients in order to detect any cancer in the earliest stages. Ulcerative colitis can be treated with a drug, but the drug is known to interfere with the absorption of folic acid from foods; so patients are often given folic acid supplements. (Even without the drug, these patients have a tendency to become deficient in folic acid.) Taking a folic acid supplement appeared to confer protection against dysplasia or cancer when the 29% of patients who took the supplement were compared with the others. Their chance of developing dysplasia or cancer was only 38% as great as in those without the supplement. A daily dose of 400 micrograms of folic acid was just as effective as 1000 micrograms. The results of this small study were not quite statistically significant; so a larger, more comprehensive study was to be undertaken.[17]

In chapter 11 I described the widespread interest in the relationship between dietary fiber and the incidence of cancer, especially colon cancer. A 1988 review from the National Cancer Institute says that thirty-two out of forty epidemiologic studies from the 1970s and early 1980s found an inverse association between dietary fiber and colon cancer risk.[18] A 1991 review from the National Cancer Institute points out that six out of seven case-control studies on breast cancer also have found an inverse relation between fiber or fiber-rich foods such as vegetables, fruits, and cereals and risk for breast cancer.[19] Many scientists believe that fiber has a protective effect against cancer, but others insist that an effect for fiber is not yet proven, that fiber-containing foods are such complex mixtures of nutrients that we cannot be sure that it is the fiber that produces the good results.

Scientists have tried to figure out which fiber-containing foods are most effective and they have speculated about which type of fiber is best. The scientists are hampered by limited knowledge of the different kinds of fiber in specific foods. "Fiber" is a general term for indigestible carbohydrates and it includes several subtypes, not all of which have been analyzed in all foods. Studies in laboratory animals have led to the conclusion that wheat bran is the most effective high-fiber supplement for reducing the incidence of colon tumors. Wheat bran has also been tested in a randomized, controlled clinical trial and was found to be effective in inhibiting the development of benign tumors (polyps) in the colon. The argument about which component of wheat bran is most effective continues, but to my knowledge, the researchers have not considered the high folic acid content of wheat bran as a possible explanation, as of 1992.

In chapter 10 I listed wheat germ as being a good source of folic acid; wheat germ contains 352 micrograms per 100 grams. (One hundred grams of wheat germ is a little less than one cup.) Wheat bran is not as high in folic acid but it still contains an appreciable amount: 79 micrograms of folic acid per 100 grams. These values are from USDA Handbook No. 8 20. Other references on folic acid content of foods give differing values for wheat bran. A 1977 compilation of data on folic acid in foods, made by scientists at the U.S. Department of Agriculture, listed 258 micrograms folic acid in 100 grams of wheat bran.[20] And a British reference lists 260 micrograms folic acid in 100 grams of wheat bran.[21]

The controlled, clinical trial that found benefits from wheat bran found evidence of improvement from consuming a supplement that gave the participants 22.5 grams of fiber per day, including the fiber from their normal diets. The participants in the four-year study all suffered from a rare, hereditary disorder that produces numerous tumors (polyps) in the colon and carries a high risk for colon cancer. Upon regular examination, those paricipants who consumed the wheat bran supplement had a decrease in the number of polyps of almost half compared to those who did not get the supplement and consumed about 11 or 12 grams of fiber a day in their normal diets. The supplemented group had this improvement after twenty-one months into the study. The study also found some evidence for more polyps in those patients who consumed more dietary fat.[22]

This trial using wheat bran and a study in rats that showed less mammary cancer in rats that were fed wheat bran stimulated considerable interest and comments in the medical journals, but apparently no one has yet suggested that the benefits from wheat bran in human and animal studies might be due to the folic acid in the wheat bran.

The researchers expect that a treatment such as wheat bran or folic acid that helps these patients who have especially high risk for cancer should also help the general population where the risk is lower. However, the costs of doing a clinical trial on the general population would be prohibitive. So, it remains for us to make our own tentative conclusions about the value of using supplements.

Both wheat germ and wheat bran are available in the supermarket in the breakfast cereals section. Some of the popular, high-fiber breakfast cereals contain wheat bran as a main ingredient and also contain extra folic acid. And of course, whole wheat bread contains both the wheat germ and the wheat bran. Scientists caution against eating excessive, unnatural amounts of fiber, as this might cause intestinal difficulties. The National Cancer Institute dietary guidelines recommend 20 to 30 grams a day of fiber, from fruits, vegetables, and whole grains.

There are many findings from the older international studies on diet and cancer incidence that are in harmony with the recommendation to include whole grains in the diet. Using the same type of 1960s data collected by the United Nations that led to the theory that a high meat or fat diet causes more cancer, Armstrong and Doll, epidemiologists at Oxford University, found in 1975 that rates of cancer mortality were inversely related to the amount of grains, or cereals, in the diet in thirty-seven countries. In addition to positive associations between cancer and meat or fat, they found an inverse correlation between cereals and colorectal cancer and inverse correlations between cereals and pulses (legumes) and cancer of the breast, uterus, ovary, prostate, testis, and kidney.[23]

More recent international surveys also show inverse associations between fiber or cereals and mortality from cancer. Diet surveys in Great Britain, Finland, and Denmark also hint that high-fiber diets are related to less colon cancer. Colon cancer became less common in the British isles and in Switzerland after the Second World War, perhaps because wartime flour milling left more bran in the flour. However, when case-control studies are done in recent years on individuals in the western countries, an association with fiber is not always found.[24] On the other hand, a case-control study in the Minneapolis-St. Paul area on cancer of the pancreas found strong inverse correlations between both whole wheat bread and cruciferous vegetables and cancer incidence.

The international studies provide clues to the cancer puzzle but they cannot provide proof for a theory involving diet. The international data are consistent with either or both of these theories and do not rule out one or the other: that fat and meat increase the incidence of cancer, or that cereals protect against development of cancer. Scientific proof for the value of a high-fiber or low-fat or high-vitamin diet must come from the randomized, controlled clinical trials that are presently under way or soon to be started.

Many of the clinical trials will no doubt continue to demonstrate some benefits for certain people at high risk for specific types of cancer. But of even greater importance than the clinical trials is the campaign by the National Cancer Institute to encourage everyone to consume at least five servings a day of fruits and vegetables. This campaign will put into practice the most consistent conclusions that have been found in the epidemiologic studies. If we can devote the attention to nutrition that our good health requires, the emphasis on vegetables and whole grains could become the way to finally bring about improvement in the cancer statistics.

Glossary

Beta-carotene. A carotenoid that can be converted to retinaldehyde in animal tissues. Most important carotenoid nutritionally because its forty carbon structure can be cleaved in the middle by an enzyme to yield, theoretically, two molecules of retinaldehyde. Color is deep orange-red.

Carcinoma. Malignant neoplasm that originated in epithelial tissue. Most common type of cancer.

Carotenoids. Polyisoprenoids with extensive conjugated double bonds. These pigments are synthesized by plants. Most contain forty carbon atoms. More than five hundred carotenoids have been identified. Approximately fifty carotenoids have nutritional value in animals; the most important of these is beta-carotene.

Folic acid. A water-soluble B vitamin, also known as folate, folacin, or pteroylglutamic acid.

Oncogenes. Genes that contribute to uncontrolled growth and malignancy. They are mutated forms of the normal proto-oncogenes.

Proto-oncogenes. Normal genes that are thought to be involved in regulation of normal growth and cell division.

Provitamin A. Carotenoid that can be converted to retinaldehyde by animals. Examples are beta-carotene, alpha-carotene, and cryptoxanthin.

Retinoic acid. A form of vitamin A that is present naturally in animal tissues in minute amounts. Has vitamin A activity except for vision.

Retinoids. A general term for retinol and related substances. Examples are retinol, retinaldehyde, retinoic acid and synthetic analogs of these compounds. Many of the synthetic analogs have been tested for pharmacologic activity.

Retinol. The form of vitamin A that is transported in the circulation complexed with retinol-binding protein. Color is pale yellow.

Retinyl ester. The predominant form of vitamin A in liver, cod liver oil, and vitamin supplements. Same as retinyl palmitate, vitamin A palmitate, retinyl acetate, vitamin A acetate.

Vitamin A. A general term for growth-restoring substances active in the rat bioassay. Synonyms are "fat-soluble A," retinol, retinaldehyde, retinyl ester. The term is also used for the carotenoids that can be used by animal tissues.

Chemical Structures

Carotenoids

beta-Carotene

$C_{40}H_{56}$

alpha-Carotene

$C_{40}H_{56}$

Cryptoxanthin

HO

$C_{40}H_{56}O$

Lycopene

$C_{40}H_{56}$

Canthaxanthin

$C_{40}H_{52}O_2$

Retinoids

Retinol

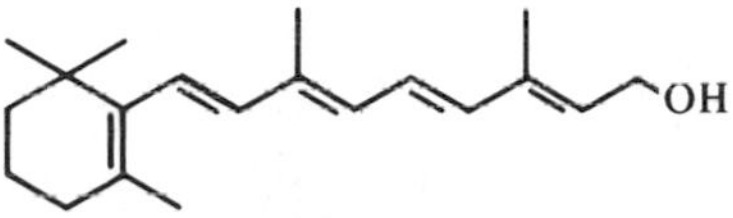

$C_{20}H_{30}O$

Retinyl ester

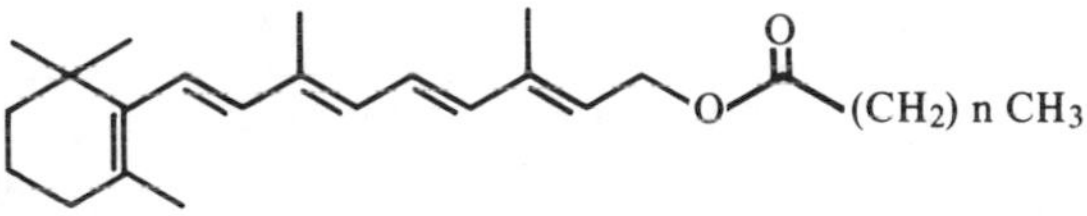

(CH_2) n CH_3

Retinaldehyde

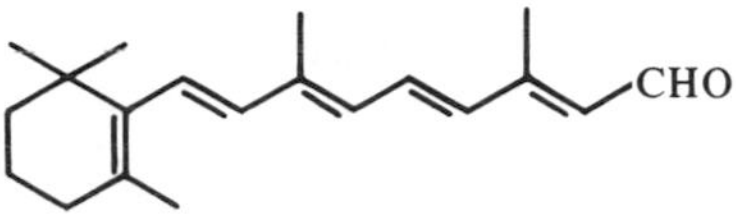

$C_{20}H_{28}O$

11-cis-Retinaldehyde

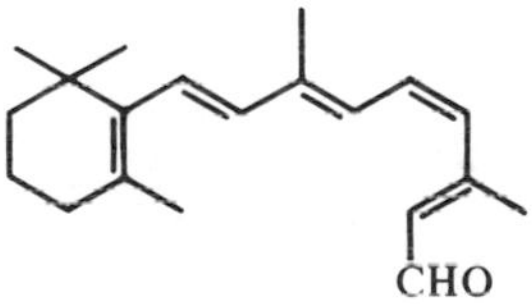

$C_{20}H_{28}O$

CHO

Retinoic acid

COOH

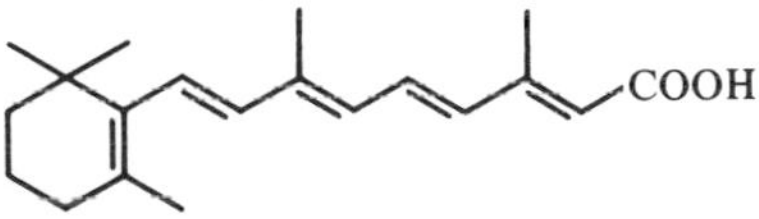

$C_{20}H_{28}O_2$

13-cis-Retinoic acid

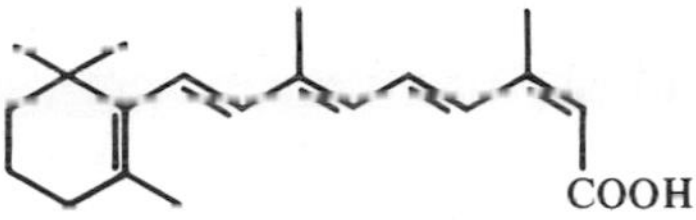

$C_{20}H_{28}O_2$

COOH

Folic acid, et cetera

Folic acid

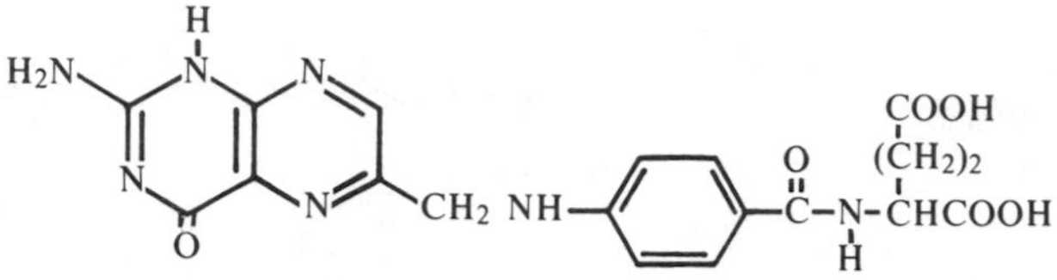

Choline

$$HOCH_2\text{-}CH_2\text{-}\overset{\oplus}{N}\text{-}(CH_3)_3$$

Methionine

$$CH_3\text{-}S\text{-}CH_2\text{-}CH_2\text{-}\overset{\overset{\displaystyle H}{|}}{C}\text{-}COOH$$
$$\underset{NH_2}{}$$

S-Adenosylmethionine

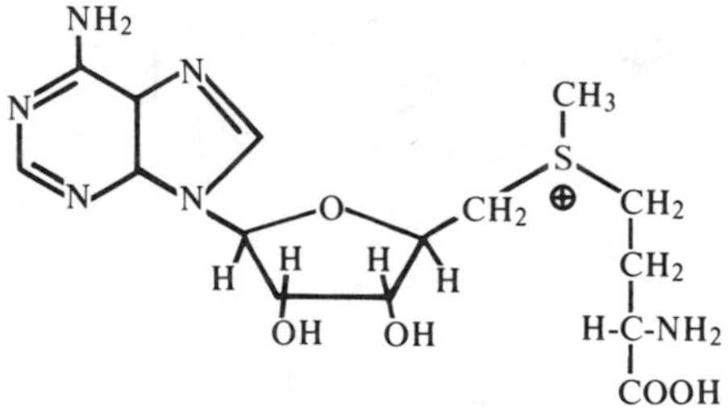

5-Methylcytosine

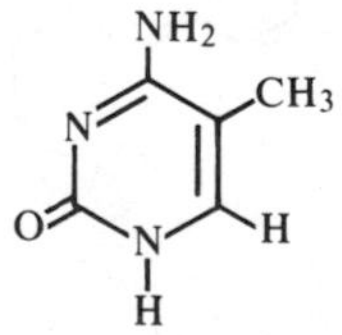

Bibliography

Chapter 2 The Hunza River Valley

1. The cover of *Science* magazine of October 7, 1988 has a photo of one of the Karakoram glaciers.
2. Emily O. Lorimer, *Language Hunting in the Karakoram*, George Allen and Unwin Ltd., London 1939.
3. John H. Tobe, *Hunza: Adventures in a Land of Paradise*, Rodale Books, Inc., Emmaus, Penna. 1960.
4. John Clark, *Hunza: Lost Kingdom of the Himalayas*, Funk & Wagnalls Company, New York 1956, and Hutchinson and Co. of London 1957.
5. Franc and Jean Shor, "The Happy Land of Just Enough," *Life Magazine*, January 30, 1950 p. 38.
6. Jean and Franc Shor, "At World's End in Hunza," *National Geographic Magazine 104 (4)*, 485–518, October 1953.
7. Tay and Lowell Thomas, Jr., "Sky Road East," *National Geographic Magazine 117*, 71–112, January 1960.
8. J.I. Rodale, *The Healthy Hunzas*, Rodale Press, Emmaus, Pa. 1948.
9. Sabina and Roland Michaud, "Trek to Lofty Hunza — and Beyond," *National Geographic Magazine 148*, 644–669, November 1975.
10. John Clark, "Hunza in the Himalayas," *Natural History 72*, 38–45, October 1963.
11. Alexander Leaf, M.D., and John Launois, "Every Day Is a Gift When You Are Over 100," *National Geographic Magazine 143 (1)*, 93–119, January 1973.

Chapter 3 The Hawthorne Works

1. In time, the plant became obsolete as a production facility, and operations ceased at the Hawthorne Works in 1983 with the breakup of AT&T. The property was converted to mini-factories, warehousing, and retail stores. More details are in the *Chicago Tribune* of December 27, 1987.
2. F.J. Roethlisberger, *Management and Morale*, Harvard University Press, Cambridge, Mass. 1941.

3. Oglesby Paul et al., "A Longitudinal Study of Coronary Heart Disease," *Circulation 28,* 20 (1963).
4. Richard B. Shekelle et al., "Diet, Serum Cholesterol, and Death from Coronary Heart Disease," *New England Journal of Medicine 304,* 65 (1981).
5. Gina Kolata, "Research News: Lowered Cholesterol Decreases Heart Disease," *Science 223,* 381 (1984).
6. R. Peto, R. Doll, J.D. Buckley and M.B. Sporn, "Can dietary beta-carotene materially reduce human cancer rates?" *Nature 290,* 201 (1981).
7. R. Doll and R. Peto, "The Causes of Cancer: Quantitative Estimates of Avoidable Risks of Cancer in the United States Today," *J. Natl. Cancer Inst. 66,* 1191 (1981).
8. R.B. Shekelle et al., "Dietary Vitamin A and Risk of Cancer in the Western Electric Study," *The Lancet 2,* 1185 (1981).
9. Vegetables in the Western Electric survey were asparagus, green beans, beets, broccoli, cabbage, carrots, cauliflower, corn, eggplant, leafy green vegetables, other green and yellow vegetables, onions, peas, and tomatoes. Fruits in the survey were avocado, apple, banana, cantaloupe, citrus fruits, other fresh or canned fruit, and dried fruit.
10. E. Bjelke, "Dietary Vitamin A and Human Lung Cancer," *Int. J. Cancer 15,* 561 (1975).
11. R. MacLennan et al., "Risk Factors of Lung Cancer in Singapore Chinese, a Population with High Female Incidence Rates," *Int. J. Cancer 20,* 854 (1977).
12. S.B. Wolbach and P.R. Howe, "Tissue changes following deprivation of fat-soluble A vitamin," *J. Exp. Med. 42,* 753 (1925).
13. D. Burk and R.J. Winzler, "Vitamins and Cancer," *Vitamins and Hormones 2,* 305 (1944).
14. U. Saffiotti et al., "Experimental cancer of the lung," *Cancer 20,* 857 (1967).

Chapter 6   The Discovery of Vitamin A

1. E.V. McCollum, "My Early Experiences in the Study of Foods and Nutrition," *Ann. Rev. Biochem. 22,* 1 (1953).
2. E.V. McCollum, *A History of Nutrition,* Houghton Mifflin Co., Boston 1957.
3. E.V. McCollum and Marguerite Davis, "The Necessity of Certain Lipins in the Diet during Growth," *J. Biol. Chem. 15,* 167 (1913).
4. E.V. McCollum, "The Supplementary Dietary Relationships Among Our Natural Foodstuffs," *J. Amer. Med. Assoc. 68,* 1379 (1917)..
5. Elmer Verner McCollum, *From Kansas Farm Boy to Scientist,* University of Kansas Press, Lawrence 1964.

6. Harry G. Day, "E.V. McCollum and Public Understanding of Foods and Nutrition," *Nutrition Today 1987*, May/June p.31.
7. H. Steenbock, "White Corn vs. Yellow Corn and a Probable Relation between the Fat-Soluble Vitamine and Yellow Plant Pigments," *Science 50*, 352 (1919).
8. H. Steenbock and P.W. Boutwell, "Fat-Soluble Vitamine. The Extractability of the Fat-Soluble Vitamine from Carrots, Alfalfa, and Yellow Corn by Fat Solvents," *J. Biol. Chem. 42*, 131 (1920).
9. Thomas Moore, "Vitamin A and Carotene. The Association of Vitamin A Activity with Carotene in the Carrot Root," *Biochem. J. 23*, 803 (1929).
10. Thomas Moore, "The Relation of Carotin to Vitamin A," *Lancet* ii, 380 (1929).
11. Thomas Moore, "Vitamin A and Carotene. The Conversion of Carotene to Vitamin A *in vivo*," *Biochem. J. 24*, 692 (1930).
12. Thomas Moore, "Vitamin A and Carotene. The Distribution of Vitamin A and Carotene in the Body of the Rat," *Biochem. J. 25*, 275 (1931).

Chapter 7   Night Blindness and Other Ills

1. Alfred Sommer, "New Imperatives for an Old Vitamin (A)," *J. Nutr. 119*, 96 (1989).
2. James A. Olson, "The Prevention of Childhood Blindness by the Administration of Massive Doses of Vitamin A," *Israel J. Med. Sci. 8*, 1199 (1972).
3. Barbara A. Underwood, "Vitamin A in Animal and Human Nutrition," in M.B. Sporn et al., eds., *The Retinoids* vol. 1, Academic Press, Inc., Orlando 1984.
4. Gregory D. Hussey and Max Klein, "A Randomized, Controlled Trial of Vitamin A in Children with Severe Measles," *N. Eng. J. Med. 323*, 160 (1990).
5. Muhilal et al., "Vitamin A-Fortified Monosodium Glutamate and Vitamin A Status: a Controlled Field Trial," *Am. J. Clin. Nutr. 48*, 1265 (1988).
6. S.B. Wolbach and P.R. Howe, "Tissue Changes Following Deprivation of Fat-Soluble A Vitamin," *J. Exp. Med. 42*, 753 (1925)
7. E.V. McCollum and N. Simmonds, "A Biological Analysis of Pellagra-Producing Diets," *J. Biol. Chem. 32*, 181 (1917).
8. H.E. Sauberlich et al., "Vitamin A Metabolism and Requirements in the Human Studied with the Use of Labeled Retinol," *Vitamins and Hormones 32*, 251 (1974).
9. Harold Jeghers, "The Degree and Prevalence of Vitamin A Deficiency in Adults," *J. Amer. Med. Assoc. 109*, 756 (1937).

Chapter 8   Metabolism and Toxicity of Vitamin A

 1. George Wald, "The Biochemistry of Vision," *Ann. Rev. Biochem. 22,* 497 (1953).
 2. Thomas Moore, *Vitamin A,* Elsevier, Amsterdam 1957.
 3. Edwin L. Sexton et al., "Studies on Carotenoid Metabolism," *J. Nutr. 31,* 299 (1946).
 4. M.R. Lakshman et al., "Enzymatic Conversion of All-trans-beta-Carotene to Retinal by a Cytosolic Enzyme from Rabbit and Rat Intestinal Mucosa," *Proc. Natl. Acad. Sci. USA 86,* 9124 (1989).
 5. DeWitt S. Goodman, "Vitamin A and Retinoids in Health and Disease," *N. Eng. J. Med. 310,* 1023 (1984).
 6. DeWitt S. Goodman and William S. Blaner, "Biosynthesis, Absorption, and Hepatic Metabolism of Retinol," in M.B. Sporn et al., eds., *The Retinoids* vol. 2, Academic Press, Inc., Orlando 1984.
 7. Charles A. Frolik, "Metabolism of Retinoids," in M.B. Sporn et al., eds., *The Retinoids* vol.2, Academic Press, Inc., Orlando 1984.
 8. F.D. Crain et al., "Biosynthesis of Retinoic Acid by Intestinal Enzymes of the Rat," *J. Lipid Res. 8,* 249 (1967).
 9. H.F. DeLuca, "Retinoic Acid Metabolism," *Federation Proc. 38,* 2519 (1979).
10. Joseph L. Napoli and Kevin R. Race, "Biogenesis of Retinoic Acid from beta-Carotene," *J. Biol. Chem. 263,* 17372 (1988).
11. Xiang-Dong Wang et al., "Enzymic Conversion of beta-Carotene into beta-Apo-carotenals and Retinoids by Human, Monkey, Ferret, and Rat Tissues," *Arch. Biochem. Biophys. 285,* 8 (1991).
12. J.A. Lucy et al., "Studies on the Mode of Action of Excess Vitamin A," *Biochem. J. 79,* 500 (1961).
13. DeWitt S. Goodman, "Plasma Retinol-Binding Protein," in M.B. Sporn et al., *The Retinoids* vol. 2, Academic Press, Inc., Orlando (1984).
14. Richard K. Miller et al., "Position Paper by the Teratology Society: Vitamin A During Pregnancy," *Teratology 35,* 267 (1987).
15. Barbara A. Underwood, "Vitamin A in Animal and Human Nutrition," in M.B. Sporn et al., eds., *The Retinoids* vol.1, Academic Press, Inc., Orlando (1984).
16. C.J. Bates, "Vitamin A in Pregnancy and Lactation," *Proc. Nutr. Soc. 42,* 65 (1983).
17. Sidney Q. Cohlan, "Congenital Anomalies in the Rat Produced by Excessive Intake of Vitamin A During Pregnancy," *Pediatrics 13,* 556 (1954).
18. Aubrey Milunsky et al., "Multivitamin/Folic Acid Supplementation in Early Pregnancy Reduces the Prevalence of Neural Tube Defects," *J. Amer. Med. Assoc. 262,* 2847 (1989).

19. L. Stange et al., "Hypervitaminosis A in Early Human Pregnancy and Malformations of the Central Nervous System," *Acta Obstet. Gynecol. Scand. 57,* 289 (1978).

20. C. Patrick Mahoney et al., "Chronic Vitamin A Intoxication in Infants Fed Chicken Liver," *Pediatrics 65,* 893 (1980).

21. Bennett A. Shaywitz et al., "Megavitamins for Minimal Brain Dysfunction—A Potentially Dangerous Therapy," *J. Amer. Med. Assoc. 238,* 1749 (1977). [Contains typographical error in measurement units for vitamin A blood levels.]

22. David J.C. Shearman, "Vitamin A and Sir Douglas Mawson," *Brit. Med. J. 1,* 283 (1978).

23. Douglas Mawson, *The Home of the Blizzard, Being the Story of the Australasian Antarctica Expedition 1911–1914,* Lippincott, Philadelphia 1914.

24. K. Rodahl and T. Moore, "The Vitamin A Content and Toxicity of Bear and Seal Liver," *Biochem. J. 37,* 166 (1943).

25. J.B. Cleland and R.V. Southcott, "Illnesses Following the Eating of Seal Liver in Australian Waters," *Med. J. Australia 1,* 760 (1969).

26. Kaare Rodahl, "Toxicity of Polar Bear Liver," *Nature 164,* 530 (1949).

27. James Allen Olson, "Provitamin A Function of Carotenoids: The Conversion of beta-Carotene into Vitamin A," *J. Nutr. 119,* 105 (1989).

28. G.B. Brubacher and H. Weiser, "The Vitamin A Activity of beta-Carotene," *Int. J. Vit. Nutr. Res. 55,* 5 (1985).

29. Maud Dagadu and Joseph Gillman, "Hypercarotenemia in Ghanaians," *Lancet 1,* 531 (1963).

30. C. Nageswara Rao and B.S. Narasinga Rao, "Absorption of Dietary Carotene in Human Subjects," *Am. J. Clin. Nutr. 23,* 105 (1970).

31. E.D. Brown et al., "Plasma Carotenoids in Normal Men After a Single Ingestion of Vegetables or Purified beta-Carotene," *Am. J. Clin. Nutr. 49,* 1258 (1989).

32. Nikolay V. Dimitrov et al., "Bioavailability of beta-Carotene in Humans," *Am. J. Clin. Nutr. 48,* 298 (1988).

33. R. Heywood et al., "The Toxicity of beta-Carotene," *Toxicology 36,* 91 (1985).

34. Adrianne Bendich, "The Safety of beta-Carotene," *Nutr. Cancer 11,* 207 (1988).

35. Food and Nutrition Board, National Research Council, *Recommended Dietary Allowances, 10th Edition,* National Academy Press, Washington DC 1989.

36. Rune Blomhoff et al., "Transport and Storage of Vitamin A," *Science 250,* 399 (1990).

Chapter 9   RDA and Vitamin A — How to Measure?

1. E.V. McCollum, Elsa Orent-Keiles, Harry G. Day, *The Newer Knowledge of Nutrition,* Macmillan, New York 1939.
2. John G. Bieri and Mary C. McKenna, "Expressing Dietary Values of Fat-Soluble Vitamins: Changes in Concepts and Terminology," *Amer. J. Clin. Nutr. 34,* 289 (1981).
3. Barbara A. Underwood, "Vitamin A in Animal and Human Nutrition," in M.B. Sporn et al., eds., *The Retinoids* vol. 1, Academic Press, Inc., Orlando (1984).
4. H.H. Inhoffen and H. Pommer, "Determination; Standardization of Activity," in W.H. Sebrell and R.S. Harris, eds., *The Vitamins,* vol. 1, 1st edition, Academic Press, New York 1954.
5. Kenneth L. Simpson and C.O. Chichester, "Metabolism and Nutritional Significance of Carotenoids," *Ann. Rev. Nutr. 1,* 351 (1981).
6. Gary R. Beecher and Frederick Khachik, "Evaluation of Vitamin A and Carotenoid Data in Food Composition Tables," *J. Natl. Cancer Inst. 73,* 1397 (1984).
7. FAO/WHO. *Requirements of Vitamin A, Thiamine, Riboflavin, and Niacin. Report of a Joint FAO/WHO Expert Committee. FAO Nutrition Meetings Series No. 41. WHO Technical Report Series No. 362.* WHO Geneva 1967.
8. Food and Nutrition Board, National Research Council, *Recommended Dietary Allowances, 9th Revised Edition,* National Academy of Sciences, Washington DC, 1980.
9. Regina G. Ziegler, "A Review of Epidemiologic Evidence that Carotenoids Reduce the Risk of Cancer," *J. Nutr. 119,* 116 (1989).
10. Food and Nutrition Board, National Research Council, *Recommended Dietary Allowances, 10th Edition,* National Academy Press, Washington DC, 1989.
11. Frederick Khachik et al., "Separation, Identification, and Quantification of the Major Carotenoids in Extracts of Apricots, Peaches, Cantaloupe, and Pink Grapefruit by Liquid Chromatography," *J. Agric. Food Chem. 37,* 1465 (1989).
12. Frederick Khachik et al., "Separation, Identification, and Quantification of the Major Carotenoid and Chlorophyll Constituents in Extracts of Several Green Vegetables by Liquid Chromatography," *J. Agric. Food Chem. 34,* 603 (1986).

Chapter 10   The Folic Acid Connection

1. Carlos L. Krumdieck et al., Synthesis and Analysis of the Pteroylpolyglutamates," *Vit. Horm. 40,* 45 (1983).

2. Arnold D. Welch, "Folic Acid: Discovery and the Exciting First Decade," *Perspect. Biol. Med. 27*, 64 (1983).
3. J.J. Pfiffner and Albert G. Hogan, "The Newer Hematopoietic Factors of the Vitamin B-Complex," *Vit. Horm. 4*, 1 (1946).
4. Victor Herbert and Kshitish C. Das, "The Role of Vitamin B12 and Folic Acid in Hemato- and Other Cell-Poiesis," *Vit. Horm. 34*, 1 (1976).
5. Clark W. Heath, Jr., "Cytogenetic Observations in Vitamin B12 and Folate Deficiency," *Blood 27*, 800 (1966).
6. Rosa C. Menzies et al., "Cytogenetic and Cytochemical Studies on Marrow Cells in B12 and Folate Deficiency," *Blood 28*, 581 (1966).
7. James Bonner et al., "The Biology of Isolated Chromatin," *Science 159*, 47 (1968).
8. Laura Manuelidis, "A View of Interphase Chromosomes," *Science 250*, 1533 (1990).
9. Grant R. Sutherland, "Heritable Fragile Sites on Human Chromosomes," *Am. J. Hum. Genet. 31*, 125 (1979).
10. Carlos L. Krumdieck and Patricia N. Howard-Peebles, "On the Nature of Folic Acid-Sensitive Fragile Sites in Human Chromosomes: An Hypothesis," *Am. J. Med. Genet. 16*, 23 (1983).
11. Jorge J. Yunis and A. Lee Soreng, "Constitutive Fragile Sites and Cancer," *Science 226*, 1199 (1984).
12. James T. MacGregor et al., "Cytogenetic Damage Induced by Folate Deficiency in Mice Is Enhanced by Caffeine," *Proc. Natl. Acad. Sci. USA 87*, 9962 (1990).
13. S. Jill James and Larry Yin, "Diet-Induced DNA Damage and Altered Nucleotide Metabolism in Lymphocytes from Methyl-Donor-Deficient Rats," *Carcinogenesis 10*, 1209 (1989).
14. Richard B. Everson et al., "Association of Marginal Folate Depletion with Increased Human Chromosomal Damage in Vivo: Demonstration by Analysis of Micronucleated Erythrocytes," *J. Natl. Cancer Inst. 80*, 525 (1988).
15. Jorge J. Yunis, "The Chromosomal Basis of Human Neoplasia," *Science 221*, 227 (1983).
16. J. Michael Bishop, "The Molecular Genetics of Cancer," *Science 235*, 305 (1987).
17. Arnold J. Levine, "Cancer, Viruses, and Oncogenes," in Richard E. LaFond, ed., *Cancer: The Outlaw Cell* 2nd edition, American Chemical Society, Washington DC 1988.
18. S. Heim and F. Mitelman, "Nineteen of 26 cellular oncogenes precisely localized in the human genome map to one of the 83 bands involved in primary cancer-specific rearrangements," *Hum. Genet. 75*, 70 (1987).

19. Janet D. Rowley, "Biological Implications of Consistent Chromosome Rearrangements in Leukemia and Lymphoma," *Cancer Res. 44*, 3159 (1984).

20. Julian Borrow et al., "Molecular Analysis of Acute Promyelocytic Leukemia Breakpoint Cluster Region on Chromosome 17," *Science 249*, 1577 (1990).

21. B. J. Barclay et al., "Genetic and Biochemical Consequences of Thymidylate Stress," *Can. J. Biochem. 60*, 172 (1982).

22. Isao Eto and Carlos L. Krumdieck, "Role of Vitamin B12 and Folate Deficiencies in Carcinogenesis," in Lionel L. Poirier et al., eds., *Essential Nutrients in Carcinogenesis*, Plenum Press, New York 1986.

23. I. Bernard Weinstein, "The Origins of Human Cancer: Molecular Mechanisms of Carcinogenesis and Their Implications for Cancer Prevention and Treatment," *Cancer Res. 48*, 4135 (1988).

24. D.H. Copeland and W.D. Salmon, "The Occurrence of Neoplasms in the Liver, Lungs, and Other Tissues of Rats as a Result of Prolonged Choline Deficiency," *Amer. J. Path. 22*, 1059 (1946).

25. Donald W. Horne et al., "Effect of Dietary Methyl Group Deficiency on Folate Metabolism in Rats," *J. Nutr. 119*, 618 (1989).

26. A.E. Schaeffer et al., "Interrelationship of Folacin, Vitamin B12, and Choline," *J. Nutr. 40*, 95 (1950).

27. Michael Potter and George M. Briggs, "Inhibition of Growth of Amethopterin-Sensitive and Amethopterin-Resistant Pairs of Lymphocytic Neoplasms by Dietary Folic Acid Deficiency in Mice," *J. Natl. Cancer Inst. 28*, 341 (1962).

28. Adrianne E. Rogers and Paul M. Newberne, "Dietary Effects on Chemical Carcinogenesis in Animal Models for Colon and Liver Tumors," *Cancer Res. 35*, 3427 (1975).

29. Paul M. Newberne, "Lipotropic Factors and Oncogenesis," in Lionel L. Poirier et al., eds., *Essential Nutrients in Carcinogenesis*, Plenum Press, New York 1986.

30. Yves B. Mikol et al., "Hepatocarcinogenesis in rats fed methyl-deficient, amino acid-defined diets," *Carcinogenesis 4*, 1619 (1983).

31. Amiya K. Ghoshal and Emmanuel Farber, "Induction of Liver Cancer by a Diet Deficient in Choline and Methionine," *Proc. Am. Assoc. Cancer Res. 24*, 98 (1983).

32. Amiya K. Ghoshal and Emmanual Farber, "The induction of liver cancer by dietary deficiency of choline and methionine without added carcinogens," *Carcinogenesis 5*, 1367 (1984).

33. Shigeaki Yokoyama et al., "Hepatocarcinogenic and Promoting Action of a Choline-devoid Diet in the Rat," *Cancer Res. 45*, 2834 (1985).

34. K.L. Hoover et al., "Profound Postinitiation Enhancement by Short-Term Severe Methionine, Choline, Vitamin B12, and Folate Deficiency

of Hepatocarcinogenesis in F344 Rats Given a Single Low-Dose Diethylnitrosamine Injection," *J. Natl. Cancer Inst. 73*, 1327 (1984).

35. Mary J. Wilson et al., "Hypomethylation of hepatic nuclear DNA in rats fed with a carcinogenic methyl-deficient diet," *Biochem. J. 218*, 987 (1984).

36. Sidney Farber et al., "The Action of Pteroylglutamic Conjugates on Man," *Science 106*, 619 (1947).

37. Sidney Farber et al., "Temporary Remissions in Acute Leukemia in Children Produced by Folic Acid Antagonist, 4-Aminopteroyl-glutamic Acid (Aminopterin)," *N. Eng. J. Med. 238*, 787 (1948).

38. T. Brailsford Robertson and Theodore C. Burnett, "The Influence of Lecithin and Cholesterin upon the Growth of Tumors," *J. Exp. Med. 17*, 344 (1913).

39. Howard H. Beard, "The Effect of Penicillin and Choline upon the Appearance, Growth and Disappearance of the Emge Sarcoma in Rats," *Exp. Med. Surg. 2*, 286 (1944).

40. R.W. Engel and D.H. Copeland, "The Influence of Dietary Casein Level on Tumor Induction with 2-Acetylaminofluorene," *Cancer Res. 12*, 905 (1952).

41. R. Lewisohn et al., "The Influence of Liver L. casei Factor on Spontaneous Breast Cancer in Mice," *Science 104*, 436 (1946).

42. Victor Herbert, "The Role of Vitamin B12 and Folate in Carcinogenesis," in Lionel L. Poirier et al., eds., *Essential Nutrients in Carcinogenesis*, Plenum Press, New York 1986.

43. Richard F. Branda et al., "Effects of Folate Deficiency on the Metastatic Potential of Murine Melanoma Cells," *Cancer Res. 48*, 4529 (1988).

44. Robert M. Hoffman, "Altered Methionine Metabolism, DNA Methylation and Oncogene Expression in Carcinogenesis," *Biochim. Biophys. Acta 738*, 49 (1984).

45. Janie J. Harrison et al., "Azacytidine-induced tumorigenesis of CHEF/18 cells: Correlated DNA methylation and chromosome changes," *Proc. Natl. Acad. Sci. 80*, 6606 (1983).

46. Shirley M. Taylor and Peter A. Jones, "Mechanism of Action of Eukaryotic DNA Methyltransferase," *J. Mol. Biol. 162*, 679 (1982).

47. Aharon Razin and Arthur D. Riggs, "DNA Methylation and Gene Function," *Science 210*, 604 (1980).

48. R. Holliday and J.E. Pugh, "DNA Modification Mechanisms and Gene Activity during Development," *Science 187*, 226 (1975).

49. A.D. Riggs, "X inactivation, differentiation, and DNA methylation," *Cytogenet. Cell Genet. 14*, 9 (1975).

50. Gary Felsenfeld and James McGhee, "Methylation and gene control," *Nature 296*, 602 (1982).

51. R. Holliday, "A New Theory of Carcinogenesis," *Br. J. Cancer 40*, 513 (1979).
52. In explaining the theory, I have omitted the technical details because I do not wish to describe the complexities of DNA repair. R. Holliday's article (reference 51) should be consulted.
53. Helen M. Blau et al., "Plasticity of the Differentiated State," *Science 230*, 758 (1985).
54. Arthur D. Riggs and Peter A. Jones, "5-Methylcytosine, Gene Regulation, and Cancer," *Adv. Cancer Res. 40*, 1 (1983).
55. Peter A. Jones and Jonathan D. Buckley, "The Role of DNA Methylation in Cancer," *Adv. Cancer Res. 54*, 1 (1990).
56. Andrew P. Feinberg and Bert Vogelstein, "Hypomethylation distinguishes genes of some human cancers from their normal counterparts," *Nature 301*, 89 (1983).
57. Andrew P. Feinberg and Bert Vogelstein, "Hypomethylation of ras Oncogenes in Primary Human Cancers," *Biochem. Biophys. Res. Comm. 111*, 47 (1983).
58. Miguel A. Gama-Sosa et al., "The 5-methylcytosine content of DNA from human tumors," *Nucleic Acids Res. 11*, 6883 (1983).
59. Susan E. Goelz et al., "Hypomethylation of DNA from Benign and Malignant Human Colon Neoplasms," *Science 228*, 187 (1985).
60. Andrew P. Feinberg et al., "Reduced Genomic 5-Methylcytosine Content in Human Colonic Neoplasia," *Cancer Res. 48*, 1159 (1988).
61. Mark T. Bedford and Paul D. vanHelden, "Hypomethylation of DNA in Pathological Conditions of the Human Prostate," *Cancer Res. 47*, 5274 (1987).
62. Kenneth W. Kinzler et al., "Identification of FAP Locus Genes from Chromosome 5q21," *Science 253*, 661 (1991).
63. Eric R. Fearon and Bert Vogelstein, "A Genetic Model for Colorectal Tumorigenesis," *Cell 61*, 759 (1990).
64. Eric R. Fearon et al., "Identification of a Chromosome 18q Gene That Is Altered in Colorectal Cancers," *Science 247*, 49 (1990).
65. Adrian L. Harris, "Telling changes of base," *Nature 350*, 377 (1991).
66. Robert Callahan and Gregory Campbell, "Mutations in Human Breast Cancer: An Overview," *J. Natl. Cancer Inst. 81*, 1780 (1989).
67. J. Mackay et al., "Molecular Lesions in Breast Cancer," *Int. J. Cancer suppl 5*, 47 (1990).
68. George C. Prendergast and Edward B. Ziff, "Methylation-Sensitive Sequence-Specific DNA Binding by the c-Myc Basic Region," *Science 251*, 186 (1991).
69. D. Heitz et al., "Isolation of Sequences That Span the Fragile X and Identification of a Fragile X-Related CpG Island," *Science 251*, 1236 (1991).

70. Michelle Hoffman, "Unraveling the Genetics of Fragile X Syndrome," *Science 252*, 1070 (1991).
71. Department of Health and Human Services, Food and Drug Administration, *Federal Register 56*, 30468. July 2, 1991.
72. Food and Nutrition Board, National Research Council, *Recommended Dietary Allowances, 10th Edition*, National Academy Press, Washington DC, 1989.
73. C.E. Butterworth, Jr. et al., "Zinc concentration in plasma and erythrocytes of subjects receiving folic acid supplementation," *Am. J. Clin. Nutr. 47*, 484 (1988).
74. Nelson A. Fernandez, "Nutrition in Puerto Rico," *Cancer Res. 35*, 3272 (1975).
75. Rafael Santini and Jose J. Corcino, "Analysis of some nutrients of the Puerto Rican diet," *Am. J. Clin. Nutr. 27*, 840 (1974).
76. Isidro Martinez et al., "Cancer Incidence in the United States and Puerto," *Cancer Res. 35*, 3265 (1975).
77. D.M. Parkin et al., "Estimates of the Worldwide Frequency of Sixteen Major Cancers in 1980," *Int. J. Cancer 41*, 184 (1988).

Chapter 11   Five Servings a Day

1. Food and Nutrition Board, National Research Council, *Diet and Health: Implications for Reducing Chronic Disease Risk*, National Academy Press, Washington DC 1989.
2. Walter Willett, "The search for the causes of breast and colon cancer," *Nature 338*, 389 (1989).
3. Barbara S. Hulka, "Dietary Fat and Breast Cancer: Case-Control and Cohort Studies," *Prev. Med. 18*, 180 (1989).
4. Curtis Mettlin, "Diet and the Epidemiology of Human Breast Cancer," *Cancer 53*, 605 (1984).
5. Denis P. Burkitt, "Epidemiology of Cancer of the Colon and Rectum," *Cancer 28*, 3 (1971).
6. James W. Orr, Jr. et al., "Nutritional status of patients with untreated cervical cancer," *Am. J. Obstet. Gynecol. 151*, 632 (1985).
7. R.W.C. Harris et al., "Cancer of the cervix uteri and vitamin A," *Br. J. Cancer 53*, 653 (1986).
8. Rolando Herrero et al., "A Case-Control Study of Nutrient Status and Invasive Cervical Cancer," *Amer. J. Epidem. 134*, 1335 (1991).

Chapter 12   Do We Eat Enough Vegetables?

1. Roger J. Williams, *Nutrition Against Disease*, Pitman Publishing Corp., New York 1971.

2. Susan Welsh, "The Joint Nutrition Monitoring Evaluation Committee," in Food and Nutrition Board, *What Is America Eating?*, National Academy Press, Washington DC 1986.

3. Faith Clark, "Recent food consumption surveys and their uses," *Fed. Proc. 33,* 2270 (1974).

4. Patricia B. Swan, "Food Consumption by Individuals in the United States: Two Major Surveys," *Ann. Rev. Nutr. 3,* 413 (1983).

5. Food and Nutrition Board, National Research Council, *Diet and Health: Implications for Reducing Chronic Disease Risk,* National Academy Press, Washington DC 1989. page 81.

6. U.S. Department of Agriculture, *Nationwide Food Consumption Survey, Continuing Survey of Food Intakes by Individuals, Women 19–50 Years and Their Children 1–5 Years, 4 Days* Report No. 85–4 (1987).

7. U.S. Department of Agriculture, *Continuing Survey of Food Intakes by Individuals, Men 19–50 Years, 1 Day* Report No. 85–3 (1986).

8. Blossom H. Patterson and Gladys Block, "Food Choices and the Cancer Guidelines," *Am. J. Public Health 78,* 282 (1988).

9. Victor Herbert et al., "Folic acid deficiency in the United States: Folate assays in a prenatal clinic," *Am. J. Obstet. Gynecol. 123,* 175 (1975).

10. Alfred J. Clark et al., "Folacin status in adolescent females," *Am. J. Clin. Nutr. 46,* 302 (1987).

11. Jean C. Tsui and James W. Nordstrom, "Folate status of adolescents: Effects of folic acid supplementation," *J. Am. Diet. Assoc. 90,* 1551 (1990).

12. L.B. Bailey et al., "Folacin and iron status and hematological findings in predominantly black elderly persons from urban low-income households," *Am. J. Clin. Nutr. 32,* 2346 (1979).

13. P.A. Wagner et al., "Comparison of zinc and folacin status in elderly women from differing socioeconomic backgrounds," *Nutr. Res. 1,* 565 (1981).

14. Philip J. Garry et al., "Nutritional status in a healthy elderly population: Dietary and supplemental intakes," *Am. J. Clin. Nutr. 36,* 319 (1982).

15. M.K. Wisehart, "What to Eat," *American Magazine 95,* 14 (1923).

Chapter 13   Another Deficiency Disease

1. Barbara Griggs, *The Food Factor,* Viking, Middlesex, England 1986.

2. Richard Doll and Richard Peto, "The Causes of Cancer: Quantitative Estimates of Avoidable Risks of Cancer in the United States Today," *J. Natl. Cancer Inst. 66,* 1191 (1981).

3. E.V. McCollum, Elsa Orent-Keiles and Harry G. Day, *The Newer Knowledge of Nutrition,* Macmillan Co., New York 1939.

4. Albert Szent-Gyorgyi, "Lost in the Twentieth Century," *Ann. Rev. Biochem. 32,* 1 (1963).

5. W. Henry Sebrell, Jr., "History of Pellagra," *Fed. Proc. 40*, 1520 (1981).
6. G. Marie Swanson, "Cancer Prevention in the Workplace and Natural Environment," *Cancer 62*, 1725 (1988).
7. Sharon K. Ostwald, "Changing Employees' Dietary and Exercise Practices: An Experimental Study in a Small Company," *J. Occup. Med. 31*, 90 (1989).

Chapter 14   Clinical Trials

1. William D. DeWys et al., "Clinical Trials in Cancer Prevention," *Cancer 58*, 1954 (1986).
2. John S. Bertram et al., "Rationale and Strategies for Chemoprevention of Cancer in Humans," *Cancer Res. 47*, 3012 (1987).
3. Winfred F. Malone, "Studies evaluating antioxidants and beta-carotene as chemopreventives," *Am. J. Clin. Nutr. 53*, 305S (1991).
4. E. Robert Greenberg et al., "A Clinical Trial of beta-Carotene to Prevent Basal-Cell and Squamous-Cell Cancers of the Skin," *N. Eng. J. Med. 323*, 789 (1990).
5. Waun Ki Hong et al., "Prevention of Second Primary Tumors with Isotretinoin in Squamous-Cell Carcinoma of the Head and Neck," *N. Eng. J. Med. 323*, 795 (1990).
6. Hans F. Stich et al., "Remission of Oral Leukoplakias and Micronuclei in Tobacco/Betel Quid Chewers Treated with Beta-Carotene and with Beta-Carotene Plus Vitamin A," *Int. J. Cancer 42*, 195 (1988).
7. Hans F. Stich et al., "Use of the Micronucleus Test to Monitor the Effect of Vitamin A, beta-Carotene and Canthaxanthin on the Buccal Mucosa of Betel Nut/Tobacco Chewers," *Int. J. Cancer 34*, 745 (1984).
8. Christopher S. Foote and Robert W. Denny, "Chemistry of Singlet Oxygen. VII. Quenching by beta-Carotene," *J. Amer. Chem. Soc. 90*, 6233 (1968).
9. Paul Knekt et al., "Vitamin E and cancer prevention," *Am. J. Clin. Nutr. 53*, 283S (1991).
10. Jeffrey R. Kanofsky, "Quenching of Singlet Oxygen by Human Plasma," *Photochem. Photobiol. 51*, 299 (1990).
11. Stephanie London and Walter Willett, "Diet and the Risk of Breast Cancer," *Hemat. Oncol. Clinics N. Amer. 3*, 559 (1989).
12. Tim Byers, "Diet and Cancer, Any Progress in the Interim?," *Cancer 62*, 1713 (1988).
13. P.J. Goodwin and N.F. Boyd, "Critical Appraisal of the Evidence That Dietary Fat Intake Is Related to Breast Cancer Risk in Humans," *J. Natl. Cancer Inst. 79*, 473 (1987).
14. D.C. Heimburger, C.L. Krumdieck, C.E. Butterworth, Jr., "Role of Folate in Prevention of Cancers of the Lung and Cervix," (abstr.) *J. Am. Coll. Nutr. 6*, 425 (1987).

15. C.E. Butterworth, Jr. et al., "Oral folic acid supplementation for cervical dysplasia: A clinical intervention trial," *Am. J. Obstet. Gynecol. 166*, 803 (1992).

16. Douglas C. Heimburger et al., "Improvement in Bronchial Squamous Metaplasia in Smokers Treated with Folate and Vitamin B12," *J. Amer. Med. Assoc. 259*, 1525 (1988).

17. Bret A. Lashner et al., "Effect of Folate Supplementation on the Incidence of Dysplasia and Cancer in Chronic Ulcerative Colitis," *Gastroenterology 97*, 255 (1989).

18. Ritva R. Butrum et al., "NCI dietary guidelines: rationale," *Am. J. Clin. Nutr. 48*, 888 (1988).

19. Sharada Shankar and Elaine Lanza, "Dietary Fiber and Cancer Prevention," *Hemat. Oncol. Clinics N. Amer. 5*, 25 (1991).

20. Betty P. Perloff and Ritva R. Butrum, "Folacin in selected foods," *J. Am. Diet. Assoc. 70*, 161 (1977).

21. B. Holland et al., *McCance and Widdowson's The Composition of Foods*, 5th edition. The Royal Society of Chemistry and Ministry of Agriculture, Fisheries and Food, 1991.

22. Jerome J. De Cosse et al., "Effect of Wheat Fiber and Vitamins C and E on Rectal Polyps in Patients with Familial Adenomatous Polyposis," *J. Natl. Cancer Inst. 81*, 1290 (1989).

23. Bruce Armstrong and Richard Doll, "Environmental Factors and Cancer Incidence and Mortality in Different Countries, With Special Reference to Dietary Practices," *Int. J. Cancer 15*, 617 (1975).

24. Gail E. McKeown-Eyssen, "Fiber Intake in Different Populations and Colon Cancer Risk," *Prev. Med. 16*, 532 (1987).

Index

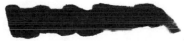